Sleep and Death lifting the body of Sarpedon (ca. 515 B.C.) by Euphronios, detail. Reprinted by permission of Metropolitan Museum of Art, New York.

MEDICAL ETHICS
IN THE
ANCIENT WORLD

PAUL CARRICK

GEORGETOWN UNIVERSITY PRESS/WASHINGTON, D.C.

Georgetown University Press, Washington, D.C.
© 2001 by Georgetown University Press. All rights reserved.
Printed in the United States of America.

10 9 8 7 6 5 4 3 2 1   2001

This volume is printed on acid-free offset book paper.

Library of Congress Cataloging-in-Publication Data

Carrick, Paul.
    Medical ethics in the ancient world / Paul Carrick.
        p. cm.—(The clinical medical ethics series)
    Includes bibliographical references and index.
    ISBN 0-87840-848-7 (cloth : alk. paper)
        1. Medical ethics–History. 2. Medicine, Ancient.
    I. Title. II. Clinical medical ethics (Washington, D.C.)

R725.5 .C37 2001
174'.209–dc21   00-047664

FOR RONALD F. HATHAWAY
1937–1991
in memoriam

O vitae philosophia dux.

Medicine heals diseases of the body;
wisdom frees the soul from passions.

—DEMOCRITUS, *Fragments*

Life is short, the art long, opportunity
fleeting, experiment treacherous,
judgment difficult.

—HIPPOCRATES, *Aphorisms*

For a physician who is lover of wisdom
is the equal of a god.

—HIPPOCRATES, *Decorum*

CONTENTS

ix

PART II
The Rise of Medical Ethics

PART III
Abortion and Euthanasia

ILLUSTRATIONS

PREFACE

In an earlier exploration of these topics, I wrote: "The pace and scope of the current biomedical revolution is not likely to redefine radically the basic relationship of mutual trust and personal autonomy between physicians and their patients any time soon."[1] I was wrong.

For example, promising neurological research into the prevention of Alzheimer's disease now leads scientists to experiment with fetal brain tissue in order to slow the devastating effects of this illness. But this use of fetal brain tissue has led critics of abortion to worry anew. They fear that in the future abortion, and possibly even infanticide, will be tacitly encouraged by the research agendas of the medical establishment. "Does the use of fetal brains stand as a morally indictable exploitation of nascent human life?" they ask. This is a fair question. The fact that the government has approved this practice for a limited and closely monitored range of medical experiments hardly settles the moral concern. It appears to some that human life is increasingly viewed as a commodity. If so, the erosion of patient trust cannot trail far behind.

At the other end of the life span, the ancient option of euthanasia—now glossed as "physician-assisted suicide"—has seldom been more contentiously argued. Here the breakdown of patient trust may occur on at least three levels. First, why would good doctors help people die? Aren't doctors dedicated to saving, nurturing, or at least compassionately caring for human life, no matter how broken? Second, given the high costs of caring for the dying in the last months of their withering lives, would the legalization of physician-assisted suicide lead finally to a felt duty to die on the part of our weakest and sickest? Third, every year over sixty thousand severely ill patients awaiting transplant surgery are lost due to a scarcity of suitable donor organs. Will the physician-patient relationship of the future be strained by this growing need to harvest spare body parts—a need bound to be more easily met if the terminally or chronically ill agree to orchestrate their deaths via physician-assisted suicide or some similar means? Given the persistent potential for moral and legal controversy inspired by these deeds, it is hardly surprising that the twin issues of abortion and euthanasia have refused to recede from our moral landscape. They represent, after all, ineliminable challenges and measures of how we value human lives and how we define human communities.

To be sure, the medical marketplace is as old as Athens. Yet added to the debates over fetal research and physician-assisted suicide, managed care has unmistakably reared its Janus-faced head. The result is that medical centers are undergoing cost-cutting pressures that also threaten to strain the quality and intimacy of the physician-patient relationship. Physicians now worry that accountants and insurance operatives, not their qualified medical peers, are second-guessing their motives and diagnostic skills. For their part, patients—over 60 percent of whom are affected by managed care—wonder whether they are still receiving the best available care or merely the cheapest. Unfortunately, this is sometimes an open question.

In revising this manuscript, I am reminded that despite dazzling advances in fighting diseases and saving lives, twenty-first-century medicine remains inextricably linked to the notion of healing as an ancient art (*techne*) based on a science. Nor is medicine yet an exact science, however difficult this fact is for its practitioners and partisans to swallow.

We live in a society seduced by the stunning accomplishments of organ transplants, impressed by the remarkable technology of embryo transfer and surrogate motherhood, and captivated by the promising evolutionary developments of bioengineering, gene therapy, and, almost inevitably, human cloning. In addition, among the public at large the expectations created by the ongoing wondrous cures and promising therapies brought by high-tech medicine are so intense that patients are demanding more and better health care for almost every imaginable malady and complaint, let alone life-threatening illnesses and crippling trauma. Hence, it is sobering indeed to picture some clinicians, under the strain of managed care reimbursement formulas, pausing to calculate the health of their bank accounts while simultaneously appraising which therapy will most efficiently restore the health of their patients. As Plato observed in his *Republic,* the excellent physician *qua* practitioner does not, properly speaking, pursue the art of healing for its monetary rewards. Medicine per se aims at curing or preventing disease. Therefore, any remuneration that the physician receives for his services is a by-product only and does not belong to the craft of medicine itself. This ancient insight deserves reflection as managed-care reform tests the current limits of the physician's sense of charity and professional responsibility toward society as a whole, a society of which approximately 20 percent go without any comprehensive health coverage.

As our inquiry into the foundations of Western medical ethics will demonstrate, financial tensions and role conflicts have long been associated with the healing arts. Still, the improvement of the patient's welfare has generally triumphed as the publicly affirmed *summum bonum.* To be sure, the much taken-for-granted triumph of this beneficent ethic was further amplified when wedded, however imperfectly, to the Judeo-Christian principle of the sanctity of human life.

So it is that we recognize a strange familiarity in the voice of the Hippocratic author of *Precepts*, practicing medicine in Athens around the first century B.C., who wrote: "And if there be an opportunity to serving one who is a stranger in financial straits, give full assistance to all such. For where there is love of man, there is also love of the art."[2]

One can hear in these distant words an admirable commitment to the importance of empathy and charity in treating the outsider, the sick, and the destitute. That this selfless response to the suffering of the stranger is also affirmed in the Hebrew Bible and Christian Gospels is remarkably coincidental. Yet, as we shall see, the similarity of these ancient pronouncements to modern notions of medical charity is more apparent than real. In his illuminating book *The Birth of Bioethics*, Albert Jonsen laments: "When health insurance became common after World War II, and when Medicaid and Medicare were initiated in the 1960s, 'charity medicine' disappeared and the duty of gratuitous care for the poor faded from the physician's ethic."[3]

Nevertheless, the love of medicine about which the Hippocratic author of *Precepts* so eloquently writes has seldom been more keenly felt than by its future practitioners and their dedicated teachers. Let no one doubt that medicine is regnant in postmodern American society—despite the admittedly hazardous social, economic, political, and ethical swamplands it must muck through in the decades ahead. This commitment to serve others competently and compassionately is especially evident in the educational covenant between first-year medical students and their demanding professors, a covenant usually witnessed by mentors, family, and friends. I personally witnessed this covenant in symbolic form when, as a visiting professor at Pennsylvania State University's College of Medicine in 1996, I and other humanities, social science, and medical faculty members were invited by the dean to attend something he called the "White Coat Ceremony." This event constituted an unforgettably moving ritual that inaugurated the opening year of studies at the Milton S. Hershey Medical Center. After marching up to the stage one-by-one to receive their brilliantly white and perfectly starched lab coats—each embroidered with the student's name—these future clinicians recited in unison a version of their own modern oath of Hippocrates. It began: "By all that I hold highest, I promise my patients competence, integrity, candor, personal commitment to their best interest, compassion, and absolute discretion and confidentiality within the law. I shall do to my patients as I would be done by . . . and shall minimize suffering whenever a cure cannot be obtained. . . ."[4] Doubtless, the father of medicine would have nodded approvingly despite the fact that these students' modern version remained silent on abortion and euthanasia. The main thing is that the patients still come first.

Given the numerous and dramatic breakthroughs in health care during the twentieth century, it is fair to ask, Why bother to explore the origins of Western medical ethics? To some, at least, it appears as if a host of lastingly important developments in both medicine and morals are uniquely occurring here and now. If so, who can afford the luxury of mounting the carousel of history for yet another ride full circle from past to present?

Having directed this volley of needling questions at myself when the present inquiry began, my answer has remained unwavering: Who can afford not to?

Consider, if you will, these observations—all of which are symptomatic of a lost sense of history:

1. We live in an era when much of the educated public still professes an almost reverential admiration for the ethical teachings of Hippocrates. At the same time, much of this same public—privately, and often unaware of their inconsistency—strongly disagrees with the Hippocratic Oath's prohibition of abortion and euthanasia as acceptable medical alternatives.
2. We live in an era when fresh attempts to define what medical ethics is all about frequently ignore the moral principles of this subject's humble beginnings. Yet new ethical theories are sometimes little more than paraphrases of traditional Hippocratic insights dressed up in the latest contemporary jargon.
3. We live in an era when a good many progressive journalists, clergy, lawyers, philosophers, physicians, and social scientists of every background are displaying an uncommon eagerness to christen themselves specialists in "bioethics." Yet not a few are doing this, sad to say, as if the entire subject came into being for the first time around 1958.

In view of the preceding evidence, there is every reason to suppose that any time devoted to recovering in a critical way the ancient foundations of medical ethics will be time well spent. Indeed, to lose our clear sense of this rich story of our bioethical heritage may cause us to stereotype the past and, worse still, under- or overvalue our humanistic and scientific accomplishments in the present. In my opinion, this is a brand of self-deception we can ill afford.

NOTES

1. Paul Carrick, *Medical Ethics in Antiquity: Philosophical Perspectives on Abortion and Euthanasia* (Dordecht and Boston: Kluwer Academic Publishers, 1985), p. xvii.
2. Hippocrates *Precepts* 6, trans. W. H. S. Jones, *Hippocrates* (Cambridge, MA.: Harvard University Press, 1962), vol. 1, p. 319.
3. Albert R. Jonsen, *The Birth of Bioethics* (New York: Oxford University Press, 1998), p. 10.
4. Roger Balger, "The Oath of Modern Hippocrates" (n. p., 1987). My thanks to Dean C. McCollister Evarts, M.D., for providing this document.

ACKNOWLEDGMENTS

No matter how elusive or cooperative the muses may be, writing is a lonely, deliberate, unforgiving process. Were it not for the pioneering works and illuminating insights of scholars whose contributions have guided and enriched my own explorations of these topics, this book would have never been written. My students, past and present, have also crystallized my thinking over the years by asking innocent-sounding questions with tricky implications that sent me back to the original texts in search of fuller meanings. For this I heartily thank them.

Specifically, I have been greatly inspired by, and am much indebted to, the studies of ancient Western medical values, practices, and traditions that were undertaken in the twentieth century by Ludwig Edelstein, W. H. S. Jones, Henry Sigerist, and, most recently, Darrel Amundsen, William Frankena, K. J. Dover, Fridolf Kudlien, Guido Majno, Owsei Temkin, Winfried Schleiner, and John Riddle.

In addition, the many constructive criticisms and lively debates on ancient philosophy, medicine, and morals supplied by my former teacher and friend, Ronald Hathaway—who died of pancreatic cancer in 1991 on his fifty-fourth birthday—stand as personal inspirations of an incalculable scale. So, too, my father, Louis Carrick, a biologist from the old school with a solid footing in the humanities, offered much encouragement throughout, as did my uncle, Lee Carrick, a physician I have long admired. Philip Lockhart rendered cheerful assistance with some of my initial translations. He also helped me negotiate the unseen perils of Scylla and Charybdis faced by all who navigate the coastal waters of classical antiquity trained mainly in philosophy. Elizabeth Beardsley, K. Danner Clouser, Michael Dockery, Jonathan Gainor, Michael Green, Joseph Margolis, George Simms, Stuart Spicker, Norman Vanderwall, Philip Weiner, and William Wisdom read all or portions of earlier drafts. They all contributed several sound suggestions. Grateful assistance was also rendered by the Clinical Medical Ethics Series coeditors, H. Tristram Engelhardt and Kevin Wildes, plus several unnamed reviewers. I owe to Darrell Amundsen a special debt of gratitude for his many detailed and perceptive comments. John Samples, Georgetown University Press, has provided persistent, incisive, and unerring advice without which this volume would never have been realized. Edmund Pellegrino has been a constant source of inspiration as physician, philosopher, and teacher.

I cannot thank these splendid individuals enough for the care and attention they have given to this project. Any flaws that may remain, despite their good counsel, must be blamed entirely on me. The first-class typing services of Barbara McDonald were invaluable in ways too numerous to count. Librarians Sandra Wood and Beverly Segina also provided unfailing assistance. Thanks, too, to Ellen and our four children for their encouragement—and the sorts of distractions that make life worth living.

Grateful acknowledgment is hereby made to the following authors, publishers, libraries, and museums for permission to reprint selections from copyrighted materials or illustrations:

Harvard University Press and Loeb Classical Library, *Seneca: Moral Essays, Volume V, Epistles 69–92,* trans. Richard M. Gummere (Cambridge, MA: Harvard University Press, 1917), reprinted by permission; Ludwig Edelstein, *The Hippocratic Oath: Text, Translation and Interpretation* (Baltimore, MD: Johns Hopkins University Press), 6, 87, © 1943; Johns Hopkins University, *Ancient Medicine,* by Ludwig Edelstein; Harvard University Press, *Ad Lucilium Epistulae Morales,* by Seneca; American Medical Association, "Code of Medical Ethics," © 1980 and Principles of Medical Ethics (Appendix A); *Management Advisory,* American Hospital Association, A Patient's Bill of Rights, reprinted by permission, © 1992 (Appendix B); World Medical Association, Declaration of Geneva, © 1994 (Appendix C) and World Medical Association Statement on Animal Use in Biomedical Research, adopted 1989 (Appendix E); International Council of Nurses, ICN Code for Nurses, reprinted by permission, © 2000 (Appendix D); Metropolitan Museum of Art, New York, Euphronios krater (1972.11.10) (frontispiece and book cover); Staatliche Museen, Berlin, detail of Achilles bandaging the wounds of Patroclus from the bowl of Sosias (Fig. 1); Harry N. Abrams, Inc., map of the ancient world (Fig. 2) and artist's reconstruction of Temple of Asclepius, detail of Tholos, originally designed by Polycleitos the Younger (Fig. 8), from *Medicine: An Illustrated History,* by Albert S. Lyons and Joseph R. Petrucelli; Louvre, Paris, detail showing Artemus and Apollo shooting arrows of death, taken from a calyx-crater by the Niobid painter (Fig. 4); National Library of Medicine, Bethesda, engraving of Hippocrates by Paulus Pontius, after Peter Paul Rubens (Fig. 5); British Museum, tombstone of the Athenian physician Jason (Fig. 6); the Royal Library, Copenhagen, illustration (codex 1653) of a fetus in utero, based on the writings of Soranus of Ephesus (Fig. 7); Martin von Wagner Museum, Wurzburg University, Germany, detail of a man vomiting, interior medallion of a cup by the Brygos Painter (Fig. 9); Musée Royaux d'Art et d'Histoire, Brussels, detail of a girl doing laundry, interior of an Athenian cup, attributed to Onesimos (Fig. 10).

Introduction

THIS BOOK EXPLORES the origins and development of medical ethics as practiced by the physicians of ancient Greece and Rome. In it I indicate the relevance of their ideas to medical debates and decision making today. For example, I identify and interpret what many of the leading Greek philosophers and physicians said and did about abortion and euthanasia. The related topics of infanticide and suicide are also discussed. Every effort is made to furnish a clear picture of how these life-and-death questions were grasped by these physicians, their patients, and the philosophers who sometimes made public their moral judgments of these matters. It is hoped that through this investigation the reader—whether a generalist, specialist, clinician, or layman interested in the problems of medicine and morals—will gain a more comprehensive understanding of just how deep the antecedents of contemporary medical ethical problems extend into the distant centuries of our scientific and humanistic heritage.

Among the questions to be explored are these: Why did some philosophers and not others judge the life of the fetus to be worth preserving? What value did the philosophers and physicians of antiquity accord to the life of the chronically or terminally ill patient? When was human life judged to begin and end? Was death, according to their religious persuasions or philosophical speculations, something one should rightfully fear?

Today, as in earlier times, it is widely known that the Hippocratic Oath disowned acts of abortion and euthanasia. But what has become increasingly clear just in the twentieth century is that, on the whole, Greek and Roman doctors ignored the Oath's opposition to these measures. This raises the question of whether the proabortion and proeuthanasia positions taken by several leading ancient philosophers contributed in any significant way toward influencing the moral thinking of physicians and others who resisted the Oath on these critical matters. If so, what practical lessons can we learn, if any, from these independently minded thinkers?

My conjecture is that philosophical opinions did play a role, then as now, in influencing both public and professional attitudes concerning the rightness or wrongness of abortion, infanticide, euthanasia, and suicide. I gauge this philosophical influence in Part III. Pythagoras, Plato, Aristotle, and the Roman Stoic Seneca constitute the center of my investigation there. In addition, relevant Greek and Roman legal developments and the powerful influences of popular morality and religious cult beliefs are consulted. Essentially, I aim at reconstructing how the Greeks, and to a lesser extent the Romans, conceived of the doctor-patient relationship in its entirety. This is the broad question to which Part I of this three-part study is specifically devoted. Yet, in a very real sense, it is the looming and unifying question with which each succeeding part is ultimately concerned.

Accordingly, Part I explores the social setting of Greek medicine. It is designed to lay the groundwork for everything that follows. This it does by examining the social and scientific milieu within which ethical judgments on abortion and euthanasia were made. Among the principal questions raised are the following: What socioeconomic, religious, or moral constraints did the average fifth- or fourth-century-B.C. Greek physician experience in his daily practice of medicine? How did these factors shape his attitudes and conduct toward his patients and his community? What did the ancient philosophers think of the physicians of their day, and vice versa?

Among my conclusions, I argue that physicians and philosophers often competed for the public's ear, just as they do to some extent in our own era: both dispensed advice on the important moral issue of how citizens *ought* to live in order to attain well-being. I further suggest that Democritus, Plato, and Aristotle, among other Greek philosophers, talked about preventive medicine issues, such as the responsibility of patients for maintaining and monitoring their own health.

On matters of death and dying, I show that at least four distinct perspectives about the afterworld are discernible in the philosophical, medical, religious, and imaginative literature of the Greeks. Furthermore, I explore medical, philosophical, and popular perspectives on (a) the moment death is said to occur and (b) attitudes toward the dying process. It becomes increasingly evident that the Greeks held myriad views on these metaphysical and eschatological questions, many of which persist in our own pluralistic society. Therefore, I caution that care must be taken not to cast the thinking of the Greeks on these subjects into a single, oversimplified mold. Nor should the many currents of Roman thought be so artificially construed.

Part II of my inquiry deals specifically with the birth of Greek medical ethics. Attention is also given to the medical values of neighboring Mediterranean cultures, including Assyria, Babylonia, Persia, and Egypt. The purpose of this comparative treatment is to gather evidence on which to base a more fully informed judgment of the alleged originality of the Hippocratic Oath. In addition, I discuss the mystery of who the historical Hippocrates really was; it remains a curious fact that little is known about the legendary Father of Medicine.

All segments of the Hippocratic Oath, then, are critically examined within the broadest social context. This includes the enigmatic prohibition against surgery and the covenant binding medical students to their teachers. Essentially, I attempt to settle the question of the Oath's true origins and purpose. The delicate distinction between medical ethics and mere medical etiquette is also traced to the complexities and mixed motives of the ancient medical marketplace, where doctors plied their healing trade at considerable risk to their own reputation and their continued economic well-being. Indeed, contemporary clinicians faced with the vagaries of managed care and the pressures of litigiously minded patients may be all too familiar with the mixed motives of medicine practiced defensively. For example, there is the temptation to anticipate whether the patient—from hindsight—will blame her doctor should her condition worsen or even remain roughly the same after costly, painful treatments. At worst, this fear of harm to one's professional reputation can affect how a doctor may proceed with medical testing, therapeutics, or charting. To be sure, a prudent physician cannot ignore altogether threats to his professional reputation or economic well-being. As I have suggested, a similar anxiety was known to the healers of Athens and Rome.

In addition, Part III will examine a variety of divergent Greco-Roman ethical views on abortion and euthanasia. Here, too, literary materials drawn from selected writings of Greek and Roman playwrights and poets, as well as anthropological, linguistic, and legal evidence, are introduced into the discussion. My intention is to supplement the philosophical arguments and medical ideas that constitute the focus of Part III in such a manner that significant social developments are never far to seek. These include ancient contraceptive practices and techniques, types and methods of suicide, and the general competition for patients among physicians, midwives, charlatans, and others. In chapter 8, I discuss the ancient physician's sense of moral responsibility in dealing with requests of patients for abortion and euthanasia. My discussion centers on the physician's social role as the primary healer of the sick and suffering. It is evident that the dominant medical ethical values expressed in the Hippocratic writings considered as a whole do *not* unequivocally oppose or condemn physicians who assist in abortion or acts of voluntary euthanasia, as some mistakenly suppose.

HAVING HIGHLIGHTED the principal topics and central conclusions of my investigation, I now would like to comment specifically on the value of the history of medical ethics to the field of clinical ethics, broadly construed. For example, just what is the connection between cultural and historical understanding and precisely formulated clinical judgment? Also, I will comment on the scope, methods, and limitations of this exploration into the medical ethics of antiquity.

To begin, it must be acknowledged that the field of "clinical ethics" is a relatively new arrival, having broken off from bioethics per se around 1987. Although there are several proposed definitions floating about, "clinical ethics" is best understood as the day-to-day moral decision making one faces while caring for particular patients suffering from particular ailments in particular (and often desperate) situations. In essence, the individual case looms larger than rarified considerations of ethical theory. Yet ethical theory and principle must finally guide conduct. How ought I treat *this* particular noncompliant cardiac patient, here and now, in a conscientious and medically effective manner? the clinician may ask herself. And, What moral principles should guide my medical judgment if this patient continues to skip his prescribed physical therapy sessions? Sometimes, there are no morally satisfactory solutions. Hence, the psychological and moral stresses on doctors and nurses, especially those with overly heavy patient workloads, threaten to undermine thoughtful ethical decision making by creating a rushed, even frenzied clinical encounter.

As the philosopher Daniel Callahan has observed, "Individual cases often give rise to great medical and moral uncertainty, and they evoke powerful emotions among those with a role in the decisions. Decision-making procedures, as well as the melding of theory and practice—what Aristotle called "practical reason"— come sharply into play."[1]

As I see it, the practical wisdom (*phronesis*) that may be gleaned by the study of the history of ancient medical ethics is for the clinician akin to taking the medical history of a patient: one wants to select the diagnostic and therapeutic interventions that are likely to be effective and appropriate, given the medical indications and the prior influences on the subject's life. But in this case, I suggest, the subject is clearly not a patient. Instead, the subject is one's own contemporary culture and the role and context of medicine therein.[2] Following this parallel reasoning, the diagnostic and therapeutic interventions represent an intellectual opportunity on the part of the clinician-historian to understand just how today's ethical norms and practices are sometimes little more than the immediately visible remnants of forgotten medical traditions long embedded in the collective consciousness of our caring communities. These distant cultural influences are seldom perceived. Nor are they even suspected of being at work in the present case, say, of the cardiac patient in examining room B who is about to be reprimanded for trying to sign himself out of the hospital against medical advice. Therefore, by better understanding the axiological foundations of the social, cultural, and ideological elements of the society that shapes our ethical norms and habits, the clinician is intellectually freed to reject, modify, or reaffirm the force of these sometimes questionable traditions. How so? Precisely because these ancient, medieval, or modern traditions no longer seem so mysterious, sacrosanct, or intimidating. In short, the clinician is in a better position to act with creativity and wisdom.

Furthermore, it must be acknowledged that the historical Hippocrates of Cos was just one man. Yet his heralded name is still invoked in a multiplicity of circumstances by a variety of disparate partisans—often with dubious or dishonest motives. This rhetorical ploy is typically adopted in order to fortify some fondly held moral principle against, for example, physician-assisted suicide. But even though this rhetorical name-dropping may sound impressive, in the absence of additional arguments it amounts to the fallacy of appeal to authority or, relatedly, question-begging. Not so is honest public policy or sound personal philosophy formulated.

As to the scope of this enterprise, my central focus extends from the sixth through the first centuries B.C. I have chosen this historical period for two reasons. First, it covers the crucial epoch during which both rational philosophy and scientific medicine first took hold on the continent of Europe. Second, though what would now be called medical ethical issues were not among the leading and recurrent topics of debate among Greek philosophers and physicians, they were nonetheless addressed by a surprising number of ancient authors. Thanks to posterity, we have some evidence of their moral positions on abortion and euthanasia, as well as on infanticide and suicide. In a few cases, what we do not possess by way of direct evidence of their writings on these particular topics, we may infer from some of their comments on related issues. To this I must add that, while my initial focus is primarily on the pre-Christian era, it is by no means rigidly confined to this period. I do not hesitate to extend the inquiry occasionally into the early Christian and Roman centuries whenever a sharper sense of the issues and arguments is thereby gained.

My method of inquiry is both historical and analytical. It is historical in the sense that my account is bound by the extant evidence of Greek literature, both philosophical and medical, that is presently at our disposal. As in almost any historical inquiry, my guiding purpose is to make sense out of the available evidence from the point of view not only of (a) the relevant subjects of that history (in this case, ancient philosophers, physicians, and patients), but also (b) contemporary students of Greco-Roman history, medicine, philosophy, and culture. In approaching these historical materials, I do not assume that one can readily interpret ancient medical ethical problems and practices in exactly the same way that these phenomena were commonly understood by people living during the distant Greek and Roman eras. But I do assume that, given sufficient evidence, an approximate picture of the values and conduct associated with these traditional bioethical problems can be responsibly secured in a manner that enriches our contemporary perspectives on these issues.

It may well be true that the categories and concepts of one's own epoch tend to influence almost any appraisal of the historical evidence, whether the evidence is medical, philosophical, theological, sociological, or anthropological. But this very tendency also invites author and reader alike to consider further the historical evidence in terms that may suggest interesting implications and parallels in regard to our present historical setting, thereby enriching, not subverting, the interpretative process. Such an opportunity, I believe, constitutes one of the most attractive justifications for pursuing almost any inquiry into the history of ideas.

There is also the related phenomenon of historical incommensurability. That is, some issues that loom large in current medical ethical debates simply have no analogue in the ancient world of Greece and Rome. Moreover, to insist otherwise in order to cleave to some fanciful kinship with a past civilization would be folly. To illustrate, consider the congeries of problems often gathered under the heading "women's health issues." Or consider the related hornet's nest of recalcitrant social justice issues referred to as medical rationing (or "the rationing of scarce medical resources"). These areas of debate have no exact ancient analogue, even though one may be tempted to think otherwise.

First, the matter of women's health issues. A growing body of clinical and experimental evidence suggests that there may be significant underlying biological differences in the hormonal, cellular, structural, neurological, immunological, and psychophysical natures of women and men. These differences may in some instances affect the accurate diagnosis and treatment of disease.[3] Furthermore, it is fair to speculate that these differences have been largely unknown, ignored, or downplayed in past centuries due to ignorance or neglect. As recently as 1980, it was usually assumed that the male subject was the fully adequate and even the preferred subject for medical testing. In fairness, this almost exclusive use of males was primarily due to an ethical concern of possibly harming female subjects during their reproductive years.[4] But ironically, this policy was in other ways detrimental to women (and indirectly to men). Let me expand.

In order to correct this imbalance of the database, since about 1991 several new avenues of medical research specifically involving women have been encouraged through generous grants issued by the National Institutes of Health. This new research is exploring such promising areas as: (1) gender-specific treatments for depression or alcoholism, (2) a more precise characterization of the vascular effects specific to women for such diseases as diabetes and heart disease, and (3) the development of so-called "designer drugs," such as anesthetics and analgesics. These drugs, if perfected, may respond more efficaciously to female hormonal and immunological needs as compared to the standard protocol of using the identical drug for both females and males.

Yet a word of caution is in order. This relatively new conjecture of the underlying biological differences between women and men may be confused with a much earlier and quite different use of the phrase "women's health issues." I am referring especially to those women's health problems associated specifically with reproduction, such as contraception, abortion, and fertility, or possibly other gynecological disorders or breast ailments. But here is the point: Since gynecological as well as reproductive health issues like contraception and abortion were known to the Hippocratic physicians and later Galen, it would be tempting to conclude that the ancients were conversant with women's health issues, too. But this was not so in the required sense. In effect, such fallacious reasoning embodies the fallacy of ambiguity. Hence one must beware of facile comparisons of this kind.

Second, the contemporary problem of fairly rationing scarce medical resources is also sui generis. That is, there really was no counterpart in Greece or Rome to the way we normally think of rationing health care resources today. For example, consider the contemporary ethical problem of procuring and distributing a limited supply of matching organs for the many patients awaiting liver transplants. Or imagine the challenge of equitably apportioning costly, labor-intensive rehabilitative care, such as speech therapy, to stroke patients.

To be blunt, what social agency in antiquity would carry out medical rationing? Surely not the Greek city-state (*polis*), which was mainly involved in military defense, maintaining the state religion, encouraging trade, and preserving lawful order. Indeed, just as there was no moral duty for professional teachers (*sophists*) to furnish an education to all youth who sought wisdom, so too there was no duty on the part of physicians to attempt to make whole all those who sought health. The family was the main unit of social organization and personal welfare. Those sick or injured individuals with means received medical care; those with little or no resources usually threw themselves on the mercy of Aesclepian priests, or bartered their goods to the itinerant physician (*iatros*), or suffered and died unattended.

Granted, by Galen's day (see Chronology, Appendix F) the Roman Imperial army looked after the medical needs of its legions with a keen sense of medical efficiency.[5] Nevertheless, there was no binding theory of social justice or medical charity that compelled serious consideration of how to distribute medical services to the masses. In fact, the dream of universal health care, and the related goal of the equitable distribution of scarce medical resources, is a largely modern notion. While it is true that Plato, in his *Republic*, criticized as futile physicians who overtreated their hopeless patients, he never saw fit to advocate health care for all. Nor did he even address the problem of scarce medical resources. Again, such sweeping notions of social justice would not have translated into the moral vocabulary of these ancient civilizations.

Finally, a word about method. My approach is analytical in the sense that I am seeking to interpret and evaluate selected aspects of the topics before us in a manner that exposes the logical relations among the key concepts that constitute the framework of ancient medical ethics. Specifically, Greek concepts dealing with health and disease, death and dying, forms of human life, and the moral responsibility of the ancient physician are of decisive importance. If the reader gains a sharper sense of how our ancient forebears struggled with some of the fundamental medical issues with which we still contend, then perhaps the over-two-thousand-year gap between the ancient and contemporary clinical scenes—which separates physicians such as Soranus and Thomas Starzl, and philosophers such as Democritus and Peter Singer—will not seem so great. Indeed, building a sturdy conceptual bridge from the present to the past and then back to the future remains my adventuresome goal.

NOTES

1. Daniel Callahan, "Bioethics," in *Encyclopedia of Bioethics*, ed. Warren T. Reich, 4 vols. (New York: Simon and Schuster Macmillan, 1995), vol. 1, p. 250 (hereafter cited *EB 1995*; the original edition [New York: The Free Press, 1979] is hereafter cited *EB*).

2. Albert R. Jonsen, Mark Siegler, and William J. Winslade, *Clinical Ethics: A Practical Approach to Ethical Decisions in Clinical Medicine,* 4th ed. (New York: McGraw Hill, 1998), pp. 8–10.
3. Kim A. McDonald, "Studies of Women's Health Produce a Wealth of Knowledge on the Biology of Gender Differences," *Chronicle of Higher Education,* 25 June 1999, sec. A19–22.
4. Carol C. Nadelson and Malkah T. Notman, "Women: Research Issues" in *EB 1995,* pp. 2572–76.
5. Guido Majno, *The Healing Hand: Man and Wound in the Ancient World* (Cambridge, U.K.: Cambridge University Press, 1975), pp. 381–403.

PART I

THE SOCIAL
AND SCIENTIFIC SETTING

1 The Status of the Physician

History is philosophy teaching by example.

—DIONYSIUS OF HALICARNASSUS

TO FULLY PENETRATE the values and conduct of the ancient Greek physician, it is necessary first to examine certain fundamental elements of his historical setting. Thus, I have selected three areas of initial inquiry that hold the key to comprehending the cultural framework within which the ancient physician practiced his craft. These three areas are best introduced in the form of three questions. First, who was the Greek physician? Second, what were some of the leading theories of health and disease that guided his care of patients? And third, what were the dominant attitudes and theories of his culture regarding death and the afterworld?

In Part I, I shall develop answers to these three important questions, with the present chapter restricted to the first among them. My primary focus throughout will be centered on cultural developments in and around the Greek mainland between the sixth through fourth centuries B.C. My secondary focus will include selected features of the Greco-Roman world up to the time of Galen in the second century A.D.

TYPES OF PHYSICIANS

Who was the ancient physician of fifth-century-B.C. Greece? What was his social rank? Ludwig Edelstein asserts that "whatever the situation may have been in prehistoric Greece, in Homer's time [ca. 725 B.C.], the physician was already the member of a lay craft; he was 'a worker for the common weal' like the maker of spears, the singer, the seer. He remained throughout antiquity a craftsman, an artist, a scientist."[1] As such, like all Hellenic craftsmen (*demiourgoi*), the physician was seen to be in the possession of the technical body of knowledge peculiar to his craft alone. He was not ordinarily confused with other tradesmen, nor was the physician equated in the public's mind with the exorcist or magician, who were common enough figures in the ancient world. Hence, by the fifth century one is hardly surprised to find the playwright Sophocles asserting that, "It is not a learned physician who sings incantations over pains which should be cured by cutting."[2] Centuries later, Roman law established that any physician who practiced by exorcisms or incantations could under no circumstances sue his patients for unpaid fees, for such methods were judged not to belong to the bona fide craft of medicine.[3]

Nor is it likely that medicine in Greece originated in the temples of the deified hero-physician, Asclepius. By the time Asclepius rose to the status of a god and temples were erected to celebrate his powers and promote his cures (most notably at Epidaurus), the physicians (iatroi) of Greece were already firmly established as independent, secular craftsmen.[4] The honorary title of "Asclepiad," by which physicians were sometimes addressed, had been a source of long-standing confusion among historians attempting to sort out the cultural roots of the Greek practitioner. But it is now emerging from the available evidence that this title did not refer to the god or to a formal religious corporation.[5] Rather, it referred to certain guilds or families of physicians who handed down medical knowledge from father to son, or master to apprentice.[6] The title of Asclepiad was, it seems, a well-chosen indirect reference to the admirable deeds and personal compassion associated with the heroic founder of medicine, Asclepius. The legacy of Asclepius was such that contemporary fifth-century physicians sought a share in it as distant descendants or "sons," as they sometimes called themselves.[7] Indeed, few physicians wished the public to lose sight of Homer's oft-repeated judgment that "a healer is man worth many men. . . ."[8]

But while the physician of Hippocratic times (ca. 450–300 B.C.) was, by definition, one who engaged in the art of preserving or restoring health, evidence exists in the writings of the philosophers Aristotle and Plato that invites the judgment that the social status of physicians varied significantly according to their training and methods. Aristotle, for example, says that "the term 'physician' means both the ordinary practitioner, and the master of the craft, and thirdly, the man who studied medicine as part of his general education."[9]

It is difficult to know whether Aristotle here intends a faithful description of well-recognized social groups within Greek medicine, as such, or whether he is supplying us with a personal evaluation of the sorts of physicians one usually encountered in the Greek city-state. I think he is rendering an evaluation. The context of his remark is a large discussion in which he is seeking to evaluate how much power a political majority should exercise over the technical affairs of the state. His mention of levels of skill among physicians is thus seen as part of a useful analogy: just as some physicians do not practice their art but acquire it as part of their general education and thereby know something about medicine, so too many citizens know something of the affairs of state though they do not personally practice the art of rulership. Additionally, when one considers the medical knowledge possessed by such pre-Socratics as Empedocles, as well as by the later sophists and generalists of Greece and Rome, it is not at all difficult to account for Aristotle's third definition of the generally educated physician.

But then, what of Aristotle's remaining distinction between "the ordinary practitioner" as opposed to "the master of the craft"? Does this refer to two distinct social classes of physicians, one the scientist-theoretician, the other the leech-practitioner?

The plausible answer is that it does not. At most it attests to Aristotle's awareness that some physicians, like Diocles of Carystus, appeared as masters of their craft in the sense that they could *explain why* their treatments worked. Others could not, though they still may have gotten helpful medical results. The former were masters, the latter ordinary practitioners. This difference in the practitioners' level of understanding, at once both detectable and significant for a theorist of knowledge like Aristotle, almost certainly constituted the basis for his threefold grouping here. This interpretation is all the more credible since, in fact, anyone in the ancient world could practice medicine; there were really no formal educational class distinctions as such. To practice medicine was a right, not a privilege. Physicians were not in the least certified or categorized by the state.

Furthermore, it is pertinent to mention that Plato distinguishes two social ranks of physicians in his *Laws*. He speaks on the one hand of the free-born physician and on the other of the slave-physician. The free-born physician "for the most part attends free men, treats their diseases by going into things thoroughly from the beginning in a scientific way"; the slave-physician generally treats fellow slaves and never gives a patient any account of his complaint.[10] He is "innocent of the theory," whereas his free counterpart can be found "talking almost like a philosopher, tracing the disorder to its source, reviewing the whole system of human physiology. . . ."[11]

Yet, despite Plato's words, it would be overly hasty to conclude that the social difference between slave and free doctors made a decisive difference in the quality of their medicine. Owsei Temkin points out that slave doctors were a known institution throughout antiquity. Highly educated persons could become slaves when they or their defeated armies became captives. So there is little warrant for supposing that physicians belonging to this slave class were automatically of inferior skill or knowledge.[12] In view of these facts, I am prepared to conclude from the *Laws* that Plato, like Aristotle, felt it instructive to distinguish those healers who studied nature in such a way that they deduced their treatments from universal principles from those less rigorous healers who acquired their skills mostly by imitation and rote. The latter were bereft of a theoretical causal framework for their medicine. The former alone were "almost like a philosopher" and stood for both men as exemplars of their craft.

Perhaps the safest conclusion to be drawn about the status of the Hellenic physician, one fully consistent with the above testimony, is that his personal status was variable. Naturally, if his cures were known to be successful and if he thereby gained a reputation as a highly capable practitioner, he would enjoy a measure of fame and status exceeding that of his more average competitors. Then, as now, there existed the country doctor, the city doctor, and the regal court physician. When the Greek physician Galen was practicing in Rome in the second century A.D., he complained that physicians treated their patients differently depending on the physician's origins, his training, and the perceived social standing of a given patient. Patients, in turn, reacted differently toward their physicians depending on the physician's perceived authority and his high or low reputation.[13]

But as to the *average* physician taken as a stereotype of fifth-century Greece, particularly Attica, I am in full accord with Edelstein's characterization:

> The Hippocratic physician is a craftsman. As a craftsman, he practices either as a resident or as an itinerant; he may also settle for awhile in some town, leave again, work in another town, or wander all over the country. When he is in a town, he works in his shop or in his patient's home. The shop is a place in which today one person, tomorrow another, plies his trade—not a hospital, not a consulting room in the physician's house. Sick people come to the shop for examination and treatment, or the physician goes to his patient's home. An itinerant physician works in the patient's house or has a booth set up in the marketplace of the town, or elsewhere, and practices there.[14]

Elsewhere, Edelstein has aptly summarized the social situation for doctors down to the time of the Roman Empire:

> About the basic social situation there can be no doubt. The medical practitioner, working for a livelihood and working with his hands, preparing drugs or performing operations, was to the ancients a craftsman and, as such, belonged to the lower strata of the social order. And this was true throughout antiquity. It did not help his standing that in the Classical and in the Hellenistic era he was usually a migratory worker, an 'out-of-towner,' and in Roman times a foreigner; in the Rome of Cicero no citizen had yet gone into medicine, while he would not scruple to become a lawyer. Nor should one forget that in the empire probably more physicians were slaves than had even been the case in Greece.[15]

Finally, it is relevant to ask: was there anything like our modern medical specialties in classical antiquity? The simple answer is no. For there was no profession as such in today's terms, and no board certification or other licensing system. But practically speaking, it may be admitted that, while there was no division between medicine and surgery (the latter then including operative surgery, setting bones, reduction of dislocations, and cauterization), evidence suggests that *some* physicians may have practiced surgery exclusively.[16] But if so, the trend toward specialization was for the most part a matter of personal convenience rather than based on any deep-seated ideological split within the craft of medicine, as some have assumed.[17]

EGYPTIAN INFLUENCES

In contrast to the comparatively unified approach to healing characteristic of fifth-century-B.C. Greek medicine (Fig. 1), the Greek historian Herodotus writes of the Egyptian physicians that "medicine is practiced among them on a plan of separation; each physician treats a single disorder, and no more: thus, the country [Egypt] swarms with medical practitioners, some undertaking to cure diseases of the eye, others of the head, others again of the teeth, others of the intestines, and some those which are not local."[18] This account raises the question: to what extent was Greek medicine influenced by the Egyptians?

To begin with, Herodotus's report of Egyptian specialization suggests that the state of the medical art in Egypt was quite advanced by ancient standards. In antiquity Egyptian physicians were much sought after in foreign lands. Indeed, the Greeks expressed admiration toward Egyptian medicine, particularly their effective use of drugs. A rich variety of these is prescribed throughout the best-preserved Egyptian medical papyri now in our possession.[19] Moreover, we know for a fact that the Greeks copied many of these Egyptian pharmaceutical formulae. They also imitated and further developed the Egyptian techniques of repeated and careful empirical examination of the patient, including both diagnosis and prognosis, which were developed by the Egyptians perhaps as early as 3000 B.C.[20] Therefore, both the testimony of the Greeks themselves and the Egyptian medical texts provide a basis for the judgment that Greek medicine was influenced by Egypt.

But how much? The jury is still out on this question. Nonetheless, opinions have been offered. The great medical historian, T. Clifford Allbutt, writing in the first quarter of the twentieth century, locates the Egyptian influence mainly in drug therapy. He discounts Egyptian anatomy as "rudimentary and pettifogging," even by Hellenistic standards. But he admits that the doctrine of the four humors may have originated in Egypt.[21]

A more generous estimate of the Egyptian contribution is provided by J. B. Saunders. Saunders credits the Egyptians with no fewer than five major accomplishments, the importance of which was not lost on the Greeks. These include: (1) the recording of reusable empirical data on the application of drugs; (2) an unusually effective causal theory of disease based on the putrefaction of digested substances within the body; (3) the development of various purgatives as an effective treatment against internal infection and swelling; (4) pregnancy and sterility tests for women; and (5) the development of a birth prognosis according to

Figure 1. Detail, the bowl of Sosias (ca. 500 B.C.). Achilles bandaging the wounds of Patroclus. The battlefield taught medical techniques to warriors and physicians alike. Reprinted by permission of Staatliche Museen, Berlin.

which the sex and condition of the developing fetus were forecast.[22] Thus, Saunders appears willing to credit the Egyptians with a causal theory of health and disease that recognizes a rational framework largely divorced from magic and supernatural explanations.

To me this seems overgenerous, based on the evidence of the five principal Egyptian medical papyri currently under study. In my view, the most one is entitled to say is this: While there are *some* empirical-rational elements to be found in the papyri (especially reasoning by analogy and going from specific cases and symptoms to general treatment rules), alongside these prescientific techniques one cannot ignore the Egyptian's reliance on magical incantations and supernatural models of disease.[23] Disease is attributed to the workings of an invading, incapacitating deity or spirit of some sort. Therefore, I am inclined to credit the Egyptians with their advanced pharmacopoeia, the lawlike rational elements in their theory of putrefaction, and their sharp clinical observations based on the methodological strategy of diagnosis and prognosis as having plausibly influenced Greek medicine. This much seems justified on the evidence.

But to the Greek physicians of the fifth century alone must go the credit for divorcing medicine from magic—something the Egyptian physicians failed to do even in Herodotus's time.[24] Thus, one must not be overenthusiastic in ascribing the beginnings of scientific medicine to Egypt without at least this very important acknowledgment.

JEWISH INFLUENCES

To be sure, the general influence of Jewish culture and, specifically, the Jews' uniquely monotheistic religious and ethical values on ancient, medieval, and modern Western civilization has been incalculably great. Yet the comparative impact of Jewish medical practices on Greco-Roman medicine per se, from the time of their exodus out of Egypt (variously dated from 1446 B.C. to 1280 B.C.) to the destruction of their Temple in Jerusalem by the Romans (A.D. 70), was relatively minor. As Darrel Amundsen and Gary Ferngren observe:

> In both Mesopotamia and Egypt, thriving medical professions existed throughout the period under consideration [3100 B.C.–70 A.D.]. In Israel a distinct medical profession appears to have developed very late (second century B.C.). If anything that could be called medical literature was produced in Israel, it was at the very end of our period. By contrast, a large body of medical literature, some of which has survived, existed in *both* Mesopotamia and Egypt.[25]

Furthermore, no evidence exists in the Hebrew Scriptures of a distinct medical profession until the second century B.C.[26] Overall, the Jewish people viewed their transcendent, omnipresent God, Yahweh, as the ultimate healer. Yahweh was worshiped as a totally moral, universal, personal deity who reigns supreme over an essentially orderly cosmos. All this stood in stark contrast to the world views of their polytheistically minded Egyptian and Mesopotamian neighbors, whose various nature gods were decidedly indifferent to human suffering and were largely linked to fertility beliefs and rituals.

> Although the Hebrew Scriptures represent Yahweh as the only healer (e.g. Exod. 15:26) and command the Israelites to refrain from resorting to magical or pagan healing practices (see, e.g., Ezek. 13:17–23), the use of natural or medical means is not discouraged, but is resorted to even in ostensibly miraculous healings (e.g. 2 Kings 20). Medical knowledge may have been limited to folk remedies, however, and there probably were no systematized therapeutics. . . . Contact with Greek civilization in the Hellenistic Age provided Jews with something that neither Mesopotamia nor Egypt could contribute: a religiously neutral theoretical framework for a rational understanding of disease and healing. . . . [This framework] allowed the co-existence of both [a] divine explanation of ultimate causality and [b] natural processes of proximate causality within Yahweh's created order.[27]

Therefore, mystical prayer and rational healing (through the application of natural remedies) were seen basically as complementary, not antithetical, within the culture of Jewish medicine. Informally, healers probably existed both inside and outside of the priesthood as medical knowledge was widely diffused.

From the Jewish perspective, then, both physician and patient must acknowledge their dependence upon God: God alone ultimately delivers the cure or takes the life. In my opinion, Owsei Temkin, Amundsen, and others correctly conclude that "Hellenistic Jews accepted rational medicine based on the Greek model as [being] fully compatible with their faith."[28] Aside from the available medical treatments—which were pathetically limited and few—cures could come only from Yahweh by confession of sin, supplication, or prayer (e.g., Job 33:19–30). The Jewish approach to healing was therefore both scientific and religious, with God ideally leading the *rofe* (Jewish physician) to a higher understanding of the patient's plight.

THE PROBLEM OF LICENSURE

One feature common to both Greek and Egyptian cultures was the absence of a system of medical licensure.[29] While little is known about the regulation of the medical profession under the Egyptian pharaohs, it is clear that compared to the freedom enjoyed by their Greek counterparts on the islands of Cnidus, Cos, and at Crotonia (in Sicily), the Egyptian physician was required to practice according to very rigid rules of treatment. One reason for this was the widely held opinion in Egypt that it was hard to improve upon the medical wisdom of older times.

Hence, the first-century-B.C. author Diodorus Siculus, who based his opinion on earlier Egyptian documents, wrote that Egyptian physicians gave treatment in accordance with strict written procedures. If their patients died, such physicians were usually absolved from any charge. But if they deviated from the traditional practices and methods in any way, they were subjected to the death penalty.[30] Aristotle in his *Politics* describes a slightly more flexible situation: "In Egypt the physician is allowed to alter his treatment after the fourth day, but if sooner, he takes the risk."[31] The risk to which Aristotle refers probably includes the death penalty, especially in the event the patient dies.

In comparison, the Greek physician was virtually immune from civil penalties if his patient died while under his care. Of course, this did not mean that he could do anything he liked to his patients. For example, he could not wantonly murder his patient and be expected to escape prosecution for homicide after charges were brought by relatives of the deceased. But he practiced his craft by and large without interference and was free to treat as best he knew how. The freedom that he enjoyed—plus the opportunity for possible harm to others as a result of this enviable freedom—did not escape the attention of his own countrymen, either. Thus, according to the comic poet, Philemon, the Greek doctor is the only person permitted to kill and not die for his crime. He is the only citizen to enjoy complete immunity for causing the death of others, the Roman Pliny would later write. For in Roman times physicians were just as free and perhaps even more taunted by their critics than they had been in Greece (Fig. 2).[32]

Figure 2. Map of the eastern Mediterranean during the time of Hippocrates. Most physicians were itinerant workers, usually working alone and moving from town to town. Reprinted by permission of Harry N. Abrams, Inc., New York.

Just how this freedom from licensure and state control led to the gradual development of medical etiquette and ethical guidelines will be addressed in Part II. The point to be made here is that the freedom enjoyed by the Hippocratic physician was at once a personal burden and an occasional source of scientific experimentation and discovery. That is, on the one hand he may have been tempted on occasion not to take a difficult case for fear that, if the unfortunate patient died, this might get around town and hurt his reputation—which was effectively his only employment credential. On the other hand, unlike the Egyptian practitioner, the Hippocratic physician was free to make adjustments in his treatments of a disease as he saw fit, which he could do at any time without civil threat or penalty. This meant that he was free to experiment to a limited extent on the particular cases before him, thus modifying established general treatments to better suit the special characteristics of each individual. This freedom to improvise and improve treatment constitutes one of the fundamental strengths of Greek medicine. It helps to explain its essentially progressive and diverse nature as well as its eventual need for *voluntarily* followed codes of conduct. These codes originated from the medical practitioners themselves, and were not (as was the case in Egypt) imposed by the state.

Thus, several of the features of the social setting in which the average Hellenic physician worked have come into view. I have argued that he was regarded as a craftsman. As such, like all Greek craftsmen, he was free to set his own fees and work for whom, when, and how he chose. He was often a stranger, wandering from village to town selling his services. Since he worked with his hands, and since medicine was excluded formally from the ancient list of liberal arts, his social status was comparable to that of other common workmen or craftsmen (*technai*), and generally below that of musicians, mathematicians, poets, and philosophers.[33] In a word, he was a businessman. In the absence of any system of licensure, he needed to protect his reputation as a wise and useful healer of the sick. Otherwise he would be confused with charlatans and quacks, of whom there were many. As I have suggested, compared to his Egyptian counterpart, the Greek doctor was freer to regulate his practice and adjust treatments as he saw fit. While usually pious in his attitude toward the gods, he was not in the habit of attributing disease to supernatural causes. Nor did he resort to magic, as did Egyptian physicians and priests (often the same person) in Pharaonic times.

Yet on balance it will also be recalled that the Greeks possessed a well-deserved reputation among the ancients for advocating the importance of a sound mind in a sound body (*mens sana in corpore sano*). Health was among their most prized values. As such, the physician, *qua* the restorer and preserver of health, was no ordinary craftsman. If he was known to be effective in his cures, he was indeed much sought after. This is why it must be underscored that, in the final analysis, the social status of a particular doctor varied with the esteem in which his public regarded him. His performance and resulting reputation were decisive to his financial success and his ability to eke out a living.

THE RELATIONSHIP BETWEEN PHYSICIANS
AND PHILOSOPHERS

The physician in antiquity was not regarded by his often skeptical public as the first and last source of medical wisdom and authority. Some will be surprised to learn that by the fifth century B.C., well into Roman times,

> . . . everybody was familiar with medicine—it was the only art or science about which everybody knew something; physicians wrote books for the general public; laymen discussed medical problems with their physicians; in short, medical knowledge was perhaps diffused more widely in Greek and Roman times than in any other period of history. . . . [34]

Philosophers, of course, exploited this common fund of public interest in and knowledge of rudimentary medical techniques for their own ends. When they wished to emphasize the peculiar tasks of the philosophical enterprise or instruct others on the nuances of their own theories, the idiom and examples of medicine often proved to be useful pedagogical tools. Hence, the atomist philosopher, Democritus, stated: "Medicine heals diseases of the body; wisdom frees the soul from passions."[35] Aristotle, himself the son of a physician, knew well the persuasive power of the medical analogy in setting forth his ethical prescriptions. The germ of his ethical doctrine of the mean is found early on in Book Two of his *Nicomachean Ethics*. There his concept of virtue is introduced in this striking medical parallel:

> . . . [I]t is the nature of such things [human actions and states of character] to be destroyed by defect and excess, as we see in the case of strength and health . . . ; both excessive and defective exercise destroys the strength, and similarly drink or food which is above or below a certain amount destroys the health, while that which is proportionate both produces and increases and preserves it. So, too, is it then in the case of temperance and courage and the other virtues.[36]

In addition, philosophers associated with the ancient Academy were especially eager to coax the public into believing that they ought to care about the health and state of their invisible soul as diligently and thoughtfully as they already cared about the health of their visible body. Aristotle shared a similar concern for the well-being of the soul. Hence, Werner Jaeger seems to me quite correct in arguing that Aristotle used the medical model to full advantage in demonstrating the details of his ethical system, as the preceding quotation illustrates.[37]

As to the related question of who held more prestige in the public's mind, the physician or the philosopher, there seems little room for doubt. The philosopher was by far more generally esteemed. Yet it must not be forgotten that the average Athenian held in high regard the practical applications of the medical craft. Health, after all, was regarded by many of the ancient Greeks and Romans as the highest good (*summum bonum*) of life; or at least, in Aristotelian terms, many regarded health as the highest external good (that is, it was necessary to the good life). This high value accorded to health suggests that the more famous and successful physicians could wield considerable power and authority. When these successful physicians spoke, people were inclined to listen. There is little reason to doubt that on some occasions, at least, philosophers and physicians competed for influence and authority before their public on moral matters relating to *the right way to live*. For this is precisely the area that the physician is likely to address in prescribing and justifying his regimen for the preservation of health. Yet the acquisition of sound habits and daily regimen is also the proper domain of the philosopher. The philosopher seeks to define what a life worth living is and may prescribe rules of conduct for achieving it.

Mindful of this potential competition for influence between physicians and philosophers on matters of personal conduct, philosophers from Plato and Aristotle on sought to reassert the supremacy of their discipline as the only proper authority on the ultimate questions of human value. This can be seen in Plato's dialogue, *Laches,* in which at one point Nicias (with Socrates' approval) asserts that Laches had just spoken falsely of physicians, ". . . because he [Laches] thinks that the physician's knowledge of illness extends *beyond* the nature of health and disease. But in fact the physician knows no more than this."[38] Elsewhere in the dialogues (e.g., *Republic*, Book Four) Plato tends to reduce the authority and role of the physician by restricting medical assistance to cases of an emergency nature only, such as the repair of broken limbs, gashes, wounds, etc. Moreover, the physician is forbidden to instruct the citizens of Plato's ideal state to seek or preserve their personal health at any cost or by any means. Such vain advice would not serve the economic interests of the state. It would instead threaten to extend human suffering beyond the limit of a useful, worthwhile life, in Plato's opinion.[39]

To sum up, the relationship between ancient philosophy and ancient medicine is both resourceful and contentious. On the one hand, the philosophers benefited from the richness and power of medical similes and analogies, casting these as useful instructional devices. On the other hand, the physician, particularly if he was renowned or well respected by the public, posed a potential threat to philosophers by trying to tell others how to live; i.e., which medical regimens were *most valuable*. The point that Plato, Aristotle, and their successors tried to make is that, at most, the physician is entitled to *describe* how one might—should one so choose—regain or preserve one's health. The physician is not entitled to *prescribe* whether one ought to try to recover or preserve one's health at any cost. In other words, the positing of ultimate aims and values was seen by most of these ancient philosophers as a task belonging to the province of philosophy alone. This task did not properly belong to the medical craft or with any other discipline, for that matter.[40]

Discussion Questions

1. Was there a true medical profession in the classical age of Greece? Were there distinct types of physicians?
2. Did Egyptian medicine influence the growing scientific tendencies of fifth-century-B.C. Greek medicine? How so? What about Jewish influences?
3. Compare the regulation of medicine by the state in Egypt to that of Greece. Which culture provided a freer climate for clinical practice?
4. What was the relationship between physicians and philosophers in ancient Greece? Does this rivalry continue today?

NOTES

1. Ludwig Edelstein, "The Distinctive Hellenism of Greek Medicine," in *Ancient Medicine: Selected Papers of Ludwig Edelstein*, ed. Owsei Temkin and Lilian C. Temkin (Baltimore: Johns Hopkins University Press, 1967), p. 376. See Homer *Odyssey* 17.383–85, trans. Richard Lattimore (New York: Harper and Row, 1967).
2. Edelstein, "The Distinctive Hellenism," p. 376.
3. *Digesta* 50.13.1:3.
4. See Ludwig Edelstein and Emma J. Edelstein, *Asclepius: A Collection and Interpretation of the Testimonies*, 2 vols. (Baltimore: Johns Hopkins University Press, 1945). See also Edwin H. Ackerknecht, *A Short History of Medicine* (New York: Ronald Press, 1955), p. 44.
5. While the Edelsteins (note 4) have done a remarkable and apparently exhaustive job of assembling (in volume one of their study) the known relevant evidence on the Asclepius religious cult, it must be acknowledged that, in general, the problems of tracing the continuity of medical developments from Homer's time to the fifth century B.C. are great. According to Henry E. Sigerist: "We would like to know what rational medicine was like between Homer and Hippocrates—that is, in the four hundred years from the ninth to the fifth century B.C.—not that it has been lost, it was never written. The writing of medical books in the fifth century was a new phenomenon." See Henry E. Sigerist, *A History of Medicine*, 2 vols. (New York: Oxford University Press, 1951 and 1961), vol. 1, p. 85.
6. Ackerknecht, *History of Medicine*, p. 44. See also chapter 8, note 8.
7. The actual sons of Asclepius were Machaon and Polalirius, both of whom Homer mentions for their bravery and service in the *Iliad*. In particular, it is Machaon who treats the wounds of Menelaus, adding further to the greatness of his family's healing skills. See Homer *Iliad* 4.192–218.
8. Homer *Iliad* 11.514, *The Iliad of Homer*, trans. Richard Latimore (Chicago: University of Chicago Press, 1961), p. 248.
9. Aristotle *Politics* 3.6.1282a, trans. H. Rackman (London: Loeb Classical Library, 1969), p. 227.
10. Plato *Laws* 4.720, trans. A. E. Taylor, *The Collected Dialogues of Plato*, ed. Huntington Cairns and Edith Hamilton (New York: Random House, 1966), pp. 1310–11.
11. Ibid., *Laws* 60.857c–e. For an alternative interpretation, see Fridolf Kudlien's monograph, "Die Sklaven in der griechischen Medizin der klassischen und hellenistischen

Zeit," *Forschungen zur antiken Sklaverei* 2 (Wiesbaden: Steiner, 1968). Kudlien questions whether Plato's distinction is between free and slave physicians in respect to their *legal* status, or between physicians who are liberal or slavish-minded in respect to their *use* of the art.

12. Owsei Temkin, "Greek Medicine as Science and Craft," *Isis* 33 (1963), p. 214.
13. Galen, *De simplicium medicamentorum temperamentis ac facultatibus* 10.22, cited in Edelstein, "Distinctive Hellenism," p. 386.
14. Ludwig Edelstein, "The Hippocratic Physician," in *Ancient Medicine*, p. 87.
15. Edelstein, "Distinctive Hellenism," p. 385. For a comparison of the classical attitude toward work and the modern concept of the nobility of toil, see Humfrey Michell, *The Economics of Ancient Greece*, 2nd ed. (Cambridge, U.K.: W. Heffer, 1963), p. 14. In general, there was a strong feeling on the part of the aristocrats of the fifth and fourth centuries B.C. (constituting a vocal minority) that working with one's hands for a living was inferior to the cultivation of intellectual skills and pursuits done for their own sake. Edelstein comments: "Completely free of any idealization of work as such, and considering it a dire necessity rather than an ennobling activity, the classical age judged all manual labor only by the standard of expertness and performance." (See Edelstein, "The Ethics of the Greek Physician," in *Ancient Medicine*, p. 326.) Cf. Aristotle *Politics* 1337b.17ff.
16. Darrel W. Amundsen, "History of Medical Ethics: Ancient Greece and Rome," in *EB*, vol. 3, p. 933.
17. Ibid., p. 933. On the topic of medical specialization in antiquity, Robert Flacelière recognizes a total of seven distinct health care practitioners of various sorts whom we would regard as medical professionals or paraprofessionals. These are (1) the *gymnastic master (paido-tribes)* "who was often a [2] *hygienist* and [3] *dietician* who could advise athletes on the best diet to follow. . . ," and could also reduce fractures, sprains, and dislocations; (4) *the pharmacist (pharmakopoles)* "who got his own supplies from the harvester of roots (*rhizotomos*)"; (5) *oculists*, whose principal method of caring for their patients' eyes was using eye washes; (6) *dentists*, who knew how to fill teeth with gold; and (7) the *midwife*, one notable child of whom was Socrates. But it was unlikely that there exists within these divisions of labor a strict recognition of one's area of competence. Thus, one must not be misled into reading contemporary medical specializations into these loosely defined ancient vocations. In addition to the seven medical functions just mentioned, there is some evidence that a few Greek city-states employed so-called *public physicians (iatros demosieuon)*. (See Robert Flacelière, "Medicine," *Praeger Encyclopedia of Ancient Greek Civilization* [New York: Praeger, 1967], pp. 288–290.) However, Louis Cohn-Haft, in his study "The Public Physicians of Ancient Greece," has raised serious doubts about the existence of such physicians in anything like a system of government-sponsored medical care. See Louis Cohn-Haft, "The Public Physicians of Ancient Greece," *Smith College Studies in History* 62 (1956): 1–99.
18. Herodotus, The Persian Wars II. 84, trans. George Rawlinson, *The Greek Historians. The Complete and Unabridged Works of Herodotus, Thucydides, Xenophon, and Arrian,* 2 vols. (New York: Random House, 1942), vol. 2, p. 123.
19. According to John W. Wilson, these are the Edwin Smith Papyrus (surgical), the Embers Papyrus, the London Papyrus, the Hearst Papyrus, and the Berlin Papyrus. See John W. Wilson, "Medicine in Ancient Egypt," *Bulletin of the History of Medicine* 32 (1962): 116.
20. Ibid., pp. 122–23.

21. T. Clifford Allbutt, *Greek Medicine in Rome* (London: Macmillan and Co., 1921), p. 133. Allbutt's claim that the humoral doctrine originated in Egypt finds little support and he supplies no evidence.

22. J. B. Saunders, *The Transitions from Ancient Egyptian to Greek Medicine* (Lawrence, KS: University of Kansas Press, 1963), pp. 15–33.

23. For evidence of clear cases of Egyptian magic alongside more rational approaches to the treatment of disease, see James H. Breasted, *The Edwin Smith Surgical Papyrus*, 2 vols. (Chicago: University of Chicago Press, Case 9, 1930), pp. 217ff.

24. W. Wilson, "Ancient Egypt," p. 123. See also Edelstein, "Distinctive Hellenism," pp. 376–77, and Owsei Temkin, "Health and Disease," *Dictionary of the History of Ideas*, ed. Philip P. Wiener, 4 vols. (New York: Charles Scribner's Sons, 1973), vol. 2, pp. 395–96.

25. Darrel W. Amundsen and Gary Ferngren, "History of Medical Ethics: Ancient Near East," in *EB 1995*, vol. 3, p. 1440. Emphasis added. For more on comparative Jewish influences, see the subheading in chapter 4, "Medical Ethics before Hippocrates."

26. Ibid., vol. 3, p. 1442. Even so, there is little doubt that the Israelites knew how to treat wounds (Isa. 3:7), set fractures (Ezek. 30:21), and treat various other ailments (Jer. 51:8). In fact, the Hebrew word for healer or physician, the participle of the verb *rapha,* can be translated "one who sews together or repairs." See also Immanuel Jacobovits, *Jewish Medical Ethics: A Comparative and Historical Study of the Jewish Religion's Attitude and Its Practice* (New York: Bloch Publishing Co., 1975), chaps. 15–20.

27. Amundsen and Ferngren, "History of Medical Ethics," vol. 3, p. 1443.

28. Ibid. See also Owsei Temkin, "The Almighty God," in *Hippocrates in a World of Pagans and Christians* (Baltimore: Johns Hopkins University Press, 1991), pp. 86–93. Nonetheless, Amundsen and Ferngren judiciously acknowledge that some Hellenistic Jews were skeptical of the motivations of those who turned to rational healing. For example, the Alexandrian philosopher Philo Judaeus (ca. 20 B.C.–A.D. 50), considered by many to be the father of Jewish philosophy, condemned those who sought medical treatment without specific reference to God, or worse—as a desperate maneuver bereft of piety.

29. Amundsen and Ferngren, "History of Medical Ethics," in *EB*, vol. 2, p. 882.

30. Ibid.

31. Aristotle *Politics* 3.1286a.12ff., trans. Benjamin Jowett, in *The Basic Works of Aristotle*, ed. Richard McKeon (New York: Random House, 1941), p. 1198.

32. Edelstein, "Distinctive Hellenism," p. 375. Cf. Philemon *Fragmenta comicorum greacorum* 14.1841, cited by Edelstein, p. 375.

33. There was no concept of "professions" in the classical age, as has been emphasized especially by Alfred E. Zimmern, *The Greek Commonwealth*, 2nd rev. ed. (Oxford: Clarendon Press, 1915), pp. 257ff. It is probably true that in Hellenistic or later times, physicians as a class continued to acquire a greater social status; that their status varied according to different schools or individual authors like Plutarch or Galen there can be no doubt. But on the whole, these were later developments. Fridolf Kudlien rightly suggests that the ancients themselves held no unanimous opinion on the classification of medicine in the system of *technai*. He writes: "One well-known and important fact is that medicine was not included in the classical canon of liberal arts; however, this does not mean that it was never counted among them. . . . " (See Fridolf Kudlien, "Medicine as a 'Liberal Art' and the Question of the Physician's Income," *Journal of the History of Medicine* 31, no. 4 [1976]: 448–59.) See also note 15.

34. Edelstein, "The Relation of Ancient Philosophy to Medicine," *Ancient Medicine*, p. 361.

35. Frag. 31, trans. Kathleen Freeman, *Ancilla to the Pre-Socratics. A Complete Translation of the Fragments in Diels, Fragmente der Vorsokratiker* (Oxford: Basil Blackwell, 1948), p. 99. Aside from Democritus, it is quite possible that many of the Pythagoreans were themselves physicians. Evidence suggests that the Pythagorean recognition symbol, the pentagram, was also used as a symbol of health. Empedocles, too, was known as a healer. Hence, early philosophical theories of the universe and early principles of medicine may have coalesced in these pre-Socratic authors. See also Plato *Gorgias* 464ff. for allusive passages hinting at loose philosophical and medical links.

36. Aristotle *Nicomachean Ethics* 2.1.1104a.1–20, trans. W. D. Ross in *Basic Works*, pp. 9353–54.

37. Werner Jaeger, "Aristotle's Use of Medicine as a Model in His Ethics," *Journal of the History of Science* 77 (1957): 54–61, especially 55–57. Cf. Diego Gracia, "The Structure of Medical Knowledge in Aristotle's Philosophy," *Sudhoffs Archiv* 62, no. 1 (1978): 17.

38. Plato *Laches* 195c-d, trans. Benjamin Jowett in *Collected Dialogues*, p. 139.

39. Plato *Republic* 4.406ff., trans. Francis M. Cornford (London: Oxford Press, 1973).

40. Edelstein, "Relation of Ancient Philosophy to Medicine," p. 360. Cf. Aristotle *Eudaemonian Ethics* 2.2.1227b.25ff.

2 Theories of Health and Disease

In all things relating to disease, credulity remains
a permanent fact, uninfluenced by civilization
or education.

—WILLIAM OSLER, M.D.

WHATEVER BENEFITS CAME to philosophy by way of Greek medicine, Greek medicine also received from the early pre-Socratic philosophers the impetus to emancipate the healing arts from magic and superstition. In this chapter, I shall explore some of the main facets of two theories of health and disease that most strongly influenced Greek physicians; namely, the humoral theory associated with Hippocrates and the eclectic theory of the best constitution associated with Galen. The pre-Socratic influence toward seeking the universal causes of phenomena in the *natural order* governed by lawlike, nonmagical forces (knowable to man through rational reflection and observation) was an influence unquestionably felt by the Hippocratic authors. However, I shall not stop to argue this point, owing both to the long digression it would entail and to the fact that scholars like Sigerist, Jaeger, and Edelstein, among others, have admirably secured this position and stand virtually unopposed. Instead, I shall be concentrating on the results of the general pre-Socratic quest for natural explanations; particular pre-Socratic philosophers will receive only the briefest mention. To promote continuity, Democritus, Plato, and Aristotle will receive additional exposure so that their theories of health and disease may be understood in relation to pertinent medical developments.

THE HIPPOCRATIC HUMORAL THEORY

It is important to recognize at the onset that, while the doctrine of the four humors is widely presupposed or explicitly mentioned by the authors of the seventy or so medical treatises that comprise the Hippocratic Collection, the basic theory about to be explored acquires various interpretations and applications, depending on the particular treatise one consults. That is, there was no single, primitive humoral theory explicitly endorsed by the Hippocratic authors. Instead one finds variations and elaborations of a recurring number of limited diagnostic, prognostic, and therapeutic principles that are often systematically linked.

Although the related question of who this person called Hippocrates really was will be pursued in a later chapter, some of the evidence indicates that Hippocrates may not have personally embraced the humoral theory. Rather, according to the testimony of Aristotle's pupil, Meno, there is reason to believe that Hippocrates himself laid disease to the generation of putrefied air that arises inside the body when the body fails to properly digest food.[1] Even so, the medical authors of the treatises with which his name is associated were influenced by Hippocrates' organistic principle according to which one cannot truly understand the nature of part of the body without first understanding the nature of the whole body. Therefore, although Hippocrates himself cannot be definitely linked with the humoral theory per se, it is fair to conclude that the systematic and holistic character evidenced by that theory would have been congenial to his medical outlook.

As to the humoral theory itself, I have modified Henry Sigerist's splendid account, based on Hippocratic sources, by casting the fundamentals of the humoral theory into seven basic principles that more fully capture the theory's explanatory power.[2] These seven principles, in the order in which they shall be discussed, are:

(1) the principle of equilibrium
(2) the principle of seasonal influence
(3) the principle of contraries
(4) the principle of innate heat
(5) the principle of natural healing
(6) the principle of *pepsis*
(7) the principle of critical days

To begin with, the *principle of equilibrium* is the most fundamental, as it asserts that health is the result of a proper balance or equilibrium within the body, whereas illness is caused by humoral imbalance. But what are humors exactly, and what substances constitute them? A treatise taken by many scholars to be one of the earliest in the Hippocratic Collection, titled *On Ancient Medicine*, identifies the humors with an *unlimited* number of forces or qualities (*dynameis*), such as heat, cold, dry, moist, sweet, bitter, etc. When the blend of these qualities is perfect, a man is in perfect health.[3] But should poor nutrition or some other cause upset the balance, disease occurs.

Yet there is little doubt that talk of forces or qualities is rather vague sounding. Accordingly, the author of another treatise, *On Breaths*, drops the humoral model in favor of an explanation of diseases based on the presence or absence in the body of the correct amount and blend of air inhaled from one's environment and drawn into the interstices of various organs. It would appear that this author sought a somewhat more tangible substance than the vague humoral qualities alluded to above; breath appeared to be real and always essential to sustaining human health.

Gradually, though, the tendency in the Hippocratic Collection was to reintroduce the terminology of the humors and, *unlike* the author of *Ancient Medicine*, limit them to just four. Thus, in *On Diseases* the humors are identified as phlegm, blood, bile, and water.[4] Moreover, in that same treatise each humor is said to originate in four specific organs: blood from the heart, phlegm from the head, water from the spleen, and bile from the gall bladder. It is also suggested that disease can be traced to three basic causes. The first cause mentioned is the excess or deficiency of any one of the four humors (usually due to an inadequate or overindulgent diet). The second is diseases stemming from violent causes, such as wounds, falls, or, on the other extreme, severe fatigue. And the third is atmospheric conditions (season, weather, climate), which can dispose people toward disease, about which more will be said later. The same author asserts that these three factors act on the humors, making them coagulate or liquify or undergo some related change. In this way, "the vitiated humor attaches itself to some part of the body and the diseases are usually named after the organ affected."[5]

However, it is in the somewhat later treatise, *The Nature of Man*, that water is replaced as a humor by black bile, which is introduced here for the first time as a normal humoral constituent of the body.[6] Sigerist designates this treatise, attributed by Aristotle to Polybus, as the starting point of the classical theory of the four humors. Along with the remaining three constituents, yellow bile, phlegm, and blood, this theory dominated medical thinking for two thousand years. In accordance with the first principle, in this treatise perfect health is said to prevail when these four humors are in equilibrium (*isonomia*) with regard to their temperature, strength, and quantity.[7] In addition, when one humor reigns supreme (what the pre-Socratic Alcmaeon called *monarchia*), isolates itself, or no longer cooperates with the other three, pain may originate in two locations within the patient: (1) the site that the humor leaves may become inflamed and (2) the site that the humor crowds may swell with pain. Similarly, the sudden or abnormal evacuation of a humor (either inside or outside the body) is said to cause considerable pain.

But what exactly, then, is a humor—at least as it is generally characterized by the Hippocratic authors?

> These are not fictitious, not mere principles, but very real. Wound the body anywhere and you will see *blood*. Give a drug that acts on phlegm and the individual will vomit *phlegm*; or [*yellow*] *bile* if you give him a cholagogic remedy. Similarly, he will evacuate *black bile* in response to certain drugs.[8]

In sum, humors were characteristically taken to be tangible substances originating in the body largely through digestive and related nutritional processes. Furthermore, they are not merely theoretical terms, for they were thought to have determinate empirical content and be spatiotemporally located within the body.

Thus, it becomes increasingly evident that the explanatory power accorded to the doctrine of the four humors owed not only to its ability to describe and classify diseases, but also to its capacity to provide physiological causal explanations.

Let us now turn to the second principle. I shall call it the *principle of seasonal influence*. Quite simply, this principle asserts that the qualities of hot, cold, moist, and dry always distributed in the four seasons are linked to the four humors always found in man in such a way that changing seasonal conditions causally determine which diseases each person is disposed to get at any given time. This means that the physician was expected to take into consideration, among other things, the climate and weather conditions when diagnosing and treating his patients. For it was suggested that the seasons, in fact, had some influence on the four bodily humors.

To illustrate, it was observed that nose bleeding occurred in the spring more than at other times—the increase of blood being related to the *hot* and *moist* seasonal conditions of spring. In contrast, summer, which is characteristically *hot* and *dry*, was thought to give rise to yellow bile in the body. This was suggested since physicians observed more bilious stools then and also observed that the skin often manifested a yellow tinge. Thus, the data of observation seemed to confirm the principle of seasonal influence.

Also adding to the wide attraction the humoral theory enjoyed in antiquity was the fact that the four qualities—hot, cold, moist, and dry—could be linked not only to the four seasons, but also to the four elements—fire, earth, water, and air—which the pre-Socratic philosopher Empedocles (495–435 B.C.) had identified as the ultimate constituents of the universe. So that part of the humoral theory expressed by the principle of seasonal influence could be elaborated easily to connect man's nature (*physis*) to the nature of the entire universe. Hence, this cosmological symmetry of qualitative, humoral, and elemental pairings lent added force to the humoral theory by physically joining the microcosm of man with the macrocosm of nature.

The third principle, which I have dubbed the *principle of contraries*, constitutes a further extension of the theory. It serves to systematize the diagnosis and treatment capabilities afforded by the humoral model by specifying that organs, diseases, and remedies likewise possess the qualities hot, cold, moist, and dry. In view of this, it prescribes that contraries should be cured by contraries.[9] A chart (Fig. 3) illustrates the relations between the four humors, the four proximal qualities, the four Empedoclean elements, and the four seasons.

What was the logic undergirding this third principle? Why and how the principle of contraries was utilized to aid in diagnosis and treatment may be seen from the following example. Suppose a patient complained of abdominal pain. Suppose further that the physician inferred from this complaint that, based on the humoral theory, its cause was probably due to a humoral imbalance associated with the patient's black bile. Black bile was thought to originate in that bodily organ known as the spleen. Furthermore, when the black bile was in proper equilibrium with the other three humors, its qualities of dryness and coldness (see Fig. 3) stood in a proportion productive of health. Now, however, suppose the patient evidenced cold

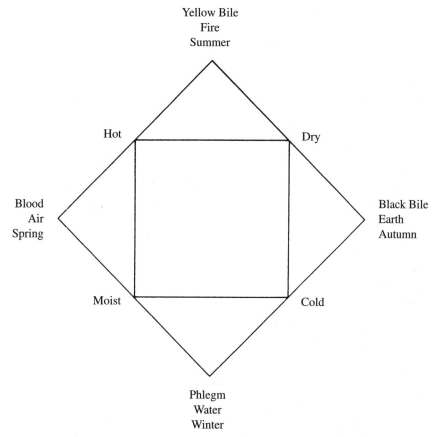

Yellow Bile
Fire
Summer

Hot

Dry

Blood
Air
Spring

Black Bile
Earth
Autumn

Moist

Cold

Phlegm
Water
Winter

Figure 3. The Humoral Square of Opposites, implying causal connections between the four basic elements, the four seasons, the four contraries, and the four bodily humors. Versions of this theory dominated Western medicine from Hippocrates' day until nearly A.D. *1650.*

chills and suffered further from constipation. These symptoms suggested an excess inside the body of the qualities cold and dry, respectively. The contraries of cold and dry are, according to the Humoral Square of Opposites, hot and moist. This information provided the basis for a treatment plan based on a seemingly rational framework.

Here, in order to remedy the abdominal pain, the patient might be prescribed periodic hot baths followed by a general increase in the intake of liquids. The aim of this particular remedy, like all similarly devised remedies, was to bring into proper balance the humoral excesses or deficiencies diagnosed as causing the affliction: the hot baths to warm the *overly cold* black bile; the increased intake of beverages to moisten the *overly dry* properties of the black bile.

As useful as the humoral theory was for supplying a causal account of the many diseases known to ancient man, the four humors alone did not seem to be able to explain the origin of life itself in the body. Some sort of driving force was thought to be involved to explain further: (a) how were the humors developed and sustained by food?; (b) what caused them to possess motion?; and (c) what blended them together in varying proportions so as to expel superfluities and regain balance? This driving force was identified as the "innate heat" (*emphyton thermon*); it is a vital force that may well have derived from Heraclitus's notion of fire as the embodiment of the dynamic motion of all existing things. In any case, innate heat was said to have its seat in the left ventricle of the heart.[10] These considerations introduce our fourth principle, the *principle of innate heat*, which states that the origin, nutritional processes, and dynamic motion of the four humors themselves are produced by the body's innate, fiery heat.

The beauty of this seemingly ad hoc principle within the humoral theory is that it furnished a convenient explanation for several other bodily phenomena that seemed to demand explanation. For example, the rapid heartbeat and higher bodily temperature of infants could *ex hypothesi* be understood as the natural result of a higher level of innate heat required to promote faster bodily growth. In contrast, that older persons have lower bodily temperatures could be explained because they are through growing and their innate heat is at a lower level. This fact also explains why older persons generally need less food than the young; i.e., their humors are fully developed and need only to be sustained. Just as neatly explained by the presence of the heart's innate heat is the whole process of respiration. It was held that the fundamental reason one must breathe is that the heart needs to be cooled lest it be damaged by excessively hot temperatures.

Having established that innate heat is an essential part of man's nature, the fifth *principle of natural healing* follows from the yet further consideration best introduced by the Hippocratic author of the treatise *Epidemics*. "Nature," he writes, "is the physician of diseases. Nature finds ways and means all by itself, not as a result of thought."[11] This observation led finally to the fifth principle, which states: (a) that nature is a cooperative force that works through each person to bring the diseased body back into that often-delicate balance that defines health and (b) the task of the physician is to understand the workings of nature, prescribe only those therapies that will support nature, and do nothing that might impede the natural healing processes.

There are two immediate implications of this fifth principle. The first is that nature was not seen to be inherently inimical to man's survival, but rather was inclined to be supportive of life. This was deduced from the fact that sometimes very sick or injured patients fully recovered on their own without seeking medical treatment. In this sense also, many Greeks (especially the Stoics) tended to view nature in a positive light and sought to live in accord with nature's laws. Second, as nature was seen to work in a regular, sometimes cooperative way, the physician sought to educate himself to nature's regular healing processes. Only then could he be effective as a cohealer and promoter of this wondrous healing power of nature (*vis medicatrix naturae*). The key to healing was a sound medical education; the best teacher was ultimately nature.

This fifth principle also helps explain why the prognosis of the Hippocratic physician was so important. To know what the likely cause and outcome of a disease would be had much to do with helping to promote the natural bodily processes in the right way, *at the right time*. But if the patient was judged beyond help owing to nature's irresistible natural course (which included, finally, decay and death), there was little point in endeavoring to begin treatment other than keeping the patient comfortable. More will be said about this decision "not to treat" in the following chapters.

The sixth and seventh principles of the humoral theory are closely related. Thus, it is profitable to discuss them together. Both are concerned with explaining and predicting the detailed physiological processes that cause disease in somewhat more precise terms than the five preceding principles do. The sixth *principle of pepsis* states that most diseases are caused by one humor dominating the others in an abnormal, excessive way; the excessive matter of the dominant humor naturally undergoes a thickening process called *pepsis* (or coction), culminating in its expulsion from the body so that humoral balance is restored.

Just what causes one humor to dominate the others in the first place is sometimes hard to specify. But the Hippocratic authors usually ascribed the imbalance to (a) improper diet; (b) lack of proper exercise; (c) bodily injury; or, more generally (d) an incorrect mode of living in relation to the seasons of the year. In any event, the excessive matter of the offending humor (later called the *materia peccans*) needed to become ripe in order to be expelled. Sigerist elaborates:

> The body mobilized all its defensive forces and attacked the raw, faulty humor which under the influence of *innate heat* became "cooked," ripe, and ready to be expelled. . . . The expulsion was quick in the form of a *crisis*; or slow and gradual—in the latter case we still speak of a *lysis*. The crisis is defined in the treatise *On Diseases* as a condition in which a disease takes a turn for the worse or for the better or changes its character or ends by being healed.[12]

In my view Sigerist has aptly termed this turning point the "decisive battle" between man's nature and the disease. Moreover, one need not look far to realize that this process called *pepsis* or thickening, which led to the expulsion of the offending matter, would seem to be supported by commonplace observations such as the increase of phlegm, sputum, and other putrid bodily fluids that often accompany a variety of diseases (including the common cold). Therefore, one can again appreciate that the theory embodied in this principle seemed well borne out by the data of experience to which the Greek physicians regularly turned.

That the *crisis* of a particular disease tends to be reached in a specifiable number of days—at which time the disease usually takes a crucial turn for better or worse—was the prognostic principle which I shall refer to as the *principle of critical days.*

One sees in this seventh and last principle an effort to mathematize medical treatment along lines that would have been quite congenial to the pre-Socratic Pythagoras and may have been inspired in part by his teaching that all phenomena are reducible to number. At any rate, the Hippocratic physician observed that many diseases—e.g., the common cold, pneumonia, malaria, etc.—appeared to have their own natural course regardless of who suffers them. If so, the effort to closely record and isolate the days associated with characteristic, marked changes in the patient's condition promised to supply predictive power based on the identification of the patient's current stage in the disease process. It also supplied a basis for classifying diseases based in part on detectible similarities or differences in the duration of the relevant symptoms.

In conformity with this last principle, the author of *Epidemics* I is quite emphatic: "One must pay attention to the crises and know that at such times they decide about the life and death or at least the changes for better or worse."[13] Also, in *Prognostics* we read:

> Fevers come to a crisis on the same days as to number, both those from which men recover and from which they die. For the mildest class of fevers, and those appearing with the most favorable symptoms prove fatal on the *fourth* day or earlier; and the most malignant and those setting in with the most dangerous symptoms prove fatal on the *fourth* day or earlier.[14]

One can discern in these words the growing tendency (now a common feature of modern medicine) to mathematize the signs and symptoms of diseases and to define more precisely diagnostic, prognostic, and therapeutic procedures. It is also possible that the emphasis on the number four in these and other passages throughout the Hippocratic Collection is indicative of Pythagorean influences.

What is more certain, however, is that though there was admittedly a strong speculative element in these attempts to link the critical days of illness to determinate disease outcomes, the bulk of the clinical observations on which such predictions rested were in themselves accurate. Indeed, in this seventh medical principle, as in almost all that have been presented, it is evident that, while from the modern medical perspective the Hippocratic physicians did not know the true causes of most diseases, they often knew the effects. These effects they diligently recorded and classified based on recurring symptom sequences from which they tried, as good empiricists, to reach general conclusions. Moreover, one finds in their inductive, systematic, and mathematical approach the embryonic beginnings of a genuinely rational and scientific medicine.

Having discussed the seven basic principles of the humoral theory, we are now in the position to notice further that it construes disease and health in basically physiological, not ontological, terms. Here a brief digression is necessary. Traditionally there have been two alternatively dominant and opposing concepts of disease theory throughout history: (1) the *physiological* and (2) the *ontological*. The former characteristically (a) construes disease as a consequence of imbalanced functions occurring within the individual; (b) emphasizes the uniqueness of each person's affliction; and (c) construes the pathological disease processes as occurring inside the whole person instead of ascribing the dysfunction or disease to outside, invading disease entities (*entia morbi*).

In contrast, the latter ontological concept of disease characteristically (a) does not construe disease as a consequence of imbalanced functions occurring within the individual; (b) emphasizes the specific reality and distinctiveness of the disease entity (*ens morbi*) in contrast to the patient harboring it; and (c) construes the disease as a discrete, usually localized entity that is external to the healthy person but that, in seating or manifesting itself inside the individual, produces the onset of disease.

Now it has been shown that, on the humoral theory, the diseased patient as a whole is regarded as sick. In the main, his illness is the result of a humoral imbalance, a dysfunction involving the entire person. For the humors were thought to run throughout the body in general, even though the faulty humor might be more concentrated in one region than another. True, some diseases were construed as localized on the humoral theory, but only roughly so and not very often. Hence, the Hippocratic authors were disinclined to view disease as a specific entity with an ontological status independent of the whole patient. For example, one such author describes what we now call mumps as "swellings in the region of the ears" (*eparmata para ta ota*).[15] But characteristically, he attaches no name to this particular disease, for the disease does not have any separate status, nor does it have a determinate seat in the anatomy of the body.

THE DEMOCRITEAN ATOMISTIC THEORY

In contrast with the physiological concept of disease that is associated with the humoral theory found in the Hippocratic Collection, the ontological concept of disease—according to which diseases are usually construed as discrete, localized entities—can be hypothetically reconstructed from the writings of Democritus (460–370 B.C.) and the later atomists. It will be recalled that Democritus sought to explain all the observable phenomena of both the macrocosm and the microcosm as the result of the size, shape, and arrangement of invisible, indestructible atoms afloat in the void. What is less widely known is that he wrote on medical topics, producing at least three books, which are lost to posterity, titled *Prognosis, On Diet,* and *On Medical Method.* In this connection, Democritus is reported to have said that one can preserve one's health through self-discipline. He wrote: "Men ask in their prayers for health from the gods, but do not know that the power to attain this lies in themselves; and by doing the opposite thing, through lack of control, they themselves become the betrayers of their own health to their diseases."[16]

Like Pythagoras before him, Democritus stresses that moderation in all things brought pleasure and well-being. Moreover, according to at least one ancient commentator, Democritus attributed mental illness to the excessive hotness or coldness of the fine round atoms that constituted a person's soul.[17] After reporting on Democritus's materialistic theory of illness, Theophrastus (ca. 370–285 B.C.) stated, "it is evident that he made thinking dependent upon the mixture of the body—which is perhaps reasonable enough in one who makes the soul a body."[18]

Reducing all psychological states to the mechanism of the material soul-atoms uniquely arranged in the void (i.e., the spaces or pores of the patient's body in this context), and construing all illness in the final analysis as the result of and identical with the body's disordered and misarranged atoms, it seems quite fitting that Democritus urged the attainment of an even, cheerful disposition. For such an ethical ideal, if realized, would on his theory keep the soul atoms free from the sort of *physical agitation* that he associated with violent passions. These violent, angry passions, having a material basis, could in turn produce unhappy, deranged thoughts. This could so affect the individual as to render him mad.

But the point at issue here is that whether a disease is termed mental or physical in our conventional usage, for Democritus all diseases are at bottom physical. Thus on his view all diseases were thought of as having a determinate seat in a localized part of the body constituted by discrete atoms. Also, the spatial relations of these atoms in the interstices and pores of the body within which they are arranged defined the separate ontological status and character of a given disease as distinct from the patient.[19] Hence, the disease may even be construed as an invading entity existing in some sense on its *own*—thus having its own ontological status.

PLATO AND ARISTOTLE

Having identified the main features of the physiological and ontological disease models associated with the humoral and atomistic theories, respectively, let us turn briefly to the way in which health and disease are interpreted by Plato (ca. 429–347 B.C.) and Aristotle (384–322 B.C.).

Neither Plato nor Aristotle supply written accounts of a full-blown theory of health. Rather, in both cases we are typically left with characterizations of healthy or diseased persons under various conditions. The more theoretically exacting premises are either tersely sketched or omitted altogether.[20] Yet, it would be a mistake to conclude from this absence of detail a lack of interest in health matters. One need only recall the fact that most educated Greeks were quite abreast of the current theories of medicine. Indeed, both Plato and Aristotle took this background knowledge for granted when they borrowed from the medical arts whatever analogies and anecdotes served their instructional ends.

That Plato's view of health is marked by Pythagorean and Empedoclean influences, very likely absorbed from Philistion during Plato's stay in Sicily (at Syracuse), has been urged by A. E. Taylor and is plausible. The Pythagorean emphasis on maintaining equilibrium, also present in the first principle of the humoral theory discussed above, is unmistakable, for example, in Plato's *Republic* 444d.3–6: "But to produce *health* is to establish the elements in a body in the natural relation of dominating and being dominated by one another, while to cause *disease* is to bring it about that one rules or is ruled by the other contrary to nature."[21]

What is the significance of this passage? In the context of the *Republic* 4, where the discussion turns on the parallel between justice in the state and justice in the individual, this passage serves mainly to establish a crucial analogy between the well-ordered body which is often called healthy, and the well-ordered soul which Plato calls just. That is, as health is the virtue (*arete*) or excellence of the body promoting its wholesomeness, beauty, and strength, so too justice is the virtue of the soul that fosters ". . . a kind of health and beauty and good condition of the soul . . . ."[22] Thus, the defect of the soul is the opposite of justice, namely injustice. What's more, injustice is pictured as a defect analogous to disease. So to ask which is more profitable, being just or unjust, is to invite the conclusion that justice *alone* is more profitable. For to choose to be just is like choosing health; to become unjust is like courting disease. Hence, it is fair to conclude that for Plato achieving a just soul is a necessary condition and, perhaps, even a sufficient condition for achieving mental health.

In addition, physical health is characterized by Plato as a proper balance among the elements of the body. (In his *Timaeus*, these elements are ultimately reducible to elementary scalene and isosceles triangles, and the four Empedoclean elements into which they are combined are given a broader explanatory role than the four humors.) Mental health is also characterized in a parallel way as a correct balance. Also in *Republic* 4, the reader is informed that the three parts of a person's soul (reason, the spirited element, and the appetitive element) must be brought into proper attunement.[23] This attunement or balance is defined as manifest in a soul whose reason, allied with the spirited element (akin to emotions), benevolently governs the appetites (akin to bodily desires). Further, the three parts of the soul must work in harmony so that each is permitted to carry out *its own function* well without interfering with each other. In other words, it is supposed that reason has as its natural function the job of restraining the appetites; if the appetites usurped the authority of reason, some sort of disorder of the soul would ensue.

However, one may wish to challenge Plato's assumption that a theory of health, whether mental or physical health, can be formulated by simply reading off the putative natural functions attendant upon each part of the soul or organ of the body. It is fair to ask how Plato can know that the natural function of reason is to rule the appetites, and not vice versa. What evidence does he provide in this regard? Ultimately, he registers his own intuitions, which are determined in the *Republic* by considerations of a normative sort regarding what form of government and what type of citizen would combine into the best possible commonwealth. But one can easily imagine another person thoughtfully submitting to his intelligence these same utopian considerations and getting a different list of "natural functions" and relations between elements of the soul or body. If so, this tends to cast doubt on there being a single, purely descriptive natural function of man, as Plato presupposes. Therefore, the starting point in Plato's theory of health—the assumption that one can discover man's natural functions—is flawed by oversimplification.

Whatever else might be said about Plato's views on health and disease, it is important to note that on his view the responsibility for carrying out a program of mental and physical hygiene rests squarely with each person. It is not the responsibility of one's physician, though the physician may make helpful suggestions. Thus, although some mental diseases in particular may have their contributing cause in (1) a defective bodily constitution inherited from one's parents or (2) a bad upbringing, a person still has the duty to pursue those endeavors that will keep him well or help him overcome either of the preceding two defects.[24] In other words, though one cannot fairly be blamed for either a defective nature or a defective nurture, one can be held accountable for remedying whatever defects of one's birth or childhood come to one's attention as an adult citizen. This is a moral obligation.

Although Plato's matchless student Aristotle went beyond his teacher by systematically defining the natural and biological sciences and pioneering the fields of comparative anatomy and physiology, there is little to be found in his writings on the explicit causes of human health and disease. Although his own father was a physician and there is every reason to believe that Aristotle was familiar with most of the medical theories of the Hippocratic Collection, not a scrap of evidence suggests that he himself practiced as a physician. But as one who directly laid the foundations of Western biology and, through Galen, indirectly influenced the course of medical thinking at least to the Renaissance, that portion of his writing that has been preserved on the topic of health deserves close attention.

One important notion that Aristotle borrowed from Plato's *Timaeus* was the conviction that nature is like an intelligent force that does nothing without a purpose. This teleological orientation looms large in the *Timaeus*, especially where it is asserted that the divine Craftsman who fashioned man was unenvious of his creatures and so aimed at what was best in creating the soul and body of man, their respective organs, activities, and functions.[25] Though as an empiricist Aristotle sought to wed his biological theories more closely to the observational data that he took pains to collect, both philosophers embraced the view (just criticized above) that at every level man manifests natural functions that may be determined by trying to discover the essential purposes of nature in designing a thing as it is.[26]

Furthermore, Aristotle fell under the influence of the Hippocratic authors to the extent that he adopted their general characterization of disease as the disequilibrium of bodily structures or parts. He also allowed that seasonal or environmental factors affected man's disposition toward certain diseases. In addition, he associated the innate heat of the body with vital nutritional processes and rejected, as did the Hippocratics, any supernatural explanations of disease.[27] Yet in his writings he does not rely on their doctrine of the four humors. Instead, he identified the four physical opposites—the hot, the cold, the moist, and the dry—as the true elements of the natural world.[28] When these dynamic elements are properly blended in the human body, health results; when they are not, disease. And so in the *Physics* Aristotle states:

> Thus bodily excellences such as health and a good state of body we regard as consisting in a blending of hot and cold elements within the body in due proportion, in relation to one another *or to the surrounding atmosphere*: and in like manner we regard beauty, strength, and all the other bodily excellences and defects. Each of them exists in virtue of a particular relation and puts that which possesses it in a good or bad condition with regard to its proper affections, where by "proper" affections I mean those influences that from *the natural constitution* of a thing tend to promote or destroy its existence.[29]

So Aristotle, like the author of the Hippocratic treatise *Regimen*, generalizes that an animal's physical blend (as constituted by these four opposing elements) determines not only that animal's physical health, but also its disposition (temperament), sensitivity, and intelligence.[30] Thus, the physical as well as the psychological characteristics of a given species and the individuals within that species are significantly determined by the unique blending of Aristotle's four elements.

My conjecture is that these four elements constituted for Aristotle the primary *material cause* of health and disease (both mental and physical). Though Aristotle does not say so explicitly, I further conjecture that he conceived the main *efficient cause* of a disease as lying in (1) the corrupting processes peculiar to the disease with which one is affected *and* (2) the choices one makes through adjustments in diet, exercise, and habits that may modify the course of the disease for better or worse. If so, both Aristotle's *formal* and *final causes* of disease can be related to the defective form of the affected organ or tissues of the diseased individual. In this sense, some diseases may be understood in Aristotelian terms as the privation or corruption of the relevant natural function properly associated with the form and purpose of the animal part in question.[31]

Given the above interpretation, an additional implication of Aristotle's theory of health may now be explored. Doubtless Aristotle wanted to resist a wholly deterministic theory of disease so that some individual responsibility could be assigned for one's own health. The individual's habits and way of life constituted part of the regimen that the individual was free to adjust in order to suit his needs, aims, and values. In other words, the individual was free to choose what foods to eat, what drugs to take, what climate to reside in, how much exercise to take, etc., to the point where he could fairly be held at least partly accountable for the state of his own health. In this sense, the agent himself had the capacity to be part of the efficient cause of his own disease and its cure.

This fact of personal accountability, in my opinion, is what Aristotle was al-luding to when he said: "Old age is a natural disease, while disease is an acquired old age."[32] That is, old age (with its normally accompanying infirmities) is the nat-ural outcome of a healthy adulthood. No one can be blamed for growing old. But disease acquired prior to old age may in some cases, at least, be viewed as having something to do with the way an individual has chosen to live. This result is also quite compatible with Aristotle's ethical teachings. He taught that with few excep-tions a person may be held accountable for his own welfare, i.e., the state of his being.

THE MEDICAL SECTS

Following the deaths of Hippocrates and Aristotle in 399 and 322 B.C., respec-tively, almost all of the medical literature of the ensuing four hundred years has been lost to posterity. But such theories as there were during this period up to the birth of Galen in A.D. 129 have been reconstructed from fragmentary remains and from the illuminating commentaries of Galen and the post-Galenic authors. What can be said with some certainty about this intermediate period between the death of Hippocrates and the rise of Galen is that philosophical differences with regard to the way medicine should be practiced intensified among the Greek physicians to the point at which four distinct medical sects gradually emerged. Listed in rough chronological order these were: the Dogmatists, Empiricists, Methodists, and Pneumatists.

As I have already suggested, there never was any such thing as a primitive Hippocratic doctrine in the first place. In other words, the Hippocratic Collection itself emphasizes a number of competing medical treatments, procedures, and theoretical assumptions. Perhaps owing in part to the general emergence of indi-vidualism associated with the Hellenistic period and the disintegration of the Greek city-states, as well as to the increasingly fashionable philosophical partisan-ship evidenced in the fragments of numerous post-Hippocratic Greek physicians, this original divergence of opinion with respect to both the theory and practice of medicine became more vocal. As to the different philosophical tendencies and treatment strategies represented by the four sects under discussion, scholars have so far reached no clear consensus on the detailed beliefs associated with each sect. Nor would it serve the basic aims of this inquiry to set forth here their conflicting assessments.

But in general it can be usefully noted that the Dogmatists emphasized in-ferring the hidden causes of disease from manifest symptoms. They were greatly influenced by the humoral theory of the Hippocratic authors as well as by the tel-eological orientation of Plato's *Timaeus*, which they quoted chapter and verse.[33]

The Empiricists reacted against what they felt was the Dogmatist obsession with overblown theories founded on an absurdly small number of observations. They emphasized instead closer observation of each individual patient and removal of the disease symptoms without necessarily trying to figure out the hidden causes of disease. They were most skeptical about being able to detect hidden causes. The Empiricists were influenced both by the skepticism of Pyrrho (fl. 340 B.C.) and, ironically, by the empirical orientation of Aristotle, though it appears they never fully appreciated the latter's respect for finding out the causes of phenomena.

The third major sect was the Methodists. They may be regarded as somewhat intermediate between the theoretical tendencies of the Dogmatists to detect hidden causes for diseases in the absence of empirical research on the one hand, and the more practical tendencies of the Empiricists to cure the patient of his suffering in the absence of ascertaining the ultimate causes of diseases on the other. The Methodists were influenced by the atomic theories of Democritus and Epicurus. They sought to understand and cure disease based on the theory that extremes of contraction or relaxation in the pores (areas of empty void) of the body caused all illness.

In contrast, the fourth major sect, the Pneumatists, were associated with the Stoics. But they were also frankly eclectic in their approach to healing. They were the strongest opponents of the Methodists in Rome, whose theory they regarded as oversimplified. Alternatively, they postulated that health and disease were determined by the condition of the pneuma, or "vital air" each person breathed. But the condition of one's pneuma (which could be monitored in the pulse) was said to be caused in turn by the imbalance of the four qualities of hot, cold, moist, and dry, plus the four humors they associated with these qualities.[34]

Finally, whatever the merits of the medical theories sponsored by these preceding four sects may have been, it is fair to conclude that the absence of any one dominant theory was due largely to the related absence of any acceptable criterion for theory selection among the various members of the medical craft. So the partisans of each sect went their separate ways, largely ignoring the theoretical objections of their opponents.

THE GALENIC CONSTITUTIONAL THEORY

Turning to the writings of Galen (A.D. 129–199) on the issue of health and disease, one is at first struck by the wide range of his contribution to medicine and philosophy in general. Benjamin Gordon states that eighty-three of Galen's works are still extant and are acknowledged to be genuine. These include fifteen books on anatomy alone, plus treatises dealing with logic, ethics, and grammar.[35] Given the sheer scope and output of the writings of this last prominent Greek physician, the most that I shall undertake in the remaining pages of this chapter is to critically discuss the eclectic nature and therapeutic implications of Galen's thought. This I shall do by highlighting some of the ideas he borrowed and refined from the previous thinkers we have encountered.

Galen was a follower of Hippocrates. All of the seven medical principles associated with the Hippocratic Collection were known to him and were by and large accepted, with various modifications. From Plato and Aristotle he revived the religious and teleological notions that, in Galen's own words, "There is nothing in the body useless or inactive, but all parts are arranged to perform their offices together and have been endowed by the creator with specific powers."[36]

Moreover, Galen's method was essentially empirical and systematic: he sought to reduce all knowledge to general, interrelated principles based on observation. At the same time, he resisted following any one medical sect or school and regarded those fellow physicians who did as slaves. Yet, notwithstanding his original contributions to experimental physiology and human anatomy (he proved that *both* arteries and veins carried blood and correctly identified for the first time many of the neurological functions of the brain and spinal cord), it must be admitted that many of Galen's anatomic concepts were flawed by his habit of reasoning by analogy. That is, he assumed that what was true of the anatomical structure of animals would be equally true of man. Galen also possessed an overzealous tendency to read into all of the structures and processes of the body the purposefulness of nature. Even so, Galen's studies of human anatomy were the best among the ancients and remained so right down to the time of Vesalius in the sixteenth century.

More specifically, Galen's writings on the causes of disease reveal a creative attempt to synthesize the physiological and the ontological concepts of disease discussed earlier. I shall argue that Galen tried to explain disease based on the natural functions of the body as well as on the determinate structure of the body's composite parts.

The physiological components of Galen's theory were borrowed from three basic sources: (1) from the various humoral doctrines of the Hippocratic and Dogmatic authors; (2) from the four Empedoclean elements and four physical opposites adopted by Plato and Aristotle, respectively; and (3) from the emphasis placed on the vital breath developed by the Pneumatist authors. These antecedents are evidenced in Galen's physiological orientation by the fact that he took the Aristotelian opposites as basic to the organizational hierarchy of the body. In addition, just above these Aristotelian opposites he postulated the Empedoclean elements. These were followed by the humors (which Aristotle had little use for). Thus, it may be said that more distinctly than Aristotle or any earlier Greek thinker, Galen emphasized the general integration (*systasis*) of all the parts of the body to compose a functional whole.[37]

In addition, the pneuma held an important place in Galenic pathology. He believed that the function of the nervous system was to carry the pneuma—which he also identified as the life-giving principle—to all the parts of the body. Moreover, like the humors, the pneuma was regarded by Galen as a physical and not merely a metaphysical substance. He did not regard pneuma as a fixed entity blown into the body at birth or conception. Rather, it was something that needed to be constantly renewed through the respiration of the inspired air of the world soul. (The Stoic influence here is obvious.) Also, he theorized that the inhaled pneuma became the *animal spirit* when it came in contact with the brain and nerves; the *vital spirit* when it reached the heart and arteries; and the *natural spirit* when it reached the liver and renal veins. Hence, in this regard he devised something like Plato's three-part division of the soul.[38]

But in other respects his psychology resembled Aristotle's. He seemed in the final analysis to count the body and soul as inseparable parts of a single integrated system. In addition, unlike Aristotle, but like Alcmaeon, Democritus, Hippocrates, and Plato, Galen linked the brain with the center of thought. Of his three postulated spirits, moreover, he said that the animal spirit lodged in the brain was the noblest. To the animal spirit, which he associated also with the reasoning faculty, he ascribed the Aristotelian efficient, formal, and final causes of the soul's motions, perceptions, and sensations. He claimed that a person's perceptions and sensations were communicated to the rest of the body through the spinal cord and its network of nerves.

Thus, for Galen health and disease can be understood on the physiological level partly in terms of the condition and natural function of the patient's pneuma. Following the Pneumatists, Galen also implied that there was some sort of soul-body causal interaction. For he allowed that the undifferentiated pneuma *originates in the blood* through the circulating action of the heart's innate heat and the lung's respiration. Hence, in this brief look at the physiological side of Galen's eclectic theory of health, we also come to appreciate his psychosomatic justification for bloodletting, which he sometimes prescribed for both physical and mental disorders (e.g., melancholy). For if the blood was suspected of being impure or defective in some way, the logic was that perhaps one's psychological condition could be altered for the better by ridding the body of any such imbalance or impurity contained in the blood. What's more, it comes as little surprise that from this partial causal dependence of mental states and processes on the bodily condition of the blood (not to mention the ascending hierarchy of opposites, elements, and humors), Galen ascribed such psychological disturbances as mania, imbecility, and dementia to somatic malfunctions of various sorts.

But Galen was not content to ascribe the processes of disease and health to the physiological functions of the body alone. The explanatory burden of Galen's system is shared by a structural analysis that focuses on the arrangement (*diaplasis*), size, and number of each of the body's constituents as well. This approach resembles what I have earlier called the ontological concept of disease. Moreover, here Galen appears to be somewhat influenced by the early Cnidian tradition and, if not by the atomists, Democritus and Epicurus, then certainly by the Methodist sect that was very active in Rome of his day.

Yet it must be acknowledged that at times[39] Galen wrote that health entailed a due proportion or blend of the four physical opposites of hot, cold, moist, and dry. This sounds like the physiological model alone. But in his treatise *On the Best Constitution of Our Body*, Galen elaborated on his theory of health in a crucial way. He clarified the point that the proper blend of the four opposites is merely a necessary and not a sufficient condition for health. In other words, the proper blend of the four opposites is at most an essential ingredient of health; it is no guarantee of health taken alone.

In addition, he wrote that the constitution of the body is determined not only by the blending of the four opposite qualities in each of the body's like-parted or homogeneous parts (e.g., tissue, blood, bones), but also by the higher *arrangement* of these homogeneous parts into heterogeneous parts comparable to those we call organs (e.g., hands, eyes, etc.).[40] The upshot of his message is that proper blend of the opposite qualities *and* proper arrangement of the body's parts are the individually necessary *and jointly sufficient conditions for health* in the body with the best constitution.

This preceding scheme led Galen to assert that the best constitution of the body is one that most efficiently resists *external* diseases due to such things as climate, excessive exercise, etc. and *internal diseases* due to such things as the *"residues of food."*[41] How, then, can one achieve the best bodily constitution? The answer is that it can be achieved when the two criteria of proper blending of the four opposites *and* proper arrangement (*diaplasis*) of the body's parts are met. The medical result of these twin criteria is that disease can be analyzed on two levels: (1) temperamentally (in terms of blending) or (2) diaplastically. Galen refers to both of these criteria simultaneously in the following passage. In speaking of the dense and rare, he is referring to the size, shape, and arrangement of the pores in the heterogeneous parts of the body as well as to the opposites of moist and dry. When these pores were open and moist, he termed them "rare"; when they were closed and dry, "dense."[42]

> Thus, we can say that the well balanced body, in addition to its other advantages, will be neither rare nor dense. It will be midway between these extremes, just as in other respects; it has the advantage in some way over each of the two excesses, for the denser body is less subject to external causes of disease, and the rarer less subject to internal ones. And, though you could not find a body that is strictly resistant to both causes, you might say that the body that is midway between all extremes is resistant to both *in a relative sense*—and we assert that such a body is the healthiest of all. . . . Thus, . . . the mean is not the most completely resistant of all conditions; but though it may be inferior to every condition in some particular way, still it is the most desirable of all.[43]

Hence, Galen formally defines an optimally constituted body as one that manifests *an intermediate position* between various excesses and deficiencies with respect to both the temperament (blending) and the arrangement (*diaplasis*) of its parts. This is so because only when these twin conditions are met (and Galen outlines the specific excesses and deficiencies in considerable detail) will the body resist disease that otherwise brings disruptions upon the body's normal functions.[44]

In sum, these disruptions can be viewed in a manner akin to the ontological disease model as having a specific location in the structure of the body. In that case, removal of the diseased part by surgery or purgation may be undertaken. Or, more typically for Galen, these disruptions may be viewed on the physiological disease model, in which adjustments in diet, exercise, or the application of drugs may correct the malfunction. It is necessary to add, however, that true to his eclectic orientation, Galen explored not one but many etiological schemes. Therefore, one must be careful not to oversimplify by casting all his ideas about health and disease in the single form just discussed.

A final point: In the preceding long quotation, as in his other writings, at least two tendencies emerge. As each of these tendencies has important therapeutic implications, I would like to digress for a moment and explore what they are.

First, from the fact that each person is regarded as having a unique temperament and a unique arrangement of bodily parts, it follows that no two people are exactly alike. This theoretical conclusion would explain the well-known fact that, given two patients with the same disease, a remedy that will work on one patient may not always work on the other. Therapeutically, these considerations led Galen to emphasize that the physician must get to know the individual characteristics of each patient *before* deciding on treatment—no matter how familiar he may be with the patient's disease. (Here Galen would agree with the Empiricist sect on the importance of closely observing the patient's traits; in general, though, he found the Empiricists' disdain for identifying the internal causes of disease totally repugnant.)

Second, Galen also appears quite willing to define health "in a relative sense." That is, health is an intermediate condition between opposing extremes. He tacitly admits that the best one can hope for is a bodily constitution that is not quite perfect since, in fact, "it may be inferior to every condition in some particular way." Furthermore, in the aforementioned treatise by Galen there is a passage in which he states: "For *absolutely perfect* functioning in every respect, so that none of the homogeneous parts and none of the organic parts is imbalanced, is not something that tends to occur very often, though *instances* may occur over longer stretches of time." He also states: "We have shown in our discussions of it that health is not something narrow and absolutely simple and indivisible, but rather capable of wide variation."[45]

What these passages point to, I am persuaded, is the relaxation of the earlier Greek Archaic and Hellenic notion of health as an absolute ideal (as Plato, for example, tended to view it in his *Republic* and *Timaeus*). Galen here moves toward a more variegated or "second best" notion of health adjusted to meet the exigencies of daily life as it was led by the average citizen. That is, only the rich and idle were in the position to follow the strict regimen of proper exercise, climate, diet, rest, etc., that was typically prescribed by the Greek physicians (especially those of the classical period). By the Hellenistic and later Roman period, economic necessity and the political pressures of being an active, involved middle-class citizen trying to earn a decent living may have combined to force *some* of the Greeks and Romans to modify their old belief in the existence of perfect health and the desirability of attaining it.

Addressing this point, Fridolf Kudlien has plausibly suggested that another factor in the relaxation of the ideal of absolute health may have been the intellectual movement associated with Protagoras's ethical relativism and, I would add, later skepticism.[46] Edelstein, moreover, has traced the trend to settle for health in the relative sense to the Hellenistic period's increasing tendency to recast health in terms of the individual's own choices. These choices are, of course, *relative to* an individual's felt needs and self-knowledge. If so, perhaps the notion of health as a delicate balance requiring the coddling of the individual outlasted its usefulness as more and more individuals increasingly sought to take charge of their own regimens. No wonder, then, that the Roman period evidences a fair amount of resentment and ridicule directed at the fawning counsel sometimes given by doctors.[47]

Whatever the specific pressures of change may have been, there is little doubt that more than simply Aristotelian language is at work in Galen's talk of the best bodily constitution in relative, not absolute terms—terms also reminiscent of Aristotle's ethical theory of the mean (virtue).

Therapeutically, the consequences of the idea of relative health seem to be helpful. On the one hand, the average patient settles for the fact that at any given time, though he may *feel* no pain or discomfort and though he may consider himself relatively healthy, he may at the same time be constitutionally disposed to get one sort of disease rather than another. If so, the physician ought to prescribe a regimen relative to the patient's own constitutional needs. The therapeutic aim would be to hold off those diseases to which the patient is more or less disposed.

On the other hand, those patients who are not able-bodied because they suffer some defect, such as loss of a limb, may yet be usefully regarded as having "sufficient health" relative to their situation. This would seem justified provided such patients are judged free of all other disease and are somehow able to cope with their defect.[48] Thus, the amputee may have been regarded as healthy in the relative sense. This way of looking at health may have lessened somewhat the stigma especially associated with such losses in antiquity when fewer restorative measures were available.

Lastly, the notion of relative health doubtless cast the doctor in a more realistically limited role: the doctor could perhaps at least improve *if not totally restore* health. And for the ancients, as for us, such relative improvement in and of itself surely has value. This, too, Galen seemed to appreciate more than did many of his predecessors.

Discussion Questions

1. From a clinical perspective, how did the humoral theory of disease provide an empirical basis for the diagnosis and treatment of illness?
2. The Hippocratic author of the treatise *Epidemics* stated that "Nature is the physician of diseases." What did this imply to the ancient clinician?
3. From the contemporary medical perspective, did the Hippocratic and Galenic doctors understand the causes of diseases? What about the effects?
4. Compare and contrast the physiological and ontological concepts of disease and health. To which model do the respective theories of Democritus, Aristotle, and Galen belong?

5. Of the four medical sects—Dogmatists, Empiricists, Methodists, Pneumatists—which was most influenced by the atomist Democritus? Which was closest to the Stoics?

NOTES

1. Ludwig Edelstein, "Hippocrates," in *The Oxford Classical Dictionary*, ed. N. G. L. Hammond and H. H. Scullard, 2nd ed. (Oxford: Clarendon Press, 1970), p. 518 (hereafter cited as *OCD*).
2. Sigerist, *History of Medicine*, vol. 2, pp. 317–38 passim.
3. Emile Littré, ed. *Oeuvres Completes d'Hippocrate*, 10 vols. (Paris: Javal et Bourdeaux, 1936–61), vol. 1, p. 602, cited by Sigerist, *History of Medicine*, vol. 2, p. 318.
4. Littré, *Oeuvres*, vol. 7, pp. 542ff., cited by Sigerist, *History of Medicine*, vol. 2, p. 319.
5. Sigerist, *History of Medicine*, vol. 2, p. 319.
6. Ibid., vol. 2, p. 320. Water was probably not as visible in the body (at least in its clear form) as were black discharges during severe illnesses. Hence, the switch to black bile probably had an observational basis.
7. Ibid., vol. 2, p. 334. Sigerist points out that the Greek word *krasis* means not only "blending" but "temperature." In medical texts, *krasis* usually translates "temperament."
8. Ibid., vol. 2, p. 321.
9. Emile Littré, *On the Nature of Man*, vol. 6, p. 53, cited by Sigerist, *History of Medicine*, vol. 2, p. 14. Benjamin Lee Gordon has pointed out that, although as a rule *contraria contratis curantur* was recommended, it was not blindly followed by the Hippocratic physicians. (See Benjamin Lee Gordon, *Medicine Throughout Antiquity* [Philadelphia: F. A. Davis Co., 1945], p. 514; see Hippocrates *On Ancient Medicine* 1, 15.)
10. Hippocrates *On the Heart* 6.6.
11. Hippocrates *Epidemics* 6.5, cited by Sigerist, *History of Medicine*, vol. 2, p. 326.
12. Sigerist, *History of Medicine*, vol. 2, p. 328, emphases added.
13. Hippocrates *Epidemics* 1, Littré, ed., vol. 2, pp. 678ff., cited by Sigerist, *History of Medicine*, vol. 2, p. 328.
14. Hippocrates *Prognostics*, Littré, ed., vol. 2, pp. 168ff., cited by Sigerist, *History of Medicine*, vol. 2, p. 329.
15. Littré, ed., *Oeuvres*, vol. 2, p. 598, cited by Sigerist, *History of Medicine*, vol. 2, p. 331. Traditionally, the medical school at Cnidus has been regarded by medical historians as having been more localistic in their description and classification of diseases than the school at Cos headed by Hippocrates. See J. H. Biggart, "Cnidus v. Cos," *Ulster Medical Journal* 41 (1971): 1–9.
16. Frag. 234, trans. Freeman, *Ancilla*, p. 112.
17. Theophrastus *De sensu* 58 (DK 58, A 133).
18. John M. Robinson, trans., *An Introduction to Early Greek Philosophy* (New York: Houghton Mifflin, 1968), p. 221.
19. The atomic theory of Leucippus and Democritus, and the modifications thereto at the hands of Epicurus, formed the basis of a later medical sect known as the Methodists. See p. 30 and R. O. Moon, *The Relation of Medicine to Philosophy* (New York: Longmans, Green & Co., 1909), chap. 2.

20. In the case of Plato, I am waiving the question of whether the medical theories found in his *Timaeus* were his own espoused views or those of a Pythagorean who is the speaker there.

21. Plato *Republic*, trans. Paul Shorey, in *Collected Dialogues*, p. 687, emphasis added. At *Timaeus* 81b–82b, Plato also distinguishes between decay (due to the natural aging process) and disease. Decay is said to be the result of the wearing out of the elementary triangles without the intervention of disease. In contrast, disease is abnormal, morbid decay occasioned by the corruption (*phthora*) and reversal of the blood currents inside the body that normally foster growth. See Francis M. Cornford, *Plato's Cosmology* (New York: Bobbs-Merrill, 1937), p. 336.

22. Plato *Republic* 445e, trans. Shorey, in *Collected Dialogues*, p. 687.

23. At *Timaeus* 69d–72d, reason, spirit, and appetite are given location in the head, heart, and liver, respectively.

24. *Timaeus* 87bff. It is interesting to note that *nosos*, which we commonly render "disease," is a Greek word that also means distress, affliction, *evil*. H. G. Liddell and R. Scott: *Greek–English Lexicon*, abridged (Oxford: Clarendon Press, 1972), p. 467.

25. *Timaeus* 29e–30b.

26. Gordon states that Aristotle mentions over five hundred different species of animals, and probably dissected at least fifty (*Medicine Throughout Antiquity*, pp. 569ff.). There is nothing in his writings to suggest that Aristotle dissected an adult human cadaver. He *may* have dissected human embryos, however.

27. See Friedrich Solmsen, "The Vital Heat, the Inborn Pneuma and the Aether," *The Journal of Hellenic Studies* 77 (1957): 119–23.

28. Aristotle *Metaphysics* 104a.26ff. See Charles H. Kahn, *Anaximander and the Origins of Greek Cosmology* (New York: Columbia University Press, 1960), p. 120.

29. Aristotle *Physics* 246b.4ff., trans. H. P. Hardie and R. K. Gay, in *Basic Works*, pp. 346–47, emphases added.

30. Charles and Peck Singer, "Zoology," in *OCD*, p. 1140. On the part played by the four Aristotelian elements in determining the biological uniqueness of each species and members thereof, see Aristotle's *Parts of Animals* 645bff. See also Thomas S. Hall, "Idiosyncrasy: Greek Medical Ideas of Uniqueness," *Sudhoffs Archiv* 58, no. 3 (1974): 283–302. Note that Aristotle regarded *the excellence of man's physical blend* as superior to all other animals as *proved* by man's higher range of intelligence, according to Singer.

31. Aristotle *Physics* 1.7–8.

32. Aristotle *Generation of Animals* 5.49.784b.33, cited by Edelstein, in *Ancient Medicine*, p. 390.

33. Moon, *Relation of Medicine to Philosophy*, pp. 17–22 passim.

34. Gordon, *Medicine Throughout Antiquity*, p. 679.

35. Ibid., p. 703.

36. M. Neuburger, trans., *History of Medicine* (London: Oxford University Press, 1910), cited by Gordon, *Medicine Throughout Antiquity*, p. 706.

37. Robert J. Penella and Thomas S. Hall, "Galen's 'On the Best Constitution of Our Body': Introduction, Translation, and Notes," *Bulletin of the History of Medicine* 47, no. 4 (1973): 283.

38. Gordon, *Medicine Throughout Antiquity*, p. 711. Like Plato, Galen attributes reason, emotion, and desire to the locations of the head (brain), heart, and belly, respectively.

39. Galen *De sanitate tuenda* 1.4–5.

40. Galen *De facultatibus naturalibus* 1.6. Galen largely adopted this hierarchical struc-
    ture of the body from Aristotle. Cf. Aristotle *On the Parts of Animals* 646b.12–27.
    Note that Aristotle, in fact, called like-parted things "homoeomerous."
41. Penella and Hall, "Galen's 'On the Best Constitution,'" p. 294.
42. Galen *De sanitate tuenda* 2.5.
43. Penella and Hall, "Galen's 'On the Best Constitution,'" pp. 294–95, emphases added.
44. Galen *De temperamentis* 1.8.
45. Penella and Hall, "Galen's 'On the Best Constitution,'" pp. 293–94, emphases added.
46. Fridolf Kudlien, "The Old Greek Concept of 'Relative Health,'" *Journal of the His-
    tory of Behavioral Sciences* 9 (1973): 58.
47. Ludwig Edelstein, "The Dietetics of Antiquity," in *Ancient Medicine*, pp. 313–14.
48. Kudlien, "The Old Greek Concept," p. 55.

3 Attitudes toward Death

Death is nothing to us, since when we are,
death has not come; and when death comes,
we are not.

—EPICURUS

NO MATTER HOW MUCH the Greeks valued health, they realized that sooner or later even the healthiest and most robust among them must die. The Greeks had no single view on the meaning of death. Rather, they held a plurality of often conflicting views, just as we do in our own culture. In this chapter, I shall illustrate some of the attitudes that the Greeks had toward death at various times in their cultural development.

Before undertaking to sketch these various attitudes, it is imperative to isolate precisely what features of this complex topic one seeks to understand. The simple expression "attitudes toward death" involves a complex of interrelated concepts that are by no means identical.[1] Attitudes may be explored on at least three levels: (a) cognitively, one may inquire how people think about death; (b) affectively, one may try to discover how people feel about death; and (c) behaviorally, one may investigate how people behave toward their own or others' impending death. My analysis will encompass primarily (a), the cognitive side of this topic. I shall ask, How did various philosophers, poets, artists, and ordinary Greek citizens conceive of death at different points in Greek culture?

Furthermore, the word "death" itself is a highly elusive and disunified concept in our ordinary usage of that term. Its standard senses in the present context include: (1) the dying process; (2) the precise moment of death; and (3) the state of being dead. I am primarily interested in (3), how the Greeks conceived of the state of being dead. The answer to this question promises to significantly contribute to our background understanding of various Greek ethical views on euthanasia, infanticide, and suicide. Yet (1) and (2) are also important to this inquiry and so will be treated here as subsidiary topics.

Moreover, for the purpose of further clarifying our focus, it will be useful to distinguish between the natural processes of aging and the actual dying process in the last days of a person's life. Otherwise, one might get ensnared by the belief that each person is dying from the moment of birth, which is at best a sensational but not very accurate appraisal. Instead, it will be assumed that the dying process entails having reached a critical and life-threatening stage in the aging process, which, if left unchecked, would normally be expected to result in death. So it is not merely Greek views on aging or growing old that will be addressed. Rather, it is how the Greeks approached dying, as just defined, that is of special interest.

Lastly, I must say a word about the inherent limitations of the evidence and method underlying the following sketch. Basically, I am confining my discussion to the treatises, poems, and fragments of selected philosophers and poets, plus secondary sources judged to be of value. Although some effort will be made to balance the main strands of thought, surely many other sources could be fruitfully included. In what follows I shall mention just a few of the pre-Socratics; and the Stoics for the moment are passed over in favor of the Epicureans. Even so, within these stated limitations, a representative picture of Greek perspectives on death may be secured.

DIVINE AND CHTHONIC PERSONAL IMMORTALITY

If one compares the depictions of the state of being dead as evidenced on the one hand by the epic poetry of the Homeric religion (725 B.C.) and on the other by the Orphic tendencies manifest in the religious doctrines of the Pythagorean Brotherhood (ca. 500 B.C.), at least one major difference in outlook is evident. The Homeric religion generally depicts death as unconquerable and terrible. The dead are shown as bloodless shadows wandering listlessly in the underworld.[2]

In contrast, the Orphic-Pythagorean religion depicts death as conquerable and promising, and claims that the best and most essential part of each person—his soul—is deathless and divine. It teaches that through purification the divine soul is destined finally to reunite with the divine cosmos from whence it originally came before becoming entombed in the inferior mortal body, which alone is subject to decay.[3]

This preceding divergence in outlook can be further characterized by calling the dominant Homeric perspective on the state of being dead *chthonic personal immortality*. By using the word chthonic (taken from the Greek *chthonios*, "of or in the earth"), I wish to emphasize the fact that the Homeric dead are essentially spirits of the underworld, mere shadows of their former selves.

The Orphic-Pythagorean perspective, on the other hand, I call *divine personal immortality*. The decisive difference between these two perspectives, it seems to me, turns on the way each characterizes (a) the initial relation of the soul to the body and (b) the further relation in which that part of each person that survives the moment of death (often called the soul) stands to the enduring order and structure of the universe.

As to (a), the initial relation of the soul to the body, Homer does not grant the soul of man divine status. Nor does he oppose the worth of the soul to the comparative worthlessness of the body. It would, however, strictly speaking be wrong to say that he makes no distinction between the two. For Homer, as for Hesiod (650 B.C.), *psyche* has two meanings. It means both "the breath of life" and "the individualized ghost." Typically, the ghost or "shade" escapes (like animating breath) from the mouth, wound, or limbs of the dying hero at the moment of death. It leaves behind the *soma*, which for Homer literally meant "corpse."[4] Then the ghost repairs to the underworld to endure a benign, joyless existence. Hence, it may be argued that there is some hint of a soul-body (or psyche-soma) dualism in Homer but only in the narrow sense that he allows some quite diminished piece of each former person, namely a ghost, to survive the body at death. After this separation of ghost and corpse, the ghost mourns for its former body as one might mourn the loss of a worthy friend.

As to (b), the relation of the ghost to the ongoing universe, with few exceptions, a former person's surviving ghost stands in a decidedly miserable and lowly relation to the rest of pulsating humanity left behind, as well as to the only truly deathless ones—the gods (Fig. 4). That is, the Homeric ghosts live a shadowy existence in a dim and dank underworld that the gods themselves cannot stand. We get some idea of the undesirable status of the dead from the *Odyssey*, Book Two. There the ghost of Achilles confronts and scolds the full-bodied Odysseus, saying: "O shining Odysseus, never try to console me for dying. I would rather follow the plow as a thrall to another man—one with no land allotted him and not much to live on—than be a king over all the perished dead."[5]

Here the judgment of Francis Cornford in his book *From Religion to Philosophy* is entirely borne out. Cornford claims that in the Homeric religion there existed a definite gulf between the divine and the merely human.[6] In this connection, I am inclined to think that the Delphic motto, "Know Thyself," which admits of many interesting interpretations, may originally have served as a reminder to mankind that this gulf was real and had to be respected at all times. It was hubris to ignore this line of demarcation and begin to think of oneself as a god.

Pythagoreanism again stands in stark contrast to the Homeric picture of man's relation to the universe. Waiving the sticky question of the origins of the three Pythagorean doctrines of (1) the essential divinity of the soul; (2) the possible purification of the soul; and (3) the transmigration of the soul, it is certain that the collective result of these three doctrines was to remove or significantly reduce the felt gap between the human and the divine. This is partly so because the Pythagorean soul is taken to be a fallen divinity. The body serves as a temporary tomb from which it can win eventual release through the study of philosophy and mathematics. Also, the soul can in this way recapture its divine purity and be restored to its full status as a truly deathless part of the harmonious cosmos.

Figure 4. Detail, "Artemis and Apollo," Niobid Painter, ca. 455–450 B.C. Popular religious belief ascribed to the gods the power of inflicting disease or death as a punishment to mankind. Here Artemis and Apollo shoot their toxic arrows bringing death. Reprinted by permission of the Musée du Louvre, Paris.

Furthermore, I suggest that, in contrast, such a sublime prospect for the deceased is not central to Homeric thought. Moreover, it is a curious fact that during the Archaic and Hellenic periods, at least, more Greeks by far adopted variants of the Homeric chthonic view of death than the competing Pythagorean divine view. Why this was so, I shall leave for others to speculate; doubtless the elitist nature of Pythagoreanism was a chief factor.

In any case, before turning to a third perspective on the prospect of survival beyond death, a brief digression to explore a few features of the grammar of the Greek word for death, namely *thanatos*, is appropriate.

Emily Vermeule suggests in her book *Aspects of Death in Early Greek Art and Poetry* that the Greeks "had no word for irreversible death; one does not die, one darkens."[7] How so? Vermeule thinks that it signifies a basic hope that the Archaic period Greeks (ca. 700–478 B.C.), at least, held for the imperishability of the *psyche*. "The *psyche*," she says, "is memory and intelligence dormant and can under proper circumstances be recalled [to life] by the grief, love, magic or poetry . . ." of the living.[8]

But this hope, however strongly felt by the Archaic period Greeks, must surely have been sensed to be in vain, even for the followers of Homer. Eventually, almost all ghosts will have been forgotten. Inevitably, the community's memories of the deceased fade from the collective consciousness of succeeding generations of mortals. The "silent majority," who after all constitute the Homeric dead, are destined—with the exception of a few remarkable heroes of old—to be recalled never again by either the eulogies or encomia of the living. Little wonder, then, that one of the favorite artistic renderings given the dead person's ghost by Archaic vase painters in the seventh and later centuries was to depict the ghost as a tiny, insignificant butterfly or soul-bird. Typically, on funeral urns the soul-bird was shown flitting about in the afterworld in assured anonymity.[9] It could almost be swatted by the living as if a bothersome mosquito.

What's more, in addition to being a common noun, *thanatos* is also a proper noun designating the personage of Death (Thanatos), who is the twin brother of Sleep (Hypnos) in the Homeric pantheon. As may be seen from the vase painting on at least one magnificently large red-figured krater dating from 515 B.C., and painted by Euphronios (see frontispiece), Thanatos is not pictured as a devouring or terrible figure. Rather, he is shown more like a resolute and avuncular escort—someone with whom one cannot argue. As he is in the present specimen, Thanatos is often rendered as a large, winged male figure cloaked in battle gear. He has piercing eyes and somewhat oversized hands and feet. On the vase mentioned above, Thanatos is shown to our right lifting the body of the Lycian prince Sarpedon at Troy, with his brother Hypnos assisting and the god Hermes overseeing their journey. Elsewhere he may be symbolized poetically as a black cloud or as a hue or mist appearing around the head of one about to die.

Moreover, Thanatos, as the personage of Death, is not a fully developed figure in the Homeric epics. He appears in the flesh only once in Homer (*Iliad* 16.671). There, the aforementioned Sarpedon is dead, stripped, looted, and surrounded by enemies. He is rescued by Thanatos, who cradles him like a fellow kinsman. The twin brothers, Sleep and Death, then escort the corpse to Sarpedon's native Lycia for proper burial. Incidentally, Thanatos is almost never characterized as a killer or as an agent of death; nor is his ally, Hades, the dreaded king of the underworld.[10] Perhaps this may be explained in part by the fact that many Greeks regarded death as the negation of life, as a cessation or an inversion of living.

NATURAL PERSONAL DISSOLUTION

If there is yet a third Greek perspective on the state of being dead, Jacques Choron may be warranted in looking for it among the early pre-Socratic philosophers of Ionia. In his book *Death and Western Thought*, Choron argues that the favored irreducible elements of the earliest monistic philosophers, such as Thales' water, Anaximander's boundless (*apeiron*), and Anaximenes' air (*aer* or *pneuma*), signify an effort on their part "to neutralize death." Furthermore, he suggests that it "may be an expression of the hope that somewhere and somehow death shall have no dominion."[11] I shall argue that Choron's interpretation with respect to these three monists is interesting but, as it stands, paradoxical. My focus will be on the lone fragment of Anaximenes, but what I have to say about Anaximenes can apply as well to Thales and Anaximander.

The only authentic fragment attributed to Anaximenes (fl. 546 B.C.) translates: "As our soul, being air [aer], holds us together, so do breath [pneuma] and air surround the whole universe."[12] Most scholars agree that for Anaximenes air is the cause of all things, for it "holds us together" and presumably controls both man and the cosmos. Further, air is the basic constituent out of which all things are born and into which they shall return. In identifying man's soul with air, Anaximenes seems at the same time to be linking air to the principle of life. It is likely that for him air was the necessary condition for life in all living creatures.

Furthermore, like Anaximander's boundless and Thales' water, Anaximenes took air to be deathless and ageless: it is the only thing that endures through change. Though it is true that he ascribes an airy quality to the soul, nothing Anaximenes or other ancient commentators say attributes to him the further crucial identification of the soul as the real, true, or essential person. This identification, though it is sometimes neglected, is crucial to any interesting notion of personal survival or immortality. That is, it serves as the necessary condition for that sort of personal immortality that links the survival of the soul with survival of the continued psychological identity of the deceased. Anthony Flew has underscored the importance of this crucial link in graphic terms. "Unless it is established that I am my soul," he writes, "the demonstration of the survival of my soul will not demonstrate *my* survival, and the news that my soul will last forever could provide me with no more justification for harboring 'these logically unique expectations' than the rather less elevated assurance that my appendix is to be preserved eternally in a bottle."[13]

Now the crux of Choron's interpretation of the early monists is this. If all things are one, as they claim, then the most shocking change of all is going from life to death. But, Choron reasons, death itself becomes less radical owing to the essential oneness of all that exists.[14] If by "less radical" he is referring to the ultimate reducibility of all phenomena (including death) to a single, underlying principle (water, the boundless, air), he may have a point. But he also implies that somehow the unified, monistic scheme provides some sort of *psychological* consolation. This it allegedly does by reducing the horror of the radical physical change each person will undergo when at death one begins to lose the unique individuality on which one's personal identity and continuity may at least partly depend. If so, was the specter of death thereby "neutralized" or made to seem "less radical" for these three pre-Socratics? It is not easy to speculate on such matters. But Choron's guess that just the thought of "the everlastingness of the Whole" somehow neutralized death finds no backing in the relevant fragments of Anaximenes, Anaximander, and Thales. Personally, I think that Choron is delivering too modern a reading of these early monists' views on death. It is just as likely that they found the finality of death, with the *prima facie* elimination of personal survival, as hapless and as perplexing a prospect as did many of their less-gifted contemporaries.

Choron's analysis of the early monists is further damaged by his use of the same word, death, in two distinct senses without being aware of it, thereby committing the fallacy of equivocation. This happens when he states that these pre-Socratics, "accepting their individual deaths, pin their hopes on the everlastingness of the whole, in which [case] death cannot be senseless perishing." The first occurrence of the word death is used in the *strict sense* to mean the exclusion of personal survival, as when we say Smith met his death in a tragic fall. But the second occurrence is used in the *loose sense* to leave open the possibility of personal survival, as when we say Jones believes in life after death.[15] That this equivocation occurs can be readily appreciated by noticing that unless the second occurrence of death leaves open the possibility of personal survival, there would be no enduring subject on which such "hopes" in the relevant sense could be "pinned."

Nevertheless, I must admit that, despite these flaws, Choron's attempt to read the early monists as if they supplied a third perspective on the state of being dead is suggestive. Hence, I shall call this third perspective *natural personal dissolution*. This label emphasizes their view that each unique person terminates at death, following which his constituents gradually dissolve and reform into various irreducible physical elements.

This perspective, with adjustments, could also characterize the basic outlook of several more pre-Socratics. The notable *exceptions* are Heraclitus, who admits no fixed boundary between the processes of life and death, since everything is changing;[16] Parmenides, who holds so fast to the notion of the imperishability of Being that death for him would have to count as a mere sensory illusion;[17] and Empedocles, who in his poem "On Nature" seems to admit natural personal dissolution, only to contradict himself in his religious poem "Purifications" by talking as if he believed in divine personal immortality.[18] Finally, if this third view of death does succeed in somehow neutralizing death, perhaps the fundamental way it accomplishes this is by replacing the frightening visages of death sometimes associated with the chthonic perspective of Homer with the seemingly more neutral notion of personal dissolution *unaccompanied* by any possible torment, loneliness, or regret in some afterworld existence.

Presently, though, I would like to leave the pre-Socratics to consider what some of the leading Greek poets and tragedians of the sixth through fourth centuries B.C. had to say about death. In addition, I intend to examine briefly some of the commonly held fifth-century beliefs about the dead.

POETIC AND POPULAR IMAGES

According to the poet Sappho (fl. 582 B.C.), death is the greatest evil. "Gods so consider it," she says, "else they would die."[19] This impeccable logic finds company in the lyric poet Anacreon (fl. 540 B.C.), who is similarly horrified by approaching death: "Death is too terrible. Frightening are the depths of Hades. There is no return."[20]

If these words of Sappho and Anacreon express the customary pessimism connected with the Homeric picture of chthonic personal survival, a far more optimistic estimate (probably inspired by Orphic ideas) is expressed by Pindar (518–438 B.C.). According to this view, which is a variant of the Pythagorean's divine personal immortality, the soul lives on after death enjoying much brighter prospects. Pindar writes: "By happy dispensation all travel to an end which sets free from woe. And the body, indeed, of all goes with mighty Death. But there remaineth alive a phantom of life; for that alone cometh from the gods."[21]

The phantom to which Pindar refers is, of course, the divine soul of man. That this soul comes from the divine gods, as Pindar says, illustrates again the tendency of this particular perspective to bridge the gulf between the gods and man–a gulf so evident in the earlier Homeric poems.

Among the works of the three major Greek tragedians, Aeschylus, Sophocles, and Euripides, there appears on the whole to be an acute death consciousness. Thus, the chorus in Sophocles' (496–406 B.C.) play *Antigone* declares: "Of all the great wonders, none is greater than man." Then, almost as an afterthought, the chorus laments: "Only for death can he find no cure."[22]

Yet Sophocles also allows us a glimpse of what might be called *the heroic attitude* toward death. According to C. M. Bowra, "the exponents of the heroic ideal regard death as the climax and completion of life, the last and most searching ideal to which a man is subject and the true test of his worth."[23] In my opinion, this heroic attitude was doubtless admired, but in actuality was probably as rare among the Greeks as true heroes were in real life. Antigone represents this heroic attitude toward death when she asks her self-righteous accusers: "Is there something more you want, or just my life?"[24] Antigone demonstrates that for the sake of preserving the high ideals of justice and honor, a worthy person should be prepared to meet death without the slightest compromise. This she did for the sake of ensuring that her outcast brother, Polyneices, would receive a proper burial as divine law, if not human law, required.

In contrast, there are some passages in Aeschylus (525/4–456 B.C.) that probably come closer to reflecting the general fifth-century-B.C. Greek attitude about death than either the Orphic or heroic visions just mentioned. It will be recalled that in the Homeric view of death there is little hope of a blessed immortality to comfort the dying or lessen the grief of surviving friends and relatives. A. W. Mair has argued that when death is spoken of as desirable at all, it is pictured merely as a refuge from evil (*kakon kataphyge*), a dreamless sleep. This is the picture of death Aeschylus presents when his chorus bewails the murder of Agamemnon in his play devoted to that tragic figure. The chorus laments: "Would that some fate might come speedy, not over painful, nor with lingering bed, bringing to us everlasting, endless sleep."[25]

But I wonder if Mair is overlooking that the Greeks also possessed the concept of euthanasia (εὐθανασια)? Probably not. For "euthanasia" was used to mean a good, easy, or noble death, a death evidenced by a minimum of pain and distress. It was not a concept that carried with it a higher or friendlier vision of the afterworld. Fundamentally, euthanasia involved the context of dying, not the state of being dead.[26] The Greek concept of euthanasia, then, includes precisely that permanent escape or refuge from the evil of relentless pain to which Mair here alludes. It does not entail any particular perspective about the afterworld.

As for the related issue of how the living tended to perceive the dead in the classical period, the primary evidence has been culled from the art, law, and literature of that age and reconstructed from the evidence found at ancient burial sites. What has crystalized from this evidence and what can be affirmed with some certainty may be summarized as follows:

(1) There was a tendency to believe that the dead could somehow perceive what is done and said in the world of the living.

(2) The presence of the dead was in some sense felt; their goodwill was valued and their contempt feared.

(3) A person who was murdered was thought to have the potential of becoming an angry ghost capable of causing sterility in crops and beasts, as well as causing other fiendish calamities.

(4) The denial of a proper burial, irrespective of the cause of death, was thought to anger the soul of the dead person and assure misfortunes for the living.[27]

Although I cannot pursue the vast implications of these four beliefs in detail, I would like to offer a few brief comments on some aspects that touch primarily on the issue of moral conscience and moral responsibility.

With respect to (1), it has not yet been positively established that belief in the capacity of the dead to perceive the affairs of the living had an effect on moral conduct. But even a wavering belief that such a possibility *might* exist may well have conditioned some of the moral reasoning and conduct of the living. At least, this possibility cannot be altogether discounted.

As to (2)–(4), it will be noticed that the alleged capacity of a bodiless ghost to influence causally the full-bodied living raises a hornet's nest of questions about just how such a causal connection would work. That is, how can a bodiless ghost impinge in any way on a thing that has body? The answer to this dilemma seems to be that it worked through some sort of supernatural agency, the full details of which were understood only by the gods. No systematic eschatology was ever established by the Greeks to explain away all the possible objections that might be prompted by considerations of logical consistency. Moreover, as K. J. Dover states, "The ghost's capacity for direct action on its own initiative and at its own discretion was regarded as limited; it was rather the gods' interests in the *rights* of the dead which mattered, an interest which extended to funeral procedures, as well as to the avenging of homicide."[28]

As to (4) in particular, the belief that the dead must receive proper burial was a longstanding one; it was a divine decree that King Creon in *Antigone* ignored only at his own peril. (For the Greeks as for the Romans, the preferred burial methods alternated between cremation or inhumation.) Homer, for example, has the ghost of the unburied Elpenor implore Odysseus to see to it that his necessary burial rites be performed, "lest I become a cause of the gods' wrath against you."[29] Also, by the fifth century the Athenian law of homicide evidences this belief in the possible ill will of the dead who are not given prompt burial. Finally, the remaining religious motivations for the urgency of ceremonial burial were chiefly these: (a) that the dead had to be cut off entirely from the sight of the gods in order to avoid polluting or offending the gods and their altars; and (b) that the dead were in need of burial as a last gesture of kindness from the living, without which the dead were not assured admission to the lower world.[30] These, then, were among the principal religious considerations, apart from considerations of public sanitation and health, that lent a strong sense of propriety and proper care on the part of the living to both the corpse and the cherished memory of their dead.

So far, I have identified three Greek perspectives on the state of being dead. These are: (1) chthonic personal immortality; (2) divine personal immortality; and (3) natural personal dissolution. In addition, some of the more common attitudes of the living toward the dead have been explored for their religious and moral implications. Attitudes toward the dying process that have come into view include the heroic attitude, plus the idea of euthanasia (about which much more will be said in chapter 7). I shall now turn to a brief examination of some of the thoughts of Plato and Aristotle on the prospect of attaining human immortality. This will be followed by a look at what some have called the death-inspired Hellenistic philosophy of Epicureanism.

PLATO AND ARISTOTLE

If I were to summarize in a few paragraphs what Plato and Aristotle had to say about the prospect of attaining human immortality, the story I would tell is this. In the case of Plato, there is every reason to believe that he regarded such a prospect as highly probable. I say "probable" because, despite the elaborate proofs for human immortality offered in his *Phaedo* and elsewhere, we are typically reminded (*Phaedo* 107b.5) that the original assumptions on which these proofs depend "still need more accurate consideration." I believe that this sort of qualification here not only signifies the Socratic habit of leaving inquiries open-ended, but also signifies the doubts still lingering in Plato's mind regarding the possibility of being able to prove *with certainty* the case for divine personal immortality. (That Plato wanted to believe in this sort of personal immortality and most assuredly did I do not dispute.[31]) If so, then what seems fair to say is that Plato regarded the divinity and personal survival of the soul (which he equated with the essential, true self) as highly plausible but not beyond all doubt.

The significance of his proofs in the *Phaedo* and elsewhere may in the final analysis lie in the fact that they served to demonstrate to many of the skeptical intellectuals of Plato's day that it was at very least reasonable for an intelligent person to adopt and defend belief in divine personal immortality. The skeptical view, which often took the form of belief in what I have termed natural personal dissolution, Plato definitely opposed. This last view is characterized by Cebes in the following speech at *Phaedo* 60a:

> ... [Y] our statement, Socrates, ... seems excellent to me, but what you said about the soul leaves the average person with grave misgivings that when it is released from the body it may no longer exist anywhere, but may be dispersed and destroyed on the very day that the man himself dies, as soon as it is freed from the body. That as it emerges it may be dissipated like breath or smoke, and vanish away so that nothing is left of it anywhere.[32]

Against this view, Plato asserts that the moment of death occurs when the immortal and imperishable soul is freed from the mortal and perishable body. Following death, Plato suggests that the soul is subject to a temporary cycle of reincarnations. The soul may be expected to acquire various kinds of bodies representing lives of lower and higher moral worth. In the *Republic*, it is suggested further that, since we dwell in an essentially just universe, those souls that attain the highest moral virtue (predicated ultimately on acquaintance with Plato's so-called Forms) may one day reside in pure and disembodied splendor among the heavenly stars.[33] Finally, for Plato, as for Pythagoras before him, doing philosophy was regarded as the best way to purify and temper the soul in preparation for that endless odyssey on which it would embark at death.[34]

Aristotle's basic thoughts on the question of human immortality are not quite so easy to interpret as Plato's. There is at least one passage in his writings, namely *De Anima* 430a.14–25, where he seems to allow the possibility that man's reason (*nous*) might in some sense survive at death. Elsewhere in that same treatise, however, he defends in unmistakable language three propositions that jointly refute the claim that Aristotle believed in personal immortality in any relevant sense. These three propositions are: (1) that the soul is inseparable from the body and is as permanently bound to it as the power of sight is to the eye;[35] (2) that the doctrines of transmigration and reincarnation, similar to those suggested by the Pythagoreans and Plato, are pure myths;[36] and (3) that man, like most other living beings, survives past death only in the narrow biological sense that he may be thought of as continuing his existence in his offspring. At *De Anima* 415a.27, Aristotle puts this last point, which I regard as his basic position, as follows:

> ... for any living thing that has reached its normal development and which is unmutilated, and whose mode of generation is not spontaneous, the most natural act is the production of another like itself, an animal producing an animal, a plant a plant, in order that, as far as its nature allows, it may partake in the eternal and divine. That is the goal toward which all things strive, for the sake of which they do whatsoever their nature renders possible. . . .

Since then no living thing is able to partake in what is eternal and divine by uninterrupted continuance (for nothing perishable can ever remain one and the same), it tries to achieve that end in the only way possible to it, and success is possible in varying degrees; so it remains not indeed as the selfsame individual but continues its existence in something *like* itself, not numerically, but specifically one.[37]

I shall call Aristotle's perspective *species survival*. This raises the question: how did Aristotle look at having to die and the dying process itself? One finds that he supplied opinions that are remarkable for their candor and psychological insight. On conquering the fear of death, he writes:

Fear may be defined as a pain or disturbance due to a mental picture of some destructive or painful evil in the future. Of destructive or painful evils . . . only such as amount to great pains or losses. And even these, only if they appear not remote but so near as to be imminent: we do not fear things that are very way off: for instance, we all know we shall die, but we are not troubled thereby because death is not close at hand.[38]

Elsewhere, in the *Nicomachean Ethics*, he admits that, while having to die may be regarded as a profound evil, it is one that can be met nobly and with dignity by the brave:

Now *death is the most terrible of all things*; for it is the end, and nothing is thought to be any longer either good or bad for the dead. But the brave man would not seem to be concerned even with death in *all* circumstances; e.g., at sea or in disease. In what circumstances, then? Surely in the noblest. Now such things are those in battle; for these take place in the greatest and noblest danger. . . . Properly, then, he will be called brave who is fearless in face of a noble death, and of all emergencies that involve death.[39]

These passages bear the marks of one who gave keen thought to what today we would call the psychology of death and dying. Nor does it escape our attention that, despite the fact that the only sort of survival Aristotle unambiguously identifies is that impersonal sort carried on by one's species, he appears to find some comfort against death by adopting the moral virtue of courage. Perhaps this is the ultimate psychological remedy against the fear of dying. But, in addition, Aristotle declares that "death is the most terrible of all things." Yet, since he also affirms that "God and nature do nothing without a purpose," it is reasonable to conclude that the fact of death did not prevent him from crediting human existence with important meaning.[40] In a word, for Aristotle as for Plato, death did not succeed in rendering life absurd, as some existentialist philosophers of this past century have harped. This is so despite the fact that, as I have argued, Aristotle dispensed with Plato's hope for divine personal immortality.

Yet one may wonder just how satisfying the average Greek or Roman found the differing answers of either Plato or Aristotle on the question of survival after death. I have suggested that if Aristotle can be said to have provided a psychological remedy to the fear of dying, it lies in the acquisition of a brave character, aided by the intellectual consolation that life and death have some definite purpose. But to the average Greek, trying to become suitably brave in middle life, say, may have seemed a rather empty piece of advice. So, too, Plato's doctrine of divine personal immortality, not to mention Homer's chthonic immortality, may have triggered in the minds of many another unsettling worry: If I survive bodily death, what torments await my soul in the afterworld?

EPICUREAN INSIGHTS

Partly in response to these unallayed fears associated with concern over existence in some afterworld, the materialistic philosopher, Epicurus (341–270 B.C.), influenced by the fifth-century doctrines of the atomists, Leucippus and Democritus, attempted to refine and popularize the logical and psychological implications of a thoroughgoing atomic theory. Like Democritus before him, Epicurus depicted being dead as an extreme form of natural personal dissolution, namely oblivion. The great strength of Epicurus's position on death was that his theory—according to which death marked the final limit of a human's experience—*prima facie* seemed to fit the universally recorded and manifest fact that "All men are mortal."

Moreover, whereas Democritus, Plato, and Aristotle had allowed that knowledge could be an end in itself, Epicurus adopted a more pragmatic and therapeutic stance. He declared that knowledge was no more than a "remedy for the soul." In fact, according to Epicurus, the soul is one and the same as the body. Given this, the entire person is ultimately comprised of tiny, invisible, indestructible pieces of matter called atoms. Thus, all functions of the human organism are explained as resulting from atomic processes, and matter is credited with somehow containing the seeds of life.[41]

Given this materialistic account of man and nature, it comes as little surprise that Epicurus defines death in purely physical terms as the dissolution and dispersion of the soul atoms into the infinite void. This happens at the exact moment at which all personal sensation permanently ceases. Following Democritus, Epicurus believed that atoms and the void are all that fundamentally exist. Even the gods, according to Epicurus, were comprised of atoms, though they were not the usual gods of Homer and were said to be totally detached from human affairs; at best, the gods were useful only as exemplars of the complete peace of mind (*ataraxia*) at which humans should aim.[42]

At the heart of his philosophy, which his contemporaries often criticized as a brand of atheism by default, Epicurus offered several fundamental doctrines. These included the so-called Four Remedies of the soul, which declared: "[1] We need not fear God; [2] Death means absence of sensation; [3] The Good is easy to obtain; and

[4] Evil is easy to bear." To these four canonical beliefs, he adds the caveat: "vain is the word of a philosopher which does not heal any suffering of man."[43]

Furthermore, the good for man is said to be pleasure, on Epicurus' view, and the highest good a life of secure and lasting pleasure. This lasting pleasure can be gotten through the cultivation of intelligent choice predicted on practical wisdom (*phronesis*). "Practical wisdom measures pleasures against pains, accepting pains that lead to greater pleasures and rejecting pleasures that lead to greater pains. It counts the traditional virtues (justice, temperance, courage, etc.) among the means for attaining the pleasant; they have no other justification."[44]

If there can be said to be a recurring impediment to the peace of mind (*ataraxia*) so valued by Epicurus in his indeterministic, mechanistic universe, it is the fear of death. This fear can tarnish whatever enjoyments one might otherwise achieve in one's life. Hence, in view of this diagnosis, Epicurus's prescription is that such fears can be intelligently removed, since in reality they are totally unfounded. In his letter to Menoecus, among his most important and characteristic thoughts on what death is and how one may end fears of dying are powerfully summarized:

> Become accustomed to the belief that death is nothing to us. For all good and evil consists in sensation, but death is deprivation of sensation. And therefore a right understanding that death is nothing to us makes the mortality of life enjoyable, not because it adds to it an infinite span of time, but because it takes away the craving for immortality. For there is nothing terrible in not living, so that the man speaks idly who says that he fears death, not because it will be painful when it comes, but because it is painful in anticipation. For that which gives no trouble when it comes is but an empty pain in anticipation. So death, the most terrifying of all ills, is nothing to us, since so long as we exist death is not with us, but when death comes, then we do not exist. It does not then concern either the living, or the dead, since the former it is not, and the latter are no more.[45]

Close inspection of the above passage reveals that the force of Epicurus's argument turns on the claim that since being dead and having sensations of any sort are mutually exclusive, and since all good and evil involve sensation, being dead is nothing to fret about. In other words, it is not intelligent to spoil one's life by harboring fears that are in reality baseless.

As seductive as this argument appears to be at first glance, I must register at least one objection. It seems to me a doubtful statement that ". . . there is nothing terrible in not living. . . ." This statement may apply for those who were not brought into existence in the first place. But the relevant case is those persons who are now fully alive and in the middle of various projects and human relationships to which they accord value.[46] Death cuts short these ongoing projects and friendships of the living. Thus, the hardship death brings is not entirely owned up to by Epicurus in the above passage. At best, he succeeds in thwarting the fears of those who worry about what will happen to them in the afterworld. But to those who highly value their ongoing projects and their friendships with the living, and so bemoan precisely having to give up what they have achieved and can never reclaim, his argument is unconvincing and oversimplified.

There were, nonetheless, many adherents who found consolation in the words of Epicurus and were attracted to his emphasis on philosophy as the medicine of the soul. Like the competing materialistic philosophy of Stoicism, which also sought to reduce the fear of death,[47] Epicureanism enjoyed wide popularity in Hellenistic and later Roman times. Its success owed not only to the renewed attention it received from the Roman poet Lucretius, but also to its promise to restore to the individual a level of personal stability and tranquility increasingly valued in the turbulent and expansive post-Alexandrian age.

SUMMARY

We have now come to the end of this investigation of Greek attitudes toward death. My research points to a plurality of perspectives rather than to any single one. As for how the Greeks pictured being dead, four distinct perspectives have been identified. There are: (1) *chthonic personal immortality* associated with the Homeric religion; (2) *divine personal immortality* associated with the philosophies of Pythagoras and Plato; (3) *natural personal dissolution* associated with Thales, Anaximander, and Anaximenes and as we have just seen, Epicurus; and what may be called (4) *species survival* associated with Aristotle.

As for Greek attitudes toward the dying process, at least four perspectives have been discovered. These are: (a) *the heroic attitude* according to which one's willingness to die is seen as the best test of one's commitment to the highest sorts of ideals; (b) *the merciful attitude* according to which a quick and easy death (euthanasia) is seen as the best solution to relentless personal suffering; (c) *the Aristotelian attitude,* according to which the personal cultivation of courage is seen as the best psychological and moral remedy for meeting death; and (d) *the Epicurean attitude,* according to which fears of death can be eliminated by recognizing the baseless and illusory character of these fears.

In addition, the moment of death was shown to receive diverse characterizations by the Greeks. In the Homeric epics, death tended to be characterized as occurring at the moment when the ghost or breath escapes from the mouth or wound of the corpse. For both Pythagoras and Plato, it occurred at the moment that the soul is released from the body. For Anaximenes, it occurred when breathing ceased. In addition, for Aristotle it occurred when the vital life functions (especially heartbeat) ceased. Lastly, Epicurus specifies the moment of death as the permanent loss of sensation.

Amidst this variety of competing beliefs concerning being dead, dying, and the moment of death, can the typical fifth-century Hellenic physician be legitimately characterized as favoring some of these beliefs over others?

With one exception, the answer appears to be no. Like other members of Greek society, physicians were free to adopt their own attitudes and beliefs on these matters. It is reasonable to infer, therefore, that almost all of the preceding perspectives were represented among the physicians. Indeed, the Hippocratic treatises, including the Oath, attest to the fact that some physicians were religious or at least respectful of the gods. No doubt a fair number held out hope for the afterworld, though few were in the habit of trying to impose their personal views on their patients. This, even though they regularly divorced their theories of health and medical treatments from supernatural explanations. The lone exception to their diverse personal views was that the moment of death was generally understood to occur when breathing, heartbeat, and sensation collectively and permanently ceased.

Thus far at least three important points have been established in Part I of this study. First, the typical Greek physician of the fifth century B.C. was an unlicensed craftsman holding a rather low social rank; he occasionally encroached on the prerogatives of philosophers by telling citizens how they ought to live. I have argued that this encroachment was resisted by most philosophers. Philosophers handily exploited the general knowledge of citizens on health matters by developing the powerful analogy that philosophers were physicians of the soul and so stood in higher authority.

Second, unlike the Egyptians, the Greeks succeeded in freeing medical theories of health and disease from magic and superstition. The impetus for this came largely from the pre-Socratic philosopher-scientists who sought to put all phenomena on a naturalistic footing and account for all processes in terms of impersonal, universal laws. In addition, the seven principles of the humoral theory of disease were shown to have influenced selected parts of Plato's, Aristotle's, and Galen's theories of health and disease. It was further argued that Galen's eclectic theory on constitutional types integrated some facets of an ontological disease model with those of a physiological disease model that remained his favorite, and which was associated with the humoral theory of health.

Finally, it has been shown that there is no warrant for the mistaken view that the Greeks possessed anything like a single, basic outlook on death and dying. Let us then turn at once to the related consideration of how Greek medical ethics came into being. For despite the fact that the Greeks themselves held a multiplicity of opinions about the nature of death and the value of life, it is puzzling to observe that the ethical values expressed in the Hippocratic Oath demonstrate a singularly high and uncompromising regard for the preservation of human life. To make sense out of this unique feature of the Oath is the task that awaits us in Part II.

Discussion Questions

1. How can one distinguish coherently between "dying" and "being dead"? How was the "moment of death" characterized by most fifth-century-B.C. Greek doctors? How is it characterized by clinicians today?

2. What were the four principal perspectives on the afterworld among the Greeks?
3. What were the four leading attitudes toward the personal process of dying? Do any of these attitudes persist in our own era?
4. Why do you think that the ancient Greeks and Romans espoused a plurality of conflicting theories about the meanings and definitions of death and dying? Are physicians or philosophers any closer to a consensus on these issues today?

NOTES

1. Richard Kalish, "Attitudes Toward Death," in *EB*, vol.1, p. 286.
2. Jacques Choron, *Death and Western Thought* (New York: Macmillan, 1963), p. 32.
3. Porphyrius *Vita Pythagorae* 19, cited by John M. Robinson, *An Introduction to Early Greek Philosophy* (New York: Houghton Mifflin, 1968), pp. 57, 58–62 passim.
4. Homer *Iliad* 16.856; 14.518. In Homer, *soma* is restricted to mean the dead body of man or beast; for a living body, Homer uses the word *demas*. After Homer's time, *soma* referred to the body of either the living or the dead (as we construe it). See Liddell and Scott, *Greek–English Lexicon*, p. 688. The word *thymos* alone Homer associates with consciousness involving thought and feeling; *psyche* he reserves to designate life and movement. On this point see F. E. Peters, *Greek Philosophical Terms* (New York: New York University Press, 1967), pp. 166–67. In general, see Bruno Snell, *The Discovery of the Greek Mind*, trans. T. G. Rosenmeyer (New York: Harper Torchbook, Harper and Row, 1953), chap. 1.
5. Homer *Odyssey* 11.488–91, trans. Lattimore, *The Odyssey of Homer,* p. 180. Hesiod shows a brighter destiny for the heroes of old, cf. Hesiod, *The Works and Days*, trans. Richard Lattimore (Ann Arbor: University of Michigan Press, 1965), p. 166.
6. Francis M. Cornford, *From Religion to Philosophy* (New York: Harper, 1967), p. xxivff.
7. Emily Vermeule, *Aspects of Death in Early Greek Art and Poetry*, The Sather Classical Lectures, vol. 66 (Berkeley, CA: University of California Press, 1979), p. 41.
8. Ibid.
9. Ibid., pp. 8–9. A fine example of the soul-bird is seen in an Attic white-ground lekythos vase of the fifth century. It depicts the boatman Charon, the messenger god Hermes, and the soul-birds in Hades. This specimen was first brought to my attention by Philip Lockhart and is photographically reproduced on p. 9 of Vermeule's book.
10. Ibid., p. 37.
11. Choron, *Death and Western Thought*, p. 35.
12. Frag. 2, trans. Freeman, *Ancilla*, p. 19.
13. Anthony Flew, "Immortality," in *Encyclopedia of Philosophy*, ed. Paul Edwards, 8 vols. (New York: Collier Press, 1967), vol. 4, p. 140, emphasis added (hereafter cited as *EP*).
14. Choron, *Death of Western Thought*, p. 33.
15. The loose sense of the word "death" is normally intended in such statements as "I believe in life after death." If the word "death" did not bend in these contexts, a whole range of perfectly understandable utterances would have to be dismissed.
16. Heraclitus frags. 36, 48, 62, and 88, *Ancilla*.
17. Parmenides frags. B8 (lines 1–25; lines 36–40) in H. Diels and W. Kranz, *Die Fragmente der Vorsokratiker,* 11th ed. (Berlin: Weidmann, 1903).

18. Cf. Empedocles frags. 8 and 9 from "On Nature" and Empedocles frags. 146 and 147 from "Purifications," *Ancilla.*
19. Choron, *Death and Western Thought*, p. 32.
20. Ibid., p. 32.
21. Pindar frag. 137. Cf. Frag. 129, cited and trans. A. W. Mair, "Life and Death: Greek," in *Encyclopedia of Religion and Ethics*, ed. James Hastings, 13 vols. (New York: Charles Scribner & Sons, 1852–1922), vol. 8, p. 30 (hereafter cited as *ERE*).
22. Sophocles *Antigone* 5.332; 360, trans. Paul Roche, *The Oedipus Plays of Sophocles* (New York: Mentor, 1958), cited by Choron, *Death and Western Thought*, p. 42.
23. C. M. Bowra, *The Greek Experience* (New York: Mentor, 1959), p. 49.
24. Paul Roche, trans., cited by Choron, *Death and Western Thought*, pp. 42–43.
25. Aeschylus *Agamemnon* 1148ff., trans. Mair in *ERE*, vol. 8, p. 30.
26. See also chapter 7.
27. For more on these four points, see K. J. Dover, *Greek Popular Morality in the Time of Plato and Aristotle* (Los Angeles: University of California Press, 1974), pp. 243–46. See also Donna C. Kurtz and John Boardman, *Greek Burial Customs* (Ithaca, NY: Cornell University Press, 1971), p. 206; and on ghosts in classical times, see E. Rohde, *Psyche*, trans. W. B. Hillis, 8th ed. (London: Paul Treuch Trubner Ltd., 1925), pp. 593–95.
28. Dover, *Greek Popular Morality*, p. 245. Cf. Plato *Laws* 10.
29. Homer *Odessey* 11.72ff., trans. Lattimore, *The Odyssey of Homer.*
30. Herbert J. Rose, "Disposal of the Dead," in *OCD*, p. 314. On pollution and purification in connection with homicide, cf. D. M. Macdowell, *Athenian Homicide Law in the Age of the Orators* (Manchester, U.K.: University of Manchester Press, 1963), chaps. 1, 12, and 14.
31. Cf. *Timaeus* 29d and *Phaedo* 107b–c. See also Plato *Letter* 7.335a–c.
32. Hugh Tredennick, trans., *Collected Dialogues*, p. 52.
33. For Plato's standard definition of death, *Phaedo* 64c-d; for a physical account of decaying and death, *Timaeus* 80c–d and chapter 2, note 21; and for his views on reincarnation, *Republic* 10.
34. I am inclined to agree with those scholars who attribute to the historical Socrates the agnostic views on immortality at *Apology* 38cff., and to Plato alone the doctrine of immortality supported in *Phaedo* and elsewhere. See chapter 7.
35. Aristotle *De Anima* 412b.5; 413a.1.
36. Ibid., *De Anima* 407b.22.
37. Ibid., *De Anima* 415a.27ff., trans. Smith, in *Basic Works*, p. 561, emphases added. Cf. Plato's *Symposium* 206–8 for a similar perspective expressed by Diotima. For a discussion of dissenting views, see Frederick Copleston, *A History of Philosophy* (New York: Image, 1962) vol. 1, pt. 2, pp. 70–73.
38. Aristotle *Rhetoric* 1382a.20–27, trans. W. Rhys Roberts, in *Basic Works*, p.1389.
39. Aristotle *Nichomachean Ethics* 3.6.1115a.26–35, emphases added, trans. W. D. Ross, in *Basic Works*, pp. 975–76.
40. Aristotle *De Caelo* 1.4.271a.33, trans. J. L. Stocks, in *Basic Works*, p. 404.
41. This last claim, called *hylozoism*, was similarly endorsed by a number of the pre-Socratics.
42. P. H. DeLacy, "Epicurus," in *EP*, vol. 2, p. 5.

43. Diogenes Laertius *De Vitis* 10.138. The caveat against untherapeutic philosophers derives from *The Stoic and Epicurean Philosophers*, ed. Whitney J. Oates (New York: Random House, 1940), p. 31, cited by Choron, *Death and Western Thought*, p. 58.
44. DeLacy, "Epicurus," in *EP*, vol. 2, pp. 4–5.
45. "Letter to Menoecus," in *Stoic and Epicurean*, ed. Oates, pp. 30–1.
46. For a possible rejoinder, see Fred Miller, "Epicurus on the Art of Dying," *The Southern Journal of Philosophy* 14, no. 2 (1976): 169–77 passim.
47. For Stoic views on death, see pp. 134–35.

PART II

THE RISE OF
MEDICAL ETHICS

4 Who Was Hippocrates?

He knew the things that were and the things that
would be and the things that had been before.

—HOMER

OF ALL THE MEDICAL WRITINGS associated with the name of Hippocrates, probably none is better known to the modern reader than the Hippocratic Oath. Since it is the explicit aim in this investigation to identify and expose ancient philosophical perspectives on abortion and euthanasia, and since the Hippocratic Oath appears to absolutely prohibit these measures, the Oath stands as a natural starting point for the present section.

A number of important questions can be raised: What, if anything, is truly unique about the Oath? How was it different from the literature produced by neighboring non-Greek cultures? Who wrote the Oath, and what purpose and influence did it exercise among physicians and laymen in pre-Christian Greco-Roman times?

In addition, it will be necessary to examine the relation of the Oath to the Hippocratic Collection as a whole. One wants to learn whether the moral imperatives expressed by the Oath are in basic accord with the medical practices and constraints expressed elsewhere in that sizeable and diverse body of writings.

To round out this investigation into the emergence of medical ethics, attention will also be given to those lesser-known Hippocratic treatises that deal primarily with medical etiquette. I shall argue that there is a distinct, logical compatibility between the Oath and these latter treatises: taken together, they display an unmistakable and sustained concern for the patient's best welfare.

MEDICAL ETHICS BEFORE HIPPOCRATES

Darrel Amundsen has written: "Medical ethics . . . is even less apt to be borrowed by members of one society, from another culturally alien to it, than are its medical theory and concomitant technique."[1] In view of the ethnocentric tendencies characteristically manifested in the moral theories of almost all cultures, no doubt Amundsen is right. But it would be an unfortunate mistake to completely ignore on this account such evidence of medical ethical values that scholars and others have culled from the Near East and Egypt, including Assyria, Babylonia, Persia, and Israel. These were neighboring Eastern cultures with medical traditions well antedating mainland Greece itself. And to the south, few can any longer seriously doubt the cross-fertilization that occurred as a result of trade between the Greek city-states and Egypt.

To overlook that the Greeks may have acquired useful ideas from their widespread commercial encounters along the Mediterranean Sea channels or on overland expeditions—ideas possibly affecting their art and medicine, if not their philosophy—is to indulge an unaffordable provincialism.[2] In fact, there is little to risk in looking at the larger ancient landscape and much to gain. For how else can one accurately gauge the originality of the Greek contribution to Western civilization, and in particular ethics, if one hesitates to survey her ancient neighbors? Essentially, then, I agree with Amundsen: the probabilities of intercultural influence in the field of medical ethics are slim. But I would insist that the moral traditions of neighboring cultures hold more than "peripheral relevance" to the fullest understanding of the unique character of Greek medical thinking.[3]

For example, unlike fifth-century-B.C. Athens, in Babylonia and Egypt medicine was practiced subject to strict state regulation. Attention has already been given to the testimony of Aristotle according to which an Egyptian physician is warned by the state not to alter a course of treatment until at least four days have passed, or else be subject to legal penalties.[4] But the legislative regulation of medicine appears to have advanced even further in ancient Babylonia. The Code of Hammurabi (dating from about 1727 B.C.) contains the first recorded attempt by any culture to protect patients from incompetent doctors.

The medical laws of Hammurabi may be divided into two broad categories. Some refer to the medical care of noblemen. Others pertain to commoners or slaves. In the case of noblemen, the Code stipulates that if a surgeon performs surgery with a bronze lancet or specifically operates with a lancet on the eye, and this results either in the loss of the eye to the patient or the patient's death, then the state shall cut off the surgeon's hand (Code no. 218).

In contrast, if the physician operates with a bronze lancet on a slave owned by a commoner and the result is that the slave dies, the physician must replace the slave by one of equal value (no. 219). Moreover, if as a result of a surgical operation on a slave's eye the slave loses his sight, the physician must pay the commoner one-half of the market value of his damaged slave (no. 220). Add to the preceding regulations those provisions of Hammurabi's Code that set differential medical fees for surgery based on the socioeconomic status of each patient (nos. 215–17; 221–23), and the picture emerges of a surprisingly comprehensive system of legislative sanctions defining the proper conduct of surgical medicine.[5] It is important to note, however, that Hammurabi's Code remains silent on most nonsurgical medical procedures. Hence, no penalties are specific for dietary and other forms of therapy. This was probably due in large part to the fact that surgery was perceived to carry more immediate and permanent risks to the patient compared to other forms of medicine known to the Babylonians (including magic). Therefore, legal sanctions against the possible abuses of surgical procedures were deemed especially necessary.

There is the related question of whether these diverse Near Eastern cultures defined the favored characteristics of their ideal physician in their medical or religious literature. All that can be said is that in the case of the Assyro-Babylonian and Egyptian cultures no such literary evidence has survived. Obviously this does not rule out the possibility that they possessed such idealized medical standards.

Investigations into the medical ethical values of ancient Persian culture have proved more fruitful. Amundsen calls attention to a sixth-century A.D. passage taken from the third book of the Sassanian Persian's encyclopedic *Dinkard*. This passage characterizes in very specific terms the qualities of the ideal physician. The importance of this passage is that some scholars think it may be based directly on a lost portion of the much older *Zend-Avesta*, of which only about one-third remains.[6] For comparative purposes in relation to the Greek ideal, it is interesting to read that according to *The Dinkard* the best physician

> . . . should know the limbs of the body, their articulations; remedies for disease; . . . should be amiable without jealousy, gentle in word, free from haughtiness; an enemy in disease, but the friend of the sick, respecting modesty, free from crime, from injury, from violence; expeditious; . . . noble in action; protecting good reputation; not acting for gain, but for a spiritual reward; ready to listen; . . . possessed of authority and philanthropy; skilled to prepare health-giving plants medically, in order to deliver the body from disease to expel corruption and impurity; to further peace and multiply the delights of life.[7]

Though one can be struck by the modern ring of the preceding description, it must be kept in mind that the "physician" to whom these words refer was a practitioner of magic in the Persian culture. That is, Persian physicians were also Zoroastrian priests. Thus, the Persians, like their Egyptian and Assyro-Babylonian counterparts, freely mixed the rational elements of medical practice with supernatural magico-religious elements. Yet it is exactly this tendency that the Hippocratic physicians opposed, for the Greeks succeeded in divorcing priestly functions from their own concept of the ideal physician.[8]

On the issue of euthanasia, there exists no direct evidence that unambiguously reveals the moral stand taken in the Near East. It *is* known that in both Egypt and Assyro-Babylonia, a person who committed suicide was thought to have irrevocably cut himself off from the gods.[9] In view of this, it seems plausible to infer that on religious grounds, physicians from these cultures may have had some serious reservations about encouraging or contributing to active voluntary euthanasia. But this is conjectural, and presupposes more than can now be proved. That is, it presupposes that the act of suicide would have been understood by these ancient peoples as morally equivalent to voluntary euthanasia. Personally, I have my doubts.

Nonetheless, it is true that in the *Edwin Smith Papyrus*, as well as in the *Papyrus Ebers*, the Egyptian physician divides his cases into three groups. If the prognosis he expected was favorable, he commented "an ailment I shall treat." On uncertain prognoses, the comment is "an ailment I shall combat." But if the prognosis is unfavorable, the notation reads, "an ailment not to be treated." Yet this last category of patients was not abandoned. As some of the cases explicitly reveal, the physicians of Egypt took steps to at least relieve the suffering; they helped the patient remain as comfortable as possible until death.[10]

As for the Persians, still less can be established. If the above passage from *The Dinkard* is carefully examined, there appears nothing in it that explicitly excludes mercy killing. Those portions of it that describe the ideal physician as the friend of the sick, free from crime, the bringer of peace, the multiplier of the delights of life, and so on, are not necessarily incompatible with a proeuthanasia perspective. This is especially so if voluntary euthanasia is viewed as a kindness to the patient; that is, as a benevolent, not a criminal act; an act that brings peace to a life judged no longer capable of delight.

In view of this possibility, I cannot agree with Amundsen's conjecture. Amundsen argues that the ancient Persian doctor, just because he was also a priest and interpreted disease as caused by the forces of evil, would probably *not* have hastened the end of hopeless patients.[11] This may be doubted. For if the patients were indeed perceived by the priest as hopeless, and if they begged for death and an end to their suffering, who can deny that the priest-physician might have been motivated by religious compassion and mercy to assist the patient in ending his torment? I do not want to press this objection, but it does serve to illustrate the ambiguity of the Persian position on this issue.

Regarding the practice of abortion, somewhat more is known. In Persia, the sacred book known as the *Vendidad* prohibited abortion. "The woman, the nurse who performed the abortion, the woman's father or the father of the fetus, if the abortion was sought at their instigation, were all held guilty of willful murder."[12]

Similarly, in Assyria there existed laws against abortion possibly as early as the fifteenth century B.C. One Assyrian law from that period provided that "if a woman had an abortion by her own act, whether or not she survived the ordeal, she was to be impaled on a stake and left unburied."[13] However, no mention is made in Assyrian law of penalties against physicians or midwives who may have aided women in their abortion attempts. This is indeed puzzling. It is possible that those who conspired with the women were implicitly covered by this edict.

In the case of Egypt, the medical papyri do contain prescriptions concerning how to induce abortions. This implies that abortions were almost certainly performed by Egyptian doctors. But whether it was entirely legal or considered moral, and to what extent and under what conditions it was understood to be medically warranted, must at present remain a matter of speculation.

What about the Israelites? Where did they stand on the issues of abortion and euthanasia? As we have seen, there existed no distinct Jewish medical literature, nor was there anything like an emerging Jewish medical profession, until the later Hellenistic period (after 150 B.C.).[14] Even so, centuries before Hippocrates came onto the ancient scene the Hebrew Bible (Torah) declared that man was created in the divine image of God (*imago dei*, in Latin; *tselem Elohim*, in Hebrew). In addition, the covenant (*berit*) relationship between the Jewish people and their monotheistic, omnipotent God (*Yahweh*) issued specific duties (*mitzvot*, Gen. 2:16), which were designed to honor and protect human life. Naturally, these life sustaining values extended to the mother and fetus, to the aged, infirm, and dying.[15] Yet the Hebrew duty to respect and protect human life is not absolute. For example, retribution against evil-doers is permitted (Ex. 21:12–17) as is sacrificing one's life for one's country or avoiding disgrace before one's God (I Sam. 31:3–4; 2 Sam. 2:12–23). The moral urgency of this life-affirming teaching is emphatically expressed at Ezekiel 18:14: "'Behold, all lives are Mine,' saith the Lord."

Envisioning human life as a sacred trust from God, which God alone can sustain or end (a view coincidentally akin to the Pythagoreans), Jewish tradition before and after the time of Hippocrates generally opposed abortion. The act of abortion was viewed as the destruction of a potential person made in the image of God. It was rarely permitted and only to protect the mother's life or health. Since self-mutilation was also proscribed, and since the act of abortion could be understood as a form of self-mutilation, elective abortion for nonhealth reasons was considered sinful.[16]

As for the moral permissibility of active euthanasia (here construed as mercy killing), Rabbi Immanuel Jakobovits clarifies that in those ancient days ". . . anyone who kills a dying person is liable to the death penalty as a common murderer."[17] The sixth commandment of the Mosaic law reads: "Thou shalt not kill." But while actively terminating the life of someone who is dying (*goses*) is blameworthy, Jewish law does permit the removal of artificial means that may otherwise prolong the dying process.[18] Therefore, passive euthanasia alone is embraced: it is viewed as a humane way of letting the person's soul escape without undue trauma. In sum, the Jews taught that care of the dying is required even when a cure was impossible. These perspectives, predicated largely on their sanctity of human life theology, were inherited and magnified by Christianity in millennia to come. Indeed, that it was wrong to abandon the dying or disrespect the elderly received further impetus from the fifth Mosaic commandment: "Honor thy father and mother that thy days may be long upon the land. . . ."

All things considered, it seems fair to conclude that the latest evidence permits only the sketchiest picture to be drawn concerning the medical ethics of the ancient Near East, Egypt, and Israel. It is worth emphasizing that, unlike the Greeks, no literature appears to have survived from the five ancient cultures under discussion that is exclusively devoted to medical ethics. If, in fact, any Assyrian, Babylonian, Persian, Egyptian, or Hebrew doctors or priests wrote an ethical code relating to medicine prior to 400 B.C., we have no evidence of it. Still, the laws and religious prescriptions at our disposal reveal an overall and varied interest in the basic welfare of the patient, whether he be freeborn or slave. Healers and priests from these neighboring cultures had a definite sense of the right and wrong way to care for those seeking their services. This sense derived mainly from the authority of their laws or their religions. But they were by no means free agents practicing their craft independently of state interference or tradition, as were their Greek counterparts.

THE PUZZLE OF HIPPOCRATES' IDENTITY

Before turning to the Hippocratic Oath, it is appropriate to comment on the puzzling fact that very little is known about Hippocrates himself (Fig. 5). The only extant ancient sources that mention him by name and that were composed near the period of his life (469–399 B.C.) are two passages in Plato. One is from Plato's *Protagoras*, the other from the *Phaedrus*. In the generation following Hippocrates' death, there exists a passing remark by Aristotle in his *Politics* and the medical writings of Meno. Lamentably, we have little to go on (even though he was the exact contemporary of Socrates).

In the *Protagoras* passage, it is attested that (a) Hippocrates was a native of the Greek island of Cos; (b) he was apparently as well known in his own day as the celebrated sculptors Phidias and Polyclitus; and (c) he accepted payment for instruction in the art of medicine.[19] In addition, the *Phaedrus* establishes that Hippocrates practiced medicine based on an organistic principle.[20] To him is attributed the principle that the nature of any component part or organ can only be properly understood after thoroughly examining the whole to which it belongs. In the *Phaedrus* passage, the discussion turns on a Socratic analogy between rhetoric and medicine. Hippocrates' organistic approach to medicine is cited approvingly by Socrates. By reference to it he reinforces his claim that both the master rhetorician and the master physician must study the whole nature of the special objects of their arts (these objects being the body and soul, respectively). Such a fundamentally comprehensive approach to inquiry was much favored by Socrates, who, in the *Phaedrus*, endorses it for anyone who ". . . mean [s] to be scientific and not content with mere empirical routine. . . ."[21]

Moreover, Aristotle mentions Hippocrates by name just once.[22] In his *Politics*, he describes Hippocrates as a great physician and implies that he was short in stature. His point is that Hippocrates' greatness stemmed from his excellence as a physician who performed well *qua* physician; Hippocrates' greatness was not merely due to noble birth or wealth or physical size. It derived rather from the quality of his work above all else.

HIPPOCRATES HIRACLIDÆ F. COVS.
Ex marmore antiquo.

Figure 5. Hippocrates, as envisioned in an engraving by Paulus Pontius (1603–1658) after a drawing by Peter Paul Rubens from an ancient marble bust. In fact, little is known of Hippocrates' true appearance. Reprinted courtesy of the National Library of Medicine, Bethesda, MD.

Furthermore, Aristotle's suggestion that Hippocrates was a man of short stature is the only reliable physical description that we have. While efforts have been made over the centuries to identify various ancient statues (mostly copies of Greek originals) with Hippocrates of Cos, no positive identification of Hippocrates' likeness so far has proved convincing. Albert Lyons has argued that some first-century A.D. Roman coins that recently have been unearthed from the island of Cos and that bear the name of Hippocrates reveal ". . . the likely appearance of Hippocrates. . . ."[23] This is extremely conjectural, however, in view of the absence of other ancient artifacts against which this alleged image may be checked. Nor will it serve in this case to argue that since numismatic specimens often obscure the true facial features of their subjects, Lyons's judgment is all the more dubious. For, in fact, before the fourth century A.D., numismatic portraiture was uncommonly realistic. So the decisive question here is, Did the first century A.D. artists themselves any longer know what Hippocrates may have looked like? This question becomes especially pertinent in the case of coins struck five hundred years after their subject's death and discovered near a site also popular to ancient collectors and travelers. So while I remain skeptical, Lyons's conjecture cannot be dismissed.

Aristotle's student, Meno, who wrote a doxographical compendium of early Greek medicine, states that Hippocrates held a theory of disease according to which badly digested or unwisely selected food produces putrid air inside the body that invades the organs and tissues, causing disease. This theory of putrefaction is attributed to Hippocrates in the so-called *Anonymous Londinensis*, a work discovered among papyri long stored in the British Museum, and one that contains some of Meno's medical writings.[24] To these few details one can add the likely facts that Hippocrates traveled widely, at least in his native Greece, as did most physicians of his day. Also that he died in Thessaly and was buried near Larissa around 399 B.C. is most probable. More about his life and personality now cannot be ascertained.[25]

In view of how little is actually known about the historical Hippocrates, how can one square this modest account with the later, unbounded fame Hippocrates acquired in antiquity as the Father of Medicine? This is a puzzling question and no simple story can be told.

In my opinion, the most credible answer appears to be this:[26] To his Greek contemporaries Hippocrates *was* regarded as a famous physician, but he was one among many. For example, in his medical history Meno discusses twenty famous Greek doctors. Hippocrates is *not* singled out as more important than the rest. Also, Plato refers to a number of other doctors in his dialogues and he seems to imply that they are also approximately as famous and well known to his readers as Hippocrates.

In addition, it is likely that scholars at the great library at Alexandria, in Egypt, began assembling and seeking out medical texts associated with the teaching of Hippocrates at Cos, along with materials from other famous Greek medical centers, sometime during the fourth century B.C. They probably began with a fair number of anonymously authored fifth- and fourth-century Greek manuscripts. When their interest in identifying the works of Hippocrates peaked on account of the latter's growing reputation among his many medical disciples, the Alexandrian scholars or their assistants probably began crediting the most impressive of these anonymous manuscripts to the physician from Cos. If the core of the Hippocratic Collection did, in fact, form in this or some related way, perhaps it continued to enlarge owing to these occasional irregularities in manuscript classification. Thus, it is not hard to imagine that in succeeding centuries the *name* of Hippocrates exceeded the fame and stature of the already prominent life that the real Hippocrates had, in fact, lived.

What is more, to this account three fortuitous developments bearing on the fame of Hippocrates must be included. First, the Romans of the Imperial period enshrined fifth-century Greece as the golden age. Greek writers and thinkers of that idealized period were regarded by most Roman intellectuals as matchless. For example, the Roman Erotian (fl. A.D. 50) ranked Hippocrates the equal of Homer as a writer.[27] This sort of romanticized Roman estimate of the Greek golden age doubtless redoubled Hippocrates' fame. Hippocrates was, after all, by Erotian's day the best known of all the fifth-century Greek physicians in Nero's Rome. Again, this owed largely to the labors of the Alexandrian scholars who aimed at amassing the entire sum of human knowledge in a single library despite the attendant risks of misattribution.

Second, while Galen himself questioned the authenticity of some of the Hippocratic manuscripts, he personally revered Hippocrates as the ideal physician. In this, he urged fellow physicians to follow his lead.[28] This was indeed fortunate. It may be said that almost any craft or profession seeks to identify an ideal hero who is the embodiment and reminder of the values and aims it holds dear. (Socrates has often been cast in such an idealized role by professional philosophers, for example.) But the personal endorsement of Galen could not have brought to the name of Hippocrates a more enduring and powerful certification of his worth for centuries to come.

Third, it cannot be overlooked that the ethical values expressed in the Hippocratic Oath conformed in many ways to the respect-for-human-life ethic that was championed by the latest of the ancient religions, namely, Christianity. To this last point I shall return in the subsequent chapter. But by way of anticipation, it is evident that the acceptability of much of the Oath popularly credited to Hippocrates by the early church fathers themselves did much to sustain his legend.

Before turning directly to explore the Oath, I must stop for a moment to consider the problem of the many stylistic and logical inconsistencies contained in the Hippocratic Collection as a whole. Because of the scarcity of evidence that has so far rendered inconclusive efforts to pinpoint any single one of the collection's more than sixty books as a genuine work by Hippocrates, a sensible convention has arisen among contemporary writers that I, too, shall employ; that is, referring to the entire collection as the product of frankly anonymous "Hippocratic authors." However, I do not wish to exclude the possibility that Hippocrates may have actually written at least some of these works. On that question I urge an open mind.[29]

Discussion Questions

1. Was Hippocrates one person or many?
2. Before Hippocrates' day in fifth-century-B.C. Greece, is there any evidence of medical, ethical, or legal norms which guided doctors in neighboring Near Eastern, Egyptian, or Jewish cultures? How unique historically is Hippocrates' insistence on practicing medicine always to benefit the patient?
3. Even though Hippocrates was a contemporary of Socrates, why do we know so comparatively little about the legendary Father of Medicine?
4. How did the name of Hippocrates become so famous by the end of the Hellenistic period? Why, in your opinion, does this fame persist today?

NOTES

1. Amundsen, "History of Medical Ethics" in *EB*, vol. 2, p. 883.
2. For a look at the contribution of Near Eastern art to later developments in Egyptian and Greek art, see Helen Gardner, *Art Through the Ages*, ed. Horst de la Croix and Richard G. Taney (New York: Harcourt Brace,1975), pp. 104, 126. On Egyptian antecedents and possible influences on Greek medicine, see Saunders, *The Transitions from Egyptian to Greek Medicine*, pp. 1ff.
3. Amundsen, "History of Medical Ethics," in *EB*, vol. 2, p. 883.
4. Aristotle *Politics* 3.15.1286a12ff., and chapter 1, pp. 18–19.
5. All the preceding features of the Code of Hammurabi are discussed by Amundsen, "History of Medical Ethics," in *EB*, vol. 2, p. 882. See also Robert Biggs, "Medicine in Ancient Mesopotamia," *History of Science* 8 (1969): 94–105.
6. Amundsen, "History of Medical Ethics," in *EB*, vol. 2, p. 883.
7. *The Dinkard* 157, 19, trans. Ratanshan Erachshah Kohiyar, ed. Peshotan dastur Behramjee Sanjana, *The Dinkard: The Original Pahlavi Text* (Bombay: Duftur Ashkara Press), pp. 1874–91, cited by Amundsen, "History of Medical Ethics," in *EB*, vol. 2, p. 883.
8. See the Hippocratic treatise *The Sacred Disease* in W. H. S. Jones, trans., *Hippocrates*, 4 vols. (Cambridge, MA: Harvard University Press, 1962), vol. 2, pp. 139–41. Prior to the emergence and influence of the pre-Socratic philosophers, there was a time when diseases were presumed by the Greeks, as they were by the Near Eastern cultures, to be sent from the gods. Homer restricted divine causes mainly to epidemic diseases. See *Iliad* 1.8–10. However, Hesiod appears to have been less restrictive and thought that the gods brought all diseases upon man. Cf. Hesiod, *The Works and Days*, pp. 103–110. See also Fig. 4, chapter 3.
9. Amundsen, "History of Medical Ethics," in *EB*, vol. 2, p. 881.
10. *The Edwin Smith Papyrus* 6.8a.20; and *The Papyrus Ebers*, pp. 108–110.
11. Amundsen, "History of Medical Ethics," in *EB*, vol. 2, p. 881.

12. Ibid., vol. 2, p. 882. See *Vendidad* 15.2.12–14, trans. James Darmesteter, *The Zend-Avesta*, 3 vols. (Oxford: Clarendon Press, 1880–83); reprint (Westport, CT: Greenwood Press, 1972).

13. Amundsen, "History of Medical Ethics," in *EB*, vol. 2, p. 882. Amundsen has located this law in Middle Assyrian Laws, A53.

14. See chapter 1, subhead "Jewish Influences."

15. David Novak, "Judaism," in *EB 1995*, vol. 3, pp. 1302–3.

16. Ibid., p. 1307. Jewish tradition has not spoken with one voice on the issue of whether moral personhood begins at conception or at birth (crowning), as Novak points out. Nevertheless, there is a *prima facie* duty to protect fetal life. As for infanticide, Jewish law considers that murder. In contrast, cf. Plato and Seneca, chapter 6, "The Problem of Abortion."

17. Immanuel Jakobovits, *Jewish Medical Ethics: A Comparative and Historical Study of the Jewish Religion and Its Practice* (New York: Bloch Publishing Co., 1975), pp. 123–24. As for the act of suicide, whether committed by the terminally ill or by others who feel they are in desperate circumstances, this is almost always considered repugnant and blameworthy. God, the giver of life, may alone take life: moral courage and religious piety are expected to see one through good times and bad.

18. Ibid., p. 124.

19. Plato *Protagoras* 331b–c.

20. Plato *Phaedrus* 170b–d.

21. Plato *Phaedrus* 270bff., trans. R. Hackforth, in *Collected Dialogues*, p. 515. The sense of the word "empirical" Socrates here intends is, of course, the superficial sense of ignoring the true causes or natures of things, which, in his view, lie beneath the surface of mere appearance.

22. Aristotle *Politics* 1326a.15.

23. Albert S. Lyons and R. Joseph Petrucelli, *Medicine: An Illustrated History* (New York: Harry N. Abrams, 1978), pp. 207–10. The Roman coins in question are now housed in the British Museum, London.

24. It is tempting to speculate on whether Hippocrates' theory of the etiology of disease was influenced by some features of the Egyptian theory of putrefaction. See chapter 1. This possibility cannot be ruled out. But just how and where Hippocrates may have gained knowledge of Egyptian medicine is a mystery. He did travel within Greece, we know, but that he visited Egypt we have no firm reason to believe. For ancient legends to the contrary and their likely misleading implications, see Sigerist, *History of Medicine*, vol. 2, p. 271.

25. Edelstein, "Hippocrates," in *OCD*, p. 518. The best known of the ancient biographies of Hippocrates is *Life of Hippocrates* by Soranus of Ephesus. The authorship of his work, however, is in doubt. For a useful evaluation of the ancient and medieval biographies on Hippocrates, see Sigerist, *History of Medicine*, vol. 2, p. 268ff.

26. Here I concur with Ludwig Edelstein, whose explanations, with a few qualifications, have won the acceptance of Henry E. Sigerist and several other leading classicists and medical historians. See Ludwig Edelstein, *Peri aeron und die Sammlung der hippokratischen Schriften* (Berlin: Weidmann, 1931), pp.116ff., cited by Sigerist, *History of Medicine*, vol. 2, pp. 266–67.

27. Sigerist, *History of Medicine*, vol. 2, p. 267.

28. Ibid. See H. Diller, "Zur Hippokratesauffassung des Galen," *Hermes* 68 (1933): 167–81.

29. Just how one goes about counting up the manuscripts belonging to the Hippocratic Collection is a matter of current controversy. According to Henry E. Sigerist, almost all the books belonging to the collection, with a few exceptions, date from the fifth and fourth centuries B.C. As I have argued, the bulk of the *Corpus Hippocraticum* represents all or most of the best medical literature from this earlier period that the Alexandrians could find. Sigerist comments: "There has been much speculation for, unlike the Hermetic books of Egypt, the *Corpus Hippocraticum* was never firmly constituted, never divided into a set number of books, never rigidly fixed. . . . Still, the best Greek manuscripts contain about sixty books which were transmitted from the fifth and fourth centuries." (See Sigerist, *History of Medicine*, vol. 2, pp. 274–75.) While Sigerist takes the position that at least *some* of the works in the collection may be genuine works by the historical Hippocrates, Ludwig Edelstein holds that none of the books preserved under the name Hippocrates is genuine. (See Edelstein, "Hippocrates," in *OCD*, p. 518.) For more on the problem, see Edelstein, "The Genuine Works of Hippocrates," in *Ancient Medicine*, pp. 133–44.

5 The Hippocratic Oath

Keep watch also on the faults of the patients,
which often make them lie about the taking of
things prescribed.

—HIPPOCRATES

AT FIRST SIGHT it is indeed ironic that the so-called Hippocratic Oath, which is the most renowned medical ethical document and the one most popularly associated with Hippocrates' name, is now judged by very few scholars to be authored by Hippocrates. What's more, it is especially doubtful that the Oath accurately reflects the ethical values and medical practices that the Hippocratic authors favored and typically followed in their practice of medicine. In what follows, I shall endorse these conclusions in two steps. First, I shall critically discuss two important contemporary positions on the date, origin, and purpose of the Oath. Then I shall argue that the Oath represents essentially an esoteric ethical code that is partly, though not exclusively, of Pythagorean origin.

The Oath itself is a very short document. It reads in full:

OATH

(P1) I swear by Apollo Physician and Asclepius and Hygieia and Panaceia and all the gods and goddesses, making them my witnesses, that I will fulfill according to my ability and judgment this oath and this covenant.

(P2) To hold him who has taught me this art as equal to my parents and to live my life in partnership with him, and if he is in need of money, to give him a share of mine, and to regard his offspring as equal to my brothers in male lineage and to teach them this art—if they desire to learn it—without fee and covenant; to give a share of precepts and oral instruction and all the other learning to my sons and to the sons of him who has instructed me and to pupils who have signed the covenant and have taken an oath according to the medical law, but to no one else.

(P3) I will apply dietetic measures for the benefit of the sick according to my ability and judgment; I will keep them from harm and injustice.

(P4) I will neither give a deadly drug to anybody if asked for it, nor will I make a suggestion to this effect. Similarly, I will not give to a woman an abortive remedy. In purity and holiness I will guard my life and my art.

(P5) I will not use the knife, not even on sufferers from stone, but will withdraw in favor of such men as are engaged in this work.

(P6) Whatever houses I may visit, I will come for the benefit of the sick, remaining free of all intentional injustice, of all mischief and in particular of sexual relations with both female and male persons, be they free or slaves.

(P7) What I may see or hear in the course of the treatment or even outside of the treatment in regard to the life of men, which on no account one must spread abroad, I will keep to myself holding such things shameful to be spoken about.

(P8) If I fulfill this oath and do not violate it, may it be granted to me to enjoy life and art, being honored with fame among all men for all time to come; if I transgress it and swear falsely, may the opposite of all this be my lot.[1]

In order to clearly refer to the several provisions of the Oath, I have assigned numbers to its eight paragraphs (hereafter P1–P8). The Oath can be usefully divided into four basic sections. These are: (1) the *preamble* (P1), involving the invocation of the appropriate health-related gods and the actual swearing of the Oath; (2) the *covenant* (P2), involving the duties of the student to his teacher, to his teacher's family, and his obligations regarding the transmission of his medical knowledge to others; (3) the *ethical code* (P3–P7), involving, among other things, prohibitions against dispensing poisons, performing abortions, performing surgery, having sexual relations with patients, and revealing to others details of a patient's private life; and (4) the *peroration* (P8), wherein the speaker expresses his belief that his own good or bad fortunes shall rest in his ability to live up to the Oath's provisions. While all four parts of the Oath have received attention in attempts to fix its date and likely origin, most discussion centers on the meaning of (2) the covenant and (3) the ethical code.

Furthermore, all interpreters of the Oath immediately face a common obstacle: some of the ethical rules embodied in the Oath are logically inconsistent with passages found in other treatises of the Hippocratic Collection. In addition, several rules are historically inconsistent with the known medical practices of the classical and later Greco-Roman period. For example, several treatises in the collection recommend surgery. Moreover, the surgical treatises are generally regarded to be the most medically precise and useful parts of the collection. As for prohibitions against aiding a patient in suicide or abortion, both were practices basically acceptable in the Greek as well as the Roman era; that is, neither religious nor legal sanctions nor moral disapprobation typically forbade such conduct.[2] Also, it is most unlikely that the Oath became a regular topic of debate among physicians or others in pre-Christian antiquity. There are no clear cross-references to it in the entire Hippocratic Collection. No known references to details of the Oath occur until the first-century-A.D. writings of Scribonius Largus.[3]

In view of these puzzling facts, modern interpreters of the Oath have characteristically adopted one of two possible interpretive strategies. On the one hand, some, like Savas Nittis, have sought to explain away various troublesome and otherwise irreconcilable features of the Oath in such a way that the Oath can still be regarded as a work genuinely authored by Hippocrates or his closest associates.

On the other hand, following a quite different strategy are scholars like Edelstein. This second strategy gives up the claim that the Oath is a typical Hippocratic writing or that it expresses typical Greek ethical values. Instead, an effort is made to show that the Oath is atypical of Greek medical literature and practice. Thus, it is argued that its origin must lie with an individual author or school whose ethical values sharply differed from those of mainstream classical society.

Edelstein's is currently the most widely discussed and comprehensive theory belonging to this second group. He argues that the Oath is not a writing of the historical Hippocrates. Rather, it is, in his opinion, plausibly understandable solely as the product of the esoteric ethical teachings of fourth-century-B.C. Pythagoreanism. Its primary purposes, he suggests, were to (a) mutually bind teacher to pupil; (b) keep the soul of the physician pure in accord with essentially Pythagorean religious values; (c) designate the proper moral duties between physician and patient; and, most important, (d) reform the practice of medicine.

To Nittis's and Edelstein's opposing interpretations I shall now turn.

THE AUTHORSHIP QUESTION

Nittis claims that the Oath was written by Hippocrates himself in Athens between March and October of the year 421 B.C.[4] His reasoning seems quite tenuous. A persistent flaw in his analysis is that Nittis inexplicably ignores the fact that the Oath is written in the Ionic dialect. Yet if, as he contends, it was likely written by Hippocrates in Athens in 421 B.C., and was used by an active medical guild founded by Hippocrates in fifth-century Athens to establish the duties and privileges that obtained between students and teachers of the medical craft, why was it not written in the Attic dialect common to Athens, as one would normally expect? This question has all the more force since Nittis also claims that the covenant (P2) originally had quasi-legal status in Athens. But, if so, it would normally have been written in Attic, as were other Athenian legal and quasi-legal documents of this sort. Nittis additionally claims that the covenant was typical of the covenants of most fraternal guilds in classical society. But he presents no evidence that in such guilds the pupil virtually adopted his teacher as a parent, as the Oath seems to imply.

In addition, on the basis of a very ambiguous piece of historical evidence taken from Thucydides' description of events in the year 421 B.C. (which may have involved no more than an arbitrary choice of words), Nittis infers that the Greek words for covenant (*xyngraphe*) and law (*nomos*) were used interchangeably in Athens between March and October, in 421 B.C.[5] He also alleges that these two words are likewise used interchangeably in the Oath's second paragraph, thereby linking its authorship to that very year. Yet this alleged equivalence is not proved or even plausibly suggested, so far as I can determine, from the relevant passages he points to in Thucydides (see *The Peloponnesian War* 7.67; 97).

Yet it must be admitted that a careful reading of these two passages does not specifically exclude Nittis's interpretation. But when one adds to this already questionable claim of word synonymity the additional dubious claim on which the second leg of Nittis's theory stands, namely, the claim that Hippocrates was probably in Athens between March and October in the year 421 B.C., it appears that Nittis's interpretation assumes too much, for Nittis apparently assumes that the brief mention of Hippocrates' name by Plato in *Protagoras* and *Phaedrus* implies that Hippocrates " . . . was living in Athens, enjoying great reputation, not only as a practicing physician, but also as a teacher of medicine . . . " in 421 B.C. But Nittis nowhere argues for the dramatic date or historical context of these two dialogues.[6] If he is aware of the controversies surrounding the exact dating of individual works from the Platonic Dialogues, he does not share his thoughts with his readers as might be hoped.

Essentially, then, Nittis's interpretation on the question of authorship is unpersuasive. This is so primarily because he appears to underrate or ignore the complexity of the very premises on which the bulk of his principal claims depend.

THE PROHIBITION AGAINST SURGERY

In a related article, Nittis tries to resolve the inconsistency between the Oath's prohibition against surgery (P5) and the outright acceptance of surgery in other Hippocratic treatises. He seeks to do this because he identifies Hippocrates as the probable author of the Oath and is at the same time sympathetic to the view that Hippocrates or his disciples authored most other treatises in the collection. This logical inconsistency involving surgery is thus an embarrassment to the unity of his theory. Nittis advocates the view, first reluctantly suggested by Littré, that the words *ou temeo*, herein translated "I will not use the knife," have a hidden meaning. These words, he argues, " . . . must in fact refer to an abomination, such as castration was considered among the Greeks, since *temnein* means also 'to castrate.'"[7]

Traditionally, scholars from the Renaissance to the nineteenth century had interpreted this troublesome fifth paragraph to signify that the Oath intended to draw a line between surgery and internal medicine. Many interpreters ascribed this separation of tasks to the supposed fact that surgery was in ancient times held to be beneath the dignity of the physician. More recent scholarship, however, has shown this last supposition to be groundless. For example, Littré argues that the ancient practitioner was a surgeon as well as a physician. Littré considered the earlier mistaken interpretation to be the result of more modern medical prejudices against surgery, and I suspect he is right.[8] Incidentally, in ancient medicine surgery included cautery, the setting of fractures, and cutting; and the Oath explicitly restricts only the last of these.

Another theory was that the operation performed in ancient times for removal of stones from the bladder, the lithotomy, was in many instances fatal. It also may have been in general morally repugnant to the Hippocratics, some argue, since it allegedly rendered men impotent. Are these the likely reasons why the Oath relegates the lithotomy to a distinct group of practitioners specializing in this procedure?

It seems that there are several reasons why such explanations fail. In the first place, all this presupposes that classical Greek medicine was for the most part divided into specialties. This I have already argued against in Part I. Also there is no evidence that suggests that lithotomies were usually fatal. In fact, they appear to have been a common operation of modest success. Yet, aside from these considerations, the decisive objection to such explanations is this: If all those who swore by the Oath harbored, for whatever reasons, definite medical or moral reservations about performing lithotomies, would it not have struck them and others as doubly reprehensible to refer their patients thereafter to " . . . such men as are engaged in this work" (P5)? I am inclined to think so. For, as in the cases of abortion and euthanasia (P4), the prohibition against surgery *could* have been made *without* directing patients toward the services of others (say, poison peddlers or perhaps some midwives). This very objection has also given Jones and Edelstein reason for doubt.[9]

To overcome it, Nittis has sought to dissolve this difficulty by translating P5 to read: "I will not cut, indeed, not even sufferers from stone, and I will *keep apart* from men engaging in this deed."[10] As mentioned, he construes the cutting to refer mainly to castration. Castration, he argues, may have been an occasional untoward consequence of lithotomies. Moreover, the second conjunction of P5 is adjusted by Nittis to escape compounding the moral dilemma just referred to of forbidding the Oath-takers to perform lithotomies, yet letting patients undergo them at the hands of others.

However, in order to justify this grammatical maneuver, Nittis must convincingly translate the verb *ekchorreso* to mean "I will keep apart from." Here he faces opposition. The standard senses of his verb do not include the preceding sense that Nittis needs.[11] Edelstein also objects because Nittis is unable to adduce *any* evidence for such an unnatural usage.[12] Therefore, despite his otherwise helpful investigation of the history of castration in Greco-Roman times, and despite the admitted possibility that lithotomy did sometimes involve the unintended consequence of castration, which the Hippocratics may have wished to avoid, Nittis's translation of P5 is not very plausible. Try as he may to salvage the alleged Hippocratic authorship and logical consistency of the Oath, these and related problems remain.

Edelstein's opposing theory can be conveniently introduced on the heels of this controversy over the prohibition against surgery. The overall form of his argument is that of a lengthy disjunctive syllogism. Arguing deductively, he examines the four main parts of the Oath (see pp. 83–84) by repeatedly proposing a string of possible cultural influences that might explain the origin of the Oath's various ethical provisions. In most cases, he *appears* to eliminate all the competing alternative sources of influence save one: the atypical values of the Pythagoreans. I find it admirable that his interpretation, unlike Nittis's, is comprehensive; it addresses all the parts of the Oath and avoids thereby the attendant risks of a fragmentary approach. Furthermore, Edelstein's interpretation has gained the endorsement of Sigerist and, more recently, the qualified assent of Amundsen.[13]

I shall argue, on the other hand, that Edelstein's proposal, while not entirely wrong, is somewhat flawed. I agree that the Oath was probably conditioned by Pythagorean influences. But I by no means share Edelstein's confidence that no other relevant influences informed its contents. Thus, it seems that Edelstein has overpressed his evidence, as I shall now show.

Consider, once again, the Oath's prohibition against surgery (P5). Edelstein reminds us in an earlier discussion of abortion and euthanasia that it was considered unethical by the Pythagoreans to knowingly take any course of action that might shed blood or lead to the destruction of human life. (I shall examine the details of their respect-for-human-life ethic in the next two chapters.) Moreover, he then introduces two additional pieces of evidence. The first, from the fourth-century-B.C. historian Aristoxenus, attests that the Pythagoreans ranked surgery last on their list of preferred therapies. Diet is given first choice; drugs second. "They believed least of all in using the knife and in cauterizing," Aristoxenus is quoted as saying.[14] The second is from Plato's *Timaeus*.[15] Adopting Taylor's view that the *Timaeus*' medical theories are essentially of Pythagorean origin, Edelstein observes that surgery and cauterization are not even mentioned in that dialogue as medical therapies. From this he infers that there must have been Pythagoreans who refused to apply *any surgical treatments whatsoever*—treatments otherwise so widely used in Greek medicine.[16]

Edelstein then concludes that the prohibition against surgery in the Oath really represents a sort of compromise. The Oath *does not allow* surgery, in the sense that the Oath-taker is strictly forbidden to perform cutting; yet it leaves open the practice of surgery to " . . . such men as are engaged in this work." Here it ostensibly disagrees with the more rigorous Pythagorean therapeutics implied by the *Timaeus*. But the Oath *does allow* cauterization, in possible agreement with the *Timaeus* and at least part of Aristoxenus's testimony (which, strictly speaking, does not specifically forbid either surgery or cauterization, but only ranks preferences). As to the longstanding and thorny problem that would remain even if all this is temporarily granted, namely, that the Oath-taker apparently does not oppose his patients' visiting the very surgeons whose operations he opposes, Edelstein supplies the following explanation:

> . . . the Pythagorean physician will allow others to help his patient in his extremity. The stipulation against operating is valid only for him who has dedicated himself to a holy life. The Pythagoreans recognized that men in general could not observe any elaborate rules of purity; in this they saw no argument against that which they considered right for themselves. To give place to another craftsman, especially in such instances where the patient might fall prey to sinful temptation; i.e, suicide, certainly was a duty demanded by philanthropy, by commiseration with those who suffered.[17]

In my opinion, Edelstein's explanation here is preferable to Nittis's. It does not depend on Nittis's unnatural translation of the text. Also, it addresses more directly the moral implications of the Oath not forbidding patients from seeking out the services of surgeons (a moral option the author of the Oath undeniably had). Yet Edelstein's preceding interpretation of P5 runs afoul of his own strong claim according to which " . . . *only* in connection with Pythagorean medicine . . ." does this prohibition against surgery make sense.[18] This seems to me doubtful.

In the first place, there is at least one other passage in the Hippocratic Collection that ranks surgery and cauterization behind other therapeutic methods (e.g., drugs). The Hippocratic *Aphorisms* 7.87 states: "Those diseases that medicines do not cure are cured by the knife. Those that the knife does not cure are cured by fire. Those that fire does not cure must be considered uncurable."[19] In general, surgery was not resorted to as a treatment of first choice by the ancients; the Pythagoreans were therefore *not alone* in ranking it behind other therapies. Hence, even taking Aristoxenus's report at face value, is not the alleged uniqueness of the Pythagorean ranking of surgery at best a matter of degree only? Have we not seen that this kind of trait is expressed by other medical writers as well?

Second, it is fair to question whether the absence of the mention of surgery in the *Timaeus* is equivalent to prohibiting this practice. It could as naturally mean that surgery was not among the *preferred* medical treatments. But, if so, the Oath's absolute stand against its adherents performing surgery is not fully equivalent to the meaning of the *Timaeus* passage, as Edelstein would have us believe.

Lastly, it is nowhere stated in the testimony Edelstein presents that the Pythagoreans *alone* excluded surgery. Indeed, it is possible that the prohibition against cutting represents a reaction on the part of some non-Pythagorean physicians against a popular fifth- and fourth-century distrust of surgical procedures.[20] For instance, we recall Heraclitus (ca. 544–484 B.C.), who, commenting on the ironic nature of the physician's craft, complained of " . . . physicians, who cut and burn, demand payment of a fee, though undeserving, since they produce the same pains as the disease."[21] By placing a personal constraint on surgery, physicians swearing the Oath might have sought to reduce the public controversy, fear, and misunderstanding generated by the most dramatic and painful therapy at their disposal. But if so, there may be more than exclusively Pythagorean influences at work in shaping the Oath's disclaimer against surgery.

THE COVENANT RECONSIDERED

Returning to the question of the covenant (P2), I find it equally doubtful that Edelstein is entirely right when he claims that " . . . all the other demands enjoined upon the pupil [by the covenant] may likewise be explained only in connection with Pythagorean views. . . . " I do not dispute his weaker claim that " . . . at least they are compatible with them."[22] On this point, I agree with C. J. DeVogel. DeVogel concurs with Edelstein's claim that in the Pythagorean school pupils regarded their teachers as adopted fathers, whose welfare they looked after, with whom they shared their possessions—if need be—and performed other special duties as the Oath seems to require. She contends, however, that Edelstein is "definitely incorrect" in claiming that, apart from the Hippocratic Oath, we possess no other non-Pythagorean indications of the existence of such an attitude in Greek culture.[23] I think, rightly, she calls attention to the evidence of Plato's *Crito* as a tacit instance of a pupil (Crito) looking out for the personal welfare of his teacher (Socrates). After all, if Socrates and a few other like-minded educators took no money for instruction (unlike the sophists, whom Socrates fiercely opposed on this issue), how, then, did they survive?

Furthermore, DeVogel reminds us that the Epicureans as well followed this pattern of mutual adoption. If so, this fact is all the more relevant. Edelstein himself assigns the Oath to the fourth century B.C., an important century to be sure for the flowering of Epicureanism. Add to these considerations the additional conjecture that popular fifth- and fourth-century mystery cults also had their novices call "father" those who introduced them to the secret cult doctrine, and one begins to suspect that Edelstein has once again made a hasty conclusion. He presses too narrowly the possible Pythagorean tendencies that appear—alongside other possible sources—to account for the special pupil-teacher duties embodied in the covenant.

THE ETHICAL CODE

Having indicated some weaknesses in Edelstein's account of the prohibition against surgery (P5), as well as in his analysis of the covenant (P2), I would like to focus attention on the Oath's ethical code per se (P3–P7). Strictly speaking, the restriction against surgery belongs to this code, but it has been convenient to discuss it separately, given its special place in most disputes about the Oath.

One may divide the ethical code into two parts. The first part concerns rules for the healing of diseases ([i]–[iv], below). The second concerns rules regulating the physician's behavior in all matters not directly connected with treatment, such as the physician's relation to the patient, the patient's family, and so on ([v]–[vi], below). Together, then, the ethical code embodies six related imperatives that the Oath-taker promises to follow:

  (i) The imperative to apply dietetic measures in accord with one's best judgment and to practice medicine so as to protect the patient from harm and injustice (P3).

 (ii) The imperative neither to give nor suggest to a patient the use of a deadly drug (P4).

(iii) The imperative not to give to a woman an abortive remedy (P4).

(iv) The imperative not to perform surgery (P5).

 (v) The imperative not to have sexual intercourse with the patient or any member of the patient's household, be they freeborn or slave, female or male (P6).

(vi) The imperative to keep secret and not divulge to others the private details of a patient's life that may be acquired during the course, or even outside the course, of treatment (P7).

Thus far, I have already addressed (iv). I shall now examine Edelstein's interpretation of (i), (v), and (vi), arguing that for the most part in these instances, too, he exaggerates the Pythagorean influence. The twin imperatives against assisting patients in abortion and euthanasia ([ii]–[iii]) I shall leave for last; they are of crowning importance and introduce the principal topics of Part III of this study.

It is Edelstein's contention that the imperative concerning (i) dietetics agrees with the dietetic practices of the Pythagoreans and " . . . acquire[s] meaning *only if* seen in the light of Pythagorean teaching."[24] Now it is well enough established that the Pythagoreans depended on elaborate dietary rules, both for the preservation of health and the treatment of disease. There is Aristoxenus's testimony, cited above. There is also the testimony of Iamblichus (A.D. 250–325), according to which the Pythagoreans " . . . approved of dietetics most of all. They practiced it with great precision."[25]

But the second half of Edelstein's contention is mistaken. For example, dietetics was in general a widely used form of therapy by the Hippocratic physicians.[26] It was not exclusively emphasized by the Pythagoreans (as Edelstein himself seems aware). On what additional grounds, then, does he see in (i) the unique impress of Pythagoreanism? His principal justification turns on the argument that the Pythagoreans had a special interest in seeing to it that no harm or injustice was done to patients (by the patients themselves, especially) owing to their adoption of immoderate or unhealthy eating habits. I do not wish to deny that for the Pythagoreans dietary practices were closely wedded to purificatory practices carrying religious and moral overtones. But, even so, the imperative to keep the patient from harm or injustice is very similar to another Hippocratic imperative found in *Epidemics* I, which says: "As to diseases, make a habit of two things— to help, or at least to do no harm."[27] Surely no conscientious Hippocratic physician would have quarreled with this basic teaching. As Edelstein himself admits, "It is the goal of all good craftsmen to seek the best for the object with which the craftsman is concerned."[28] Hence, I must also differ with Edelstein's tendency to see this injunction to protect the patient as referring to Pythagorean dietetics alone. It seems to me better understood as a pledge to protect the patient from harm and injustice in *other* areas of medical treatment as well, not just dietetics. Read in this equally plausible way, Edelstein's argument loses force.

In addition, consider (v), the imperative not to have sexual intercourse with the patient or any member of the patient's household—freeborn or slave, female or male. Here, too, Edelstein fails to establish that this unconditional prohibition expresses uniquely Pythagorean values or is understandable *only* in connection with Pythagorean doctrine. I do think he makes a good case for the view that the Pythagoreans probably judged sexual relations in terms of just or unjust conduct. There is little doubt that they condemned adultery and sodomy and that they had high praise for marital fidelity. Moreover, in their performance of moral duties the Pythagoreans taught that one should not discriminate between freeborn persons and slaves.[29]

Nevertheless, DeVogel is right in resisting Edelstein's characteristically exclusive claims here on behalf of Pythagoreanism.[30] Did the Pythagoreans alone oppose adultery, sodomy, and sexual injustices, among all the Greeks? It appears not. The Stoics, for example, were among those who shared in the condemnation of adultery.[31] It is equally questionable, as Edelstein seems to imply, that both homosexuality and adultery were opposed by no other fourth century philosophers except the Pythagoreans. Plato, for one, condemns both in his *Laws*.[32] In addition, one discovers in the Hippocratic treatise, *The Physician*, which primarily addresses matters of proper medical etiquette, the following passage:

> *In every social relation* he will be fair, for fairness must be of great service. The intimacy also between physician and *patient* is close. Patients in fact put themselves into the hands of their physician, and at every moment he meets women, maidens, and possessions very precious indeed. So towards all these self-control must be used. Such then should the physician be, both in body and in soul.[33]

Edelstein is, of course, aware of this preceding Hippocratic parallel. But he labors to discredit it as different in kind from (v) because (a) the preceding passage speaks only of the avoidance of injustice, whereas (v) includes the avoidance of "mischief" (consult the Oath [P6], p. 84); and because (b) the preceding passage, unlike (v), literally refers only to women (not men or slaves).

I do not wish to minimize these differences. But it seems fair to conclude that we are faced here with at most a difference in the stated degree of the prohibition only. In fact, the preceding passage also includes such introductory phrases as "in *every* social relation" and refers to "patients" in general—without qualification. Therefore, it is a bit hasty to regard it as intended for women or the freeborn alone, as Edelstein would have us think. Thus, here again, the singularity of his Pythagorean thesis does not fit the facts.

On the matter of protecting the privacy of patients, it is of no small significance that the Oath includes the imperative (vi) that the physician not gossip about his patients. He is sworn to silence, both at home and abroad, about information he acquires " . . . in the course of treatment or even outside of the treatment in regard to the life of men . . . " (P7).

In this connection, Edelstein reminds us that the Pythagoreans greatly valued reticence. Silence was part of the Pythagorean way of life. The Pythagoreans were not in the habit of imparting their knowledge to others; they did not divulge everything to everybody. Moreover, for their secrecy and frugality they were sometimes made the butt of ridicule in ancient comedy.[34] Presumably the Pythagoreans considered reticence a high moral duty, not merely a matter of convention. Also, they apparently held that the scientist or aspiring pupil ought to acquire a quiet, attentive demeanor in order to attain a clear state of mental concentration receptive to fresh discoveries. To be able to consistently demonstrate such reticence was considered a sure sign of moral self-control.[35]

Here I must concur with Edelstein that P7 is also imbued with a similarly strict moral tone. It is an unconditional pledge. It is strongly implied that to violate this pledge would amount to a serious violation of duty. Moreover, it is not hard to imagine that there were those in Greek culture, as in our own, who sought to secure some advantage for themselves by learning from a physician the details of a patient's physical or mental condition, or about other such personal matters. If so, the author of this Oath deemed such an indiscretion "shameful." Thus, the Oath, in (vi) as elsewhere, establishes in no uncertain terms the primary moral duties and responsibilities that define a good medical relationship between doctor and patient.

Against Edelstein, Kudlien has argued that this Pythagorean tendency to value silence and eschew gossip (which seems mirrored in the Oath) was not unique.

> First, the command to observe the *aporrheta* [state secrets] is very common in other Greek oath-formulations as sworn by citizens and officials. Second, it is an old command of Greek popular ethics (or polis ethics) to avoid the uttering of *aporrheta*, a command that may have been still current in later epochs, at least in professional and political (civic) ethics if this latter were enforced in the rigid, and traditionally solemn, form of the oath.[36]

However, Kudlien's evidence in support of these claims is tenuous. He cites, in particular, some of the proverbial passages attributed to the so-called seven wise men of antiquity. Also, it is far from clear whether such pledges to secrecy as he cites, especially those associated with the popular (i.e., nonphilosophical) ethics common to the Hellenistic area, were much more than guides to social etiquette. In contrast, the pledge to remain silent (P7) is absolute and carries unmistakable

moral overtones of a sort unmatched by Kudlien's allegedly parallel examples.
Hence, I do not take Kudlien's assertions here as proven.

ABORTION AND EUTHANASIA

Finally, we come to the all-important imperative against aiding a patient either in
abortion or euthanasia ([ii] and [iii], respectively). Edelstein again attempts to narrow the alternatives in such a way that Pythagoreanism emerges as the best explanation of the source of these two moral constraints. In addition, Edelstein argues that these expressed constraints do not agree with either the dominant moral
outlook or actual practices of the ancient physicians of Greece and Rome. That
is, not until Christian values became dominant during the last century and a half
of the Roman Empire (particularly the Judeo-Christian value of respect for human
life) did the prohibitions against abortion and euthanasia gain support in ancient
medical circles. Therefore, at best, Edelstein contends, the prohibitions in question long represented a small segment of Greek opinion.

Is Edelstein right in identifying the Pythagoreans as the likely authors of
these two prohibitions? It will be helpful to directly consider the premises of his
argument.

> Ancient jurisdiction did not discriminate against suicide; it did not attach
> any disgrace to it, provided that there was sufficient reason for such an act.
> And self-murder as a relief from illness was regarded as justifiable, so much
> so that in some states it was an institution duly legalized by the authorities.
> Nor did Greek or Roman law protect the unborn child. If, in certain cities,
> abortion was prosecuted, it was because the father's right to his offspring
> had been violated by the mother's action. Ancient religion [i.e., Homeric re-
> ligion] did not proscribe suicide. It did not know of any eternal punishment
> for those who voluntarily ended their lives. Likewise, it remained indiffer-
> ent to foeticide. Its tenets did not include the dogma of an immortal soul for
> which men must render account to their creator. Law and religion then left
> the physician free to do whatever seemed best for him.
>
> From all these considerations it follows that a specific philosophical con-
> viction must have dictated the rules laid down in the Oath. Is it possible to
> determine this particular philosophy? To take the problem of suicide first:
> Platonists, Cynics, and Stoics can be eliminated at once. They held suicide
> permissible for the diseased. . . . Aristotle, on the other hand, . . . and Epi-
> curus [were opposed to suicide but this] . . . did not involve moral censure.
> If men decided to take their lives, they were within their rights as sovereign
> masters of themselves.
>
> Pythagoreanism, then, remains the only philosophical dogma that can
> possibly account for the attitude advocated in the Hippocratic Oath. For in-
> deed, of all the Greek thinkers, the Pythagoreans alone outlawed suicide and

did so without qualification. . . . Most of the Greek philosophers even commended abortion. For Plato, foeticide is one of the regular institutions of the ideal state. . . . Aristotle reckons abortion the best procedure to keep the population within the limits which he considers essential for a well-ordered community.[37]

What I shall try to show in the remainder of this section is that Edelstein's exclusive singling out of the Pythagoreans as the *only* plausible source for the prohibitions against abortion and euthanasia is not fully justified. The Pythagorean influence cannot be ruled out, I shall argue, but neither can it be fairly seen as the only likely one operating here. Hence, I shall postpone until Part III a detailed examination of selected philosophical perspectives and ancient medical practices associated with abortion and euthanasia in the Greco-Roman era. My present task is to clarify in a preliminary way the likely meaning of these twin prohibitions for those who may have taken the Oath.

It will be recalled that the paragraph in question (P4) is this:

Ou doso de oude pharmakon oudeni aitetheis thanasimon oude hyphegeso-mai xymboulien toiende; homoios de oude gynaiki pesson phthorion doso. Agnos de kai hosios diatereso bion emon kai technen emen.

I will neither give a deadly drug to anybody if asked for it, not will I make a suggestion to this effect. Similarly, I will not give to a woman an abortive remedy. In purity and holiness I will guard my life and my art.

As to the first sentence, it becomes tempting to ask whether we have here something more than a prohibition against assisting in euthanasia or suicide. That is, can this sentence be plausibly understood in a somewhat wider sense to formally prohibit, in addition, the ancient physician from involvement in any sort of murder plot as the supplier of effective poisons? Edelstein denies this. But in so doing, I think he is oversimplifying the full meaning of this constraint. He needs to deny this wider meaning. If it is admitted that other, non-Pythagorean elements may have shaped this proviso of the Oath, it becomes increasingly difficult for him to make his exclusively Pythagorean thesis stick.

I hold that the author of this proviso may have intended at least a tacit reminder to the physician that under no circumstances does his profession morally permit him to be an accomplice to murder. There are several considerations that render this wider meaning acceptable. First, it is a documented fact that in the Greco-Roman era it was popularly believed that the physician who is skillful at curing was, in virtue of this knowledge, also peculiarly well suited to know how to kill. One can find Plato echoing this suspicion in his *Republic*. In Book One, Socrates asks Polemarchus: "Who then is the most able when they are ill to benefit friends and *harm enemies* in respect to disease and health?" To which Polemarchus correctly replies, "The physician."[38]

Moreover, in Book Eleven of his *Laws*, Plato specifies that any physician who is found guilty of willfully attempting to poison another (whether the attempt is fatal to the victim or not), " . . . *must* be punished by death."[39] It is worth noting that, in contrast, the *Laws* dictates that any *layman* found guilty of the identical crime need not face capital punishment. "The court is to decide the proper penalty or *fine* to be inflicted in his case."[40] This passage shows, I think, the special contempt (if not veiled popular prejudice) that Plato felt toward the Greek doctor who plied his trade in vicious ways. Such a person, by dint of the special knowledge embodied in his craft, in some sense knows (in the way a layman ordinarily cannot) the outcome and special effects of drugs on the body. Hence, the doctor is all the more responsible for his crime: his crime is at once all the more vicious.

Edelstein's attempt to discredit the possibility that Plato's *Laws* may here share a common element of disapproval, paralleled in this wider reading of the Oath's stricture against poisoning, is hardly convincing. Edelstein says that the stricture under discussion would then represent a useless or absurd duplication of existing Greek laws.[41] But suppose there was just such a duplication. If so, it is hard to see why this would therefore prove useless. Such a reinforcement of the aforementioned Hippocratic value to "at least do no harm"[42] may plausibly have stood as a very useful moral supplement to the homicide laws of the Greek city-states. In fact, ancient oaths sometimes did incorporate various features of contemporary legal or religious norms. So it would be overhasty to exclude the influence of popular suspicion against the potential power of physicians to do harm in either medical or nonmedical contexts. Thus, we must not rule out the possibility that the Oath's proviso against poisoning represents in the broadest sense a conservative reaction to such suspicions and popular prejudices.[43] The author of the Oath may therefore not have been a Pythagorean, even though his *prima facie* respect for human life would have admittedly proved congenial to Pythagorean physicians and philosophers.

To this I must add that there is no evidence that it was illegal under the laws of the Greek city-states for physicians to supply a person who wished to commit suicide with a suitable drug. Nor during the Roman Empire was this a criminal act.[44] As Plato's *Laws* suggest, it *was* a criminal act for any person, physician or layman, to poison another citizen in a murderous plot. Why, then, should such an obviously wrong deed as murder by poisoning receive mention in a doctor's code of ethics? Again, it is worth emphasizing that times were different then. Anyone could practice medicine, and many who did were quacks and charlatans. Money and greed were powerful motives for complicity in murder. As P4 itself presupposes, ancient physicians themselves dispensed pharmaceuticals and so were in the position to sell the necessary poisons in order to enrich themselves.

In addition, it is very much in doubt whether the Greeks possessed sufficient knowledge of pathology and postmortem medical diagnosis to be able to detect death by poisoning, or deduce by chemical analysis the likely person or persons who slipped the deadly compound to the victim.[45] This ignorance of forensic and postmortem medicine may have redoubled the temptation of unscrupulous doctors to peddle their knowledge and their drugs for ill-gotten gain.[46] If so, then this supplies all the more reason to think that the prevention of murder, as well as suicide or euthanasia, may have been relevantly addressed in this single and elusive sentence of the Oath.

As for the next sentence of P4, which, as it is rendered here absolutely prohibits abortion, some may wish to challenge whether Edelstein's translation of this sentence is correct.[47] Personally, I am convinced that it is. This, despite the fact that his rendering of *pesson phthorion* as "an abortive remedy" goes significantly beyond what the Greek literally says. Literally translated, one gets "a poisonous pessary." The point is that pessaries (vaginal suppositories) were but one of several methods then used for inducing abortion. Given this, a case can be made that, at most, the Hippocratic Oath prohibited just one type of abortion, not all—as it has commonly been interpreted to do.[48] But is such a literal translation sound? Since so much of our ensuing investigation depends on getting this passage straight, it will be necessary to consult the pertinent internal and external evidence.

What counts most against what I shall call the literalist interpretation, in view of the internal evidence of the Oath itself, is the parallel logic which is implied in the first two sentences of P4. For example, the Greek word *homoios* means "in like manner," or "similarly."[49] *Homoios* introduces the restriction in question concerning abortion immediately following a sentence that all agree unconditionally prohibits the Oath-taker from assisting in acts of active euthanasia (whatever else that sentence may accomplish). Consider: does it make good sense to suppose that the author of the Oath would introduce his second major restriction by employing the strong adverbial modifier "similarly," if, as the literalist insists, the author intended merely a conditional prohibition here? A prohibition that *ex hypothesi* singled out and excluded just one of the several abortion methods at the physician's disposal?

The point is that any literalist translation of this sentence faces the burden of explaining on what grounds partisans of the Oath (so construed) held abortifacient pessaries to be morally objectionable, but not such related abortion methods as the manual puncturing of the womb; the drinking of allegedly abortifacient potions; or forms of violent bodily exercise. In fact, external evidence drawn from contemporary and subsequent medical sources in antiquity suggests that these alternative methods were widely known to physicians, midwives, and others.[50] What, then, made these remaining kinds of abortion methods morally unobjectionable in the Oath-taker's mind? For did these not aim at the identical result, i.e., the willful termination of the life of the fetus?

One possible answer is that abortifacient pessaries were capable of being so powerfully concocted that they sometimes led not only to the intended death of the fetus, but to the unintended death of the pregnant woman (by infection?).[51] But, if so, how odd that there is scarcely a whisper of evidence to this effect in the ancient medical writings. One might well expect to find some mention of such a tragic outcome in the writings of the first-century-A.D. gynecologist, Soranus, if anywhere.[52] After all, he warns of many other treatment hazards that he would have his peers and his patients eschew.

Yet, notwithstanding these difficulties, the literalist still has at least one seemingly powerful rejoinder. He can remind us that *pesson phthorion* unequivocally means "a poisonous pessary." The text does not say "an abortive remedy," as Edelstein contends. Nor, by any reasonable stretch of the imagination, can it be legitimately so read. Granted, he continues, a literal reading of *pesson phthorion* may cause us to confront a whole web of loose ends that betray a coherent grasp of the ancient problem of abortion. But let us not invent a reading of the text in a vain effort to rescue our preconceived notions about what Hippocratic medical ethics does or does not permit.

This last-ditch literalist defense is not persuasive. To insist that the text can be reasonably understood only in the literalist case on the grounds that no other interpretation is eligible is manifestly question-begging. Alternatively, I speculate that by the time physicians were enlisted for their help in procuring an abortion, the patient (in conjunction with compliant midwives, old family nurses, or other confidantes) usually had tried in vain to dislodge the fetus using mechanical methods that were generally known to experienced women at that time. The prepared pessary was probably the most common abortifacient remedy dispensed by physicians; and for it there were recipes of variable effectiveness and safety. Typically, going to a physician for an abortion was the last resort: the proper preparation and insertion of the pessary required something more than the ordinary layman's knowledge of first aid.

Seen against this background, I further conjecture that the Oath's literal prohibition against giving poisonous pessaries had the symbolic moral force of excluding the physician from *all other* modes of inducing abortion. Mention of the deadly pessary functioned linguistically to signal opposition to the entire range of abortive remedies in roughly the same way that, today, a person's explicit statement that he opposes the hanging of criminals is usually taken to mean that he opposes all forms of capital punishment. If so, the poisonous pessary prohibited in P4 functioned linguistically to announce an absolute restriction on the entire class of abortion techniques. Hence, because he tacitly embraced a version of the respect-for-human-life principle,[53] any one of these life-destroying maneuvers was morally repugnant to the Oath-taker, no less so than the termination of human life involved at the other end of the spectrum in the equally prohibited act of active euthanasia. I conclude that no alternative translation of this passage coheres so well with the fuller text of the Oath, nor explains measurably more so concisely.

As for the next sentence of P4, which prohibits dispensing drugs for the purpose of inducing abortion, it is a questionable premise whether this prohibition represents, as Edelstein holds, an *exclusively* Pythagorean value. I do not wish to dispute that the Pythagoreans saw the fetus as an animate human life unconditionally worthy of preservation from the moment of conception. It is also undeniable that children were greatly valued by the Pythagoreans on religious, and not merely socioeconomic, grounds. That is, Pythagoreans viewed it as each man's duty to beget children so as to leave behind at death another earthly worshiper of the gods. Even so, here doubts arise about whether the Pythagoreans *alone* resisted abortion, as Edelstein needs to demonstrate. William Frankena, for one, has questioned this assumption, though he fails to supply any damaging counterexamples.[54]

More importantly, Kudlien has argued that there is some evidence that non-Pythagorean Hellenistic cult laws also viewed miscarriage or abortion with distaste. These bloody events were seen as possible sources of ritual uncleanliness and impurity. As such, they were condemned as cult taboos among some of the very religious.[55] If Kudlien is right, as I am inclined to think, then Edelstein's thesis is again weakened. As I have argued all along, it is too narrowly conceived. In the present case, it is equally possible, I submit, to understand the origins of the Oath's constraint against abortion as the product of a religiously minded person with a particular fondness for cult rules and institutions. Such an understanding also fits in well with the last sentence of P4: "In purity and holiness I will guard my life and my art." The Greek words *hagnos kai hosios* ("in purity and holiness") do signal, as Edelstein correctly argues, a distinctly devout attitude on the part of the author. But versions of this phrase were generally used in cult oaths and rituals—a fact Edelstein does not share with his readers.

THE OATH'S DATE AND ORIGINS RECONSIDERED

My final departure from Edelstein's account concerns his attempt to locate the Oath specifically in the fourth century B.C. In view of the dearth of evidence at our disposal, I do not claim to know the approximate date of the Oath's authorship. If pressed, I would say it probably was written between the sixth and third centuries B.C. Already I have shown that Nittis's attempt to date it within a six-month span in the year 421 B.C., in Athens, is overdetermined and unpersuasive. And, for different reasons, I find Edelstein's judgment equally unpersuasive. Edelstein's argument for narrowing the Oath to the fourth century turns on a false dilemma. Suppose, for the sake of argument, that the Oath is entirely of Pythagorean origins. Even so, it is overhasty to infer, as he does, that owing to our ignorance of Pythagorean developments in the two prior centuries, the Oath is therefore not a very likely product of the sixth or fifth centuries. It is also overhasty to exclude the third century just because the Pythagorean movement held less sway over Greek and Roman intellectuals during that later Hellenistic period. As DeVogel has aptly pointed out:

> The [Pythagorean] School flourished during the 6th and the first half of the 5th centuries, and if there is still a tradition of Pythagorean forms of behavior during the 4th century, this is due to the things that were handed down by previous generations. The Pythagorean principles . . . —not to kill,

not to dispose of one's own or someone else's life, the reverence for life even if it is not yet born, the avoidance of surgery even in cases where others commonly used it, the reverence for the human person—all these were doubtless of ancient standing.[56]

All things considered, then, the conclusion I am willing to support regarding the Oath's origins, date, and purpose is this: Edelstein is at best half-right about the date of the Oath. It may have been written in the fourth century. But I see no reason why it could not have originated a century later, or during the two previous centuries, for that matter.

As to its origins, the Oath does contain moral and religious elements, in its covenant and ethical code especially, that are fully compatible with a Pythagorean influence. This much I grant. But I have also demonstrated that it is likely that additional influences—from Greek religious cults, homicide laws, and popular ethics—may have affected the form and content of the Oath as well.

As to its purpose, there is probably some substance to Edelstein's suggestion that the Oath served as the tool of a reform movement in Greek medicine that broke away from the more dominant ethical values and medical practices of classical times. But it is far from certain that the Oath was therefore an esoteric document, though I do not rule this out. Indeed, at least some of the evidence introduced in this section implies that the Oath may have reflected a broader and more diverse range of popular, religious, and social sentiments than one might have at first supposed. In any case, it does seem likely that at best only a small number of physicians in antiquity actually swore and abided by the Oath's moral directives. Those who did were nonconformists. Whether they acted as individuals or were part of a secret medical fraternity devoted to a blend of Pythagorean and other ideals is hard to say. Personally, I think that the Oath may have been used by some ancient medical fraternities or guilds. Nothing we have discovered so far excludes this possibility.

MEDICAL ETIQUETTE

To complete the present account of the rise of Greek medical ethics, we turn now to explore four additional Hippocratic works that promise to shed more light on the values and conduct of the ancient physician. Among the things these four Hellenistic works have in common is that, while their exact origins are unknown, they all specify in some detail the good manners that the ideal Hippocratic physician should display in the practice of his craft. Since they address such topics as professional conduct between physicians, bedside manners, proper decorum, and handling difficult patients, these four works are traditionally counted as the basic Hippocratic guide to sound medical etiquette. In contrast, the Hippocratic Oath may be characterized as a more substantive and unified work. As the preceding section suggests, its ethical code appears to be founded on moral principles of the highest sort. I shall show in what follows that, while the four works in question do primarily involve lessons in etiquette, they also manifest a sincere concern for the patient's welfare. This concern goes beyond the ancient physician's understandable inclination to promote his own professional reputation and secure his own pecuniary self-interest by the cultivation of patronizing bedside manners.

The Greek word for etiquette, *euschemosyne*, literally means "being graceful, elegant, manifesting good form or bearing." This word can be usefully compared with the Greek *ethika*, meaning "of or for morals."[57] For what is done for morals or out of moral concern was ordinarily taken by the Greeks to involve something more like the performance of duties (to oneself or others) than the mere display of good form, though it may have incidentally involved that, too. This subtle difference between ethics and etiquette is confirmed by observing that *euschemosyne*, not *ethika*, carried with it a derogatory sense meaning good in outward show; i.e., specious. I begin by calling attention to the Greek grammar of these two concepts because some ambiguity exists in recent discussions of ancient professional ethics regarding what sets medical ethics apart from medical etiquette. The tendency has been to conflate any distinction between ethics and etiquette, or ignore it altogether. The safest line of demarcation, and one fully borne out by the four Hippocratic texts about to be examined, is that, in general, a concern for etiquette and for doing the right thing morally do very often overlap. But etiquette concentrates primarily on the outward show of correct behavior; thus it is usually associated with courtesy and what is popularly termed "good breeding." In contrast, moral prescriptions are primarily concerned with making the right choice and doing the right thing based on some favored principles of human duty; thus moral prescriptions ultimately transcend a mere concern for outward show and ceremony.

In addition, it is worth recalling that for the Greek physician the rules of etiquette (as well as ethics) were followed not through fear of civil punishment, for there was no regulation of medicine. Ideally, the physician was motivated to acquit himself well partly out of a love for his craft. Also, he was motivated by a somewhat more egoistic concern to acquire and preserve a good reputation. For reputation was the only professional credential of the ancient physician. Rules of etiquette, as such, had nothing to do with the application of categorical imperatives. One gets the impression that, at most, they were rules of thumb that implied "should" or "ought," never the unequivocal "must." Yet etiquette was nonetheless of considerable importance to the successful practice of medicine (Fig. 6). For, in the absence of medical licensure, the financial success of one's practice depended almost entirely *on the patients' perceptions of the physician* (regardless of what medical skill the physician, in fact, possessed).

Having considered all this, let us begin with the oldest and shortest of the manuals of Hippocratic etiquette, the very brief tract titled *Law*. My intention throughout is to let these excerpts speak for themselves, except for my mention of a few background details on each piece.

Law was known to the compiler and physician Erotian (fl. A.D. 50) but is mentioned by no other ancient author. Both Jones and Edelstein date *Law* between

Figure 6. Tombstone of the Athenian physician Jason (second century B.C.) examining a young patient by palpating his abdomen. Copyright © The British Museum.

the fifth and fourth centuries. Whether it is a fragment or a complete work (it runs only about three hundred words), no one is sure. Jones suggests that its name derives from the fact that it lays down the law for a good medical education. He further speculates that *Law* may have been a short address by the head of a medical school to graduating physicians.[58] At any rate, our interest in it here is that it begins by complaining of the lack of any state regulation over those who practiced medicine. Incidentally, the lament that the art of medicine is a noble profession but much maligned owing to the quacks in its ranks is echoed by physicians throughout antiquity.

> Medicine is the most distinguished of all the arts, but through the ignorance of those who practice it, and of those who casually judge such practitioners, it is now of all the arts by far the least esteemed. The chief reason for this error seems to me to be that medicine is the only art which our states have made subject to no penalty save that of dishonor, and dishonor does not wound those who are compacted of it. Such men in fact are very like the supernumeraries in tragedies. Just as these have the appearance, dress and mask of an actor without being actors, so too with physicians; many are physicians by repute, very few are such in reality.[59]

The author continues to sketch what natural abilities and type of education are required for becoming a competent physician. Moreover, consistent with the author's joint concern for advancing his profession's interest, as well as meeting the genuine needs of patients, he lectures the reader to acquire a *real knowledge* of medicine—not just a good outward show. This must be done " . . . before we travel from city to city, and win the reputation of being physicians not only in word, but also in deed."[60]

A second, somewhat later work, is titled *The Physician*. It probably dates from about 350–300 B.C., and like *Law* and the remaining *Precepts* and *Decorum*, it was probably intended as prudent advice for young doctors. Unlike the other three tracts, however, this piece proceeds in its later chapters to address methods of bandaging and surgery. The book ends by advising students of medicine to try to find work caring for mercenary troops in order to acquire valuable experience in the practice of surgery.[61] All this is consistent with the fact that war-related injuries supplied a prime source for the study of human anatomy and physiology in the ancient world. Galen himself was a former physician of gladiators, and he alluded to the valuable use of combatants for the gain of medical knowledge.[62]

It will be recalled that I have already quoted from the first chapter of *The Physician* to demonstrate the author's general concern for fairness in social relations along with his stated opposition to the sexual exploitation of patients (above, p. 92). Yet there are passages of another sort to be found in that same chapter that reveal a more personal, egoistic concern for the physician's reputation alone. These directives have to do with such comparatively mundane matters as the proper deportment, dress, and demeanor of the socially correct doctor.

The dignity of a physician requires that he should look healthy, and as plump as nature intended him to be; for the common crowd consider those who are not of this excellent bodily condition to be unable to take care of others. Then he must be clean in person, well dressed, and anointed with sweet smelling unguents that are not in any way suspicious. This, in fact, is pleasing to patients. The prudent man must also be careful of certain moral considerations—not only to be silent, but also of a great regularity in life, since thereby his reputation will be greatly enhanced; . . . . In appearance, let him be of a serious but not harsh countenance; for harshness is taken to mean arrogance and unkindliness, while a man of uncontrolled laughter and excessive gaiety is considered vulgar, and vulgarity especially must be avoided.[63]

Turning finally to *Precepts* and *Decorum*, which are longer works and probably date to the first century B.C., their origins are still uncertain. Both appear Stoic in influence. But, unfortunately, attempts to convincingly link any of the four manuscripts to specific philosophical schools have been fraught with difficulty.[64] They are too widely eclectic and so do not reveal a clear moral ideology. What's more, it is probably misleading to infer that these works were widely read and faithfully followed by the run-of-the-mill Greek or Roman doctor. Collectively, these works represent a considerable commitment to the best that medicine could then reasonably offer to patients in need. Any one at all could practice medicine. Many apparently unsavory characters did so without the slightest regard for the welfare of their patients, let alone the nuances of etiquette. When their reputations caught up with them, they traveled on.

Notwithstanding these considerations, *Precepts* and *Decorum* are philosophically important along with the others. They serve to demonstrate the higher road that Greco-Roman medicine was capable of taking. They also demonstrate an understandable *tension* between furthering the self-interests of the practitioner, on the one hand, and providing sound medical care aimed at the best interests of patients, on the other. This mediation between egoistic and altruistic interest is evident in the following excerpt from *Precepts*. Dealing essentially with fee-setting, it admonishes the physician to consider the wealth of his patients in seeking the fullest possible payment for services rendered; at the same time, the physician is reminded not to practice without compassion and attention to the needy.

I urge you not to be too unkind, but to consider carefully your patient's superabundance or means. Some times give your services for nothing, calling to mind a previous benefaction or present satisfaction. *And if there be an opportunity of serving one who is a stranger in financial straits, give full assistance to all such.* For where there is *love of man*, there is also love of the art. For some patients, though conscious that their condition is perilous, recover their health simply through their contentment with the goodness of the physician. And it is well to superintend the sick to make them well, to care for the healthy to keep them well, *but also to care for one's own self,* so as to observe what is seemly.[65]

In *Decorum*, as in the other three works on etiquette, disapprobation is expressed against the vulgar and untutored quacks who masquerade as physicians and so threaten to spoil the reputations of all. Characteristic of these works on etiquette, every effort is made to remind the young physician of the grand ideals to which medicine at its best aspires. Here, as elsewhere, there is no explicit mention of the Hippocratic Oath. Nor is there a sustained discussion of moral principles. There is, however, what appears to be a utilitarian emphasis throughout that attempts to balance the doctor's needs with the needs of his patient. These next four passages may suffice to give the flavor of the author's three central aims. These are: (1) to proclaim the exemplary intellectual and moral ideals of the medical art; (2) to provide for his patients' best interests; and (3) to secure for himself the best reputation and greatest financial success he can.

> For a physician who is a lover of wisdom is equal of a god. Between wisdom and medicine there is no gulf fixed; in fact, medicine possesses all the qualities that make for wisdom. It has disinterestedness, shamefastness, modesty, reserve, sound opinion, judgment, quiet pugnacity, purity, sententious speech, knowledge of the things good and necessary for life, selling of that which cleanses, freedom from superstition, pre-excellence divine.[66]
>   . . .
> Make frequent visits; be especially careful in your examinations, counteracting the things wherein you have been deceived at the changes. . . .[67]
>   . . .
> Keep watch also on the faults of the patients, which often make them lie about the taking of things prescribed. For through not taking disagreeable drinks, purgative or other, they sometimes die. What they have done never results in a confession, but the blame is thrown upon the physician.[68]
>   . . .
> On entering [the patient's room] bear in mind your manner of sitting, reserve, arrangement of dress, decisive utterance, brevity of speech, composure, bedside manner, care, replies to objections, calm self-control to meet the troubles that occur, rebuke of disturbance, readiness to do what has to be done.[69]

It is worth noting that to the extent that *Law, The Physician, Precepts,* and *Decorum* do express a commitment to protect the best interests of the patient, these works may be said to be logically consistent with the patient-benefitting ethic found in the ethical code of the Hippocratic Oath. Yet there is a marked difference in emphasis. The ethical code of the Oath is manifestly bereft of a concern for mere manners and outward deportment. It speaks of " . . . remaining free of all *intentional* injustice."[70] In general, the Oath expresses a pledge to define and preserve the right conduct of the physician-patient relationship, based ultimately on ethical principles and concern for the intentions of the *inward*-reflecting person. Anything to be gained by *mere outward show* and the ready cultivation of clever manners is at best a secondary consideration to the Oath-taker. Strictly speaking, in swearing the Oath he gives no notice to these things.

A decidedly different emphasis, however, pervades the four Hippocratic works just discussed. The guiding and persistent interest here is unabashedly that of doctors who would choose to live prudently. The tone and content of these writings is generally more practical than the Oath. Yet it would be harsh, I think, to judge such repeated concerns for proper bedside manners and deportment out of the context of the ancient medical marketplace. There, cultivating a sound medical reputation in the absence of any system of licensure was especially critical. Notwithstanding this fact, I have shown that the welfare of the patient is never really completely subordinated to the physician's more selfish interests. Nor is it ignored. Rather, the patient is again and again taken into consideration, and, very often, not without evidence of sustained human compassion.

SUMMARY

If we return now to reconsider the principal questions with which Part II began, the evidence and analysis of the preceding pages can be summarized as follows:

The Hippocratic Oath is a unique medical ethical document from at least two fundamental perspectives: (1) the pan-Mediterranean and (2) the pan-Hellenic. Seen in the broader context of the pan-Mediterranean world, the Oath stands without parallel or precedent in Egypt, Assyria, Babylonia, Israel, and Persia. If these neighboring and more ancient cultures produced an oath, prayer, treatise, or philosophical-religious document of any sort devoted exclusively to the ethics of medicine, there is no record of this in their literature, art, or science.

As for their laws, the Babylonians may be credited as the first civilization on record to create laws designed, among other things, to regulate medical practice. The Babylonian Code of Hammurabi set forth stiff fines against malpractice more than a thousand years before the Hippocratic Oath came into being. But these laws were confined to surgical procedures alone. Also, patients did not receive equal protection under the laws of Hammurabi: the degree of legal protection one received against medical malpractice varied in proportion to the social status of the patient. Therefore, only a fraction of Babylonian medicine was brought under the legal jurisdiction of the state, and individuals seeking surgical treatments, at least, were apparently not deemed to be of equal worth.

This stands in marked contrast to the Hippocratic Oath (and, also, it would seem, the later Hippocratic treatises concerned with etiquette). In the Oath, a single standard of medical care is proposed for all patients, protecting even the slave. In addition, the Oath is probably not a legal document. It was not created by any legislature, nor was it made legally binding on any Greek physician throughout antiquity, so far as we know. How the Oath specifically came into existence is a puzzle. But one fact is beyond doubt: It arose largely as a response by its author or authors to the free and unrestrained marketplace that Greek medicine enjoyed. It was very likely the result of a felt need by a handful of Greek physicians to fill a void that had been created by the absence of any legal constraints on the practice of medicine. Thus, the Oath was *voluntarily* obeyed by those few who chose to adopt it; it emerged out of the precondition of a relatively high degree of personal and professional freedom. None of this can be said of the state-imposed regulations of medicine found among the neighboring Babylonians, Assyrians, and Egyptians.

Furthermore, while there is evidence to suggest that, on either legal or religious grounds, abortion was probably once opposed by the Assyrians and Persians, if not the Egyptians, we are not privy to the moral reasoning behind this opposition. As to the moral, legal, or religious stands these cultures took against euthanasia, it *is* known that in Egypt and Assyro-Babylonia, the act of suicide was thought to cut one off from the gods. But no evidence indicates their specific condemnation of euthanasia.

Quite the opposite is true when one considers the Hippocratic Oath. Both abortion and euthanasia are unequivocally opposed (P4). And to the extent that this opposition may have been founded on something akin to a respect-for-human-life ethic, at least some hint of the moral reasoning behind these powerful prohibitions may be secured. Clarifying the premises of this reasoning is part of the task that awaits us in Part III.

Equally significant, even though the ancient cultures of Egypt, Assyria, Babylonia, Israel, and Persia gave at least *some* thought to the proper conduct of their physician-priests, no evidence suggests that their medical ethical values in any way influenced either the form or content of the Hippocratic Oath. The same may be said for the Hippocratic treatises on medical etiquette.

On the other hand, when the Oath is seen in the narrower context of the pan-Hellenic world alone, its uniqueness becomes apparent in at least two ways. First, the Hippocratic Oath stands as the only Greek medical ethical document of its kind. If there were other such medical oaths, we lack any evidence of their existence. One is left with the distinct impression that craft-related documents like this were in any case quite rare.[71] Second, although the Oath was not legally binding, it is fair to say that the power over men's minds that it exercised derived mainly from the practitioner's sense of moral duty and personal conscience. Whether or not the Oath is entirely a Pythagorean manifesto, as Edelstein has argued, or, as I think, only partly so, the primary duties it involves can be reduced to two fundamental kinds: first and foremost, the duty to protect the patient from harm and to rid him of disease. This is a duty to others. Second, the duty to preserve and promote the good reputation of the medical craft by adopting practices designed to ensure the integrity and competency of its members. This is primarily a duty to oneself (though it also affects others). Hence, the Oath is unique in formally defining for some Greeks the proper conduct of the physician-patient relationship. It goes a long way toward putting this relationship on a *prima facie* moral and religious footing. Even so, as I have implied, the Oath may have been influenced by more prudential considerations as well. The latter may include the desire to avoid public controversy (in regard to surgery, abortion, and euthanasia, especially) and the desire to win the lasting admiration of both gods and men (P8). But even these aims, taken in context, were considered praiseworthy. For, to quote from the *Precepts*: "Where there is love of man, there is also love of the Art."[72] Perhaps the same may be said for the effects of love of the health-related gods like Apollo, Asclepius, and the latter's two daughters, Hygieia and Panaceia, before whom the Oath is specifically sworn. For did they not likely motivate the Oath-taker to higher aspirations for both himself and his patients, too?

Lastly, if the riddle of the Oath's opposition to the widespread ancient practices of abortion and euthanasia has not been altogether solved, then perhaps it may now be dissolved. For if the Oath is, as I have argued, a possibly esoteric document partly informed by Pythagorean tendencies, and if, in addition, it does represent some sort of reform movement in Greek medical practice, then it is plausible to infer that its adherents constituted a relatively small group of physicians. This does not mean that those who refused to join them were regarded by the Oath's adherents to be practicing bad medicine. But it does mean that these dissenters, who were in the majority, were likely influenced by somewhat different ethical values. Hence, in Part III, to which we now turn, I shall isolate and analyze just what some of these competing philosophical perspectives on abortion and euthanasia may have been.

Discussion Questions

1. Is there any conclusive evidence that casts doubt upon the claim that Hippocrates wrote the Oath that bears his name?
2. What are the six major parts of the Hippocratic Oath?
3. How can the prohibition against surgery in the Oath be understood? Were there sound reasons medically for banning surgery?
4. Was the Hippocratic Oath very well known among most ancient medical practitioners? Why or why not?
5. How does medical ethics differ from medical etiquette?

NOTES

1. Ludwig Edelstein, trans., "The Hippocratic Oath," in *Ancient Medicine*, p. 6. For the Greek text, see *Hippocratis Opera*, ed. I. L. Heiberg, Corpus Medicorum Graecorum 1.1.4–5. The text is also reproduced in full by Edelstein, "The Hippocratic Oath," p. 5.
2. For the general evidence on the prevalence of abortion and suicide in the ancient world, see A. E. Crawley, "Foeticide," in *ERE*, vol. 6, pp. 54bff.; A. W. Mair, in "Suicide," in *ERE*, vol. 12, pp. 31–32; and Edelstein, "Hippocratic Oath," pp. 9–20. A full

discussion of the prevalence of abortion, euthanasia, and suicide in Greek times is addressed in Part III.

3. Scribonius Largus, *Professio Medici.*
4. Savas Nittis, "The Authorship and Probable Date of the Hippocratic Oath," *Bulletin of the History of Medicine* 8 (1940): 1020.
5. See Thucydides, *The Peloponnesian War* 8.67, 97; and Nittis.
6. Nittis, "Authorship of the Hippocratic Oath," p. 1020. On the question of the dramatic date of the *Protagoras*, see Gregory Vlastos's introduction to Plato's *Protagoras*, ed. G. Vlastos (New York: Bobbs-Merrill, 1957). On the *Phaedrus*, see Thomas More's article in *Patterns in Plato's Thought*, ed. Julies M. Moravcsik, Synthese Historical Library, no. 6 (Boston: Kluwer, 1973).
7. Savas Nittis, "The Hippocratic Oath in Reference to Lithotomy: A New Interpretation with Historical Notes on Castration," *Bulletin of the History of Medicine* 7 (1939): 721.
8. Littré, *Oeuvres,* vol. 4, pp. 616–17.
9. W. H. S. Jones, *The Doctor's Oath* (London: Cambridge Press, 1924), p. 48, and Edelstein, "Hippocratic Oath," p. 27.
10. Nittis, "Oath in Reference to Lithotomy," p. 721.
11. According to H. G. Liddell and R. Scott, *Greek-English Lexicon*, p. 213, *ekchorreso*, ordinary means (1) to go out and away; (2) to slip out of or be dislocated; and (3) to give way, to give place to.
12. Edelstein, "Hippocratic Oath," p. 27, note 80.
13. Sigerist, *History of Medicine*, vol. 2, p. 303. See also Darrel Amundsen, "The Physician's Obligation to Prolong Life: A Medical Duty without Classical Roots," *Hastings Center Report* (1978): 26.
14. Aristoxenus 58d.1, trans. Edelstein, "Hippocratic Oath," p. 30.
15. Plato, *Timaeus* 87cff., especially 89d.
16. Edelstein, "Hippocratic Oath," p. 31.
17. Ibid., p. 32. Some commentators suggest that distress from kidney or bladder stones was a contributing cause of suicide, so painful are its unrelieved effects.
18. Ibid., emphasis added.
19. W. H. S. Jones, trans., *Hippocrates*, vol. 4, p. 217.
20. This alternative is explored in Fridolf Kudlien, "Medical Ethics and Popular Ethics in Greece and Rome," *Clio Medica* 6 (1970): 103–4.
21. Frag. 58, trans. Freeman, *Ancilla*, p. 28.
22. Edelstein, "Hippocratic Oath," p. 44. Edelstein's evidence here is that the Pythagorean Epaminondas is said to have honored his teacher as a father. See Diodorus 10.11.2.
23. C. J. DeVogel, *Pythagoras and Early Pythagoreanism* (The Netherlands: Royal Van-Gorcum Ltd., 1966), p. 240. See Plato's *Symposium* for related cases of personal devotion, if not adoption.
24. Edelstein, "Hippocratic Oath," p. 26, emphases added.
25. Iamblichus, *De Vita Pythaegorica* 163. DeVogel, *Pythagoras*, p. 234.
26. The prominent role played by carefully calculated dietary therapies was suggested in chapter 1 in connection with the *principle of contraries*. The Greeks tried to identify which foods engendered the qualities hot, cold, wet, and dry in order to restore humoral balance to the sick patient. The Hippocratic author of *Regimen* 1.2 states that knowledge of the qualities of all foods and drink must be acquired by anyone aspiring to practice good medicine.

27. *Epidemics* I 11, trans. Jones, *Hippocrates*, vol. 1, p. 165.

28. Edelstein, "Hippocratic Oath," p. 22. Cf. Plato *Republic* 1, concerning the crafts—including medicine—and the proper objects at which they aim.

29. Ibid., p. 35. In saying that the Pythagoreans alone judged sexual relations in terms of justice, Edelstein means that such conduct was *not* merely judged in accord with what was allowed by human laws or conventions. Justice here refers to a higher moral principle, ultimately mathematical in nature, that transcends human law.

30. DeVogel, *Pythagoras*, pp. 237–38.

31. To be unfaithful to one's spouse was to live in disharmony with nature (reason). The Stoics counted neither pleasure as good, nor pain as evil. Thus, one was expected to endure the possible hardships of marriage.

32. Plato *Laws* 8.842a–848c; see also *Laws* 1.636c. Cf. Socrates' attitude according to Alcibiades' speech in the *Symposium*, and what DeVogel has rightly inferred is Plato's implicit disapproval of homosexuality there.

33. Jones, trans., *Hippocrates*, vol. 2, p. 313, emphases added.

34. Edelstein's evidence for these claims includes Diogenes Laertius *Aristoxenus* 8.15 and a fragment from Aexis in Diels and Kranz, *Die Fragmente*, 5th ed., p. 464.

35. In contrast with the Pythagoreans' motivation for cultivating silence, which ultimately had a moral basis going beyond good manners, we read in the Hippocratic work, *The Physician* (also discussed above, p. 103), "The prudent man must also be careful of certain moral considerations—not only to be silent, but also of a great regularity of life, *since thereby his reputation will be greatly enhanced.*" (See Jones, trans., *Hippocrates*, vol. 2, pp. 311–12.)

36. Kudlien, "Medical Ethics and Popular Ethics," p. 110. Kudlien cites as evidence for these two points Ziebarth, *Pauly-Wissowa Realencyclopadie*, 1905 ed., vol. 2, p. 2080; and Diogenes Laertius *Aristoxenus* 1.3.69; 1.7.98.

37. Edelstein, "Hippocratic Oath," pp. 15–18 passim.

38. Plato *Republic* 1.332d-4, trans. Shorey, in *Collected Dialogues*, pp. 581–82, emphases added. That physicians were ready targets for the charge of harming their patients is frequently commented on in the Hippocratic Collection. See, e.g., *The Art* 7; *Decorum* 14, 17; *On Joints* 67.

39. Plato *Laws* 11.932eff., trans. Trevor J. Saunders, *The Laws* (New York: Penguin Books, 1970), p. 480.

40. Ibid., p. 480, emphases added.

41. Edelstein, "Hippocratic Oath," p. 10, note 11.

42. See pp. 91–92.

43. This possibility is also discussed by Fridolf Kudlien, who, along with Emile Littré before him, basically supports my wider reading of the proviso against supplying poison. Cf. Kudlien, "Medical Ethics and Popular Ethics," pp. 97ff., and Littré, *Oeuvres*, vol. 4, pp. 662ff.

44. Darrel W. Amundsen, "Romanticizing the Ancient Medical Profession: The Characterization of the Physician in the Greco-Roman Novel," *Bulletin of the History of Medicine* 48, no. 3 (1974): 323, note 14.

45. This claim is admittedly open to debate. Edelstein contends that the Greeks were confident that they could detect such crimes as poisoning by getting a confession through torturing prime suspects, if need be. (See Edelstein, "Hippocratic Oath," p. 10.) Louis Lewin discusses ancient methods of investigating alleged cases of poisoning in his *Die Gifte in der Weltgeschichte* (Berlin: J. Springer, 1920), pp. 37ff. Kudlien concurs with

my judgment, against Edelstein, that the Greeks during this period possessed neither a pathological anatomy nor a legal medicine in the modern sense. (See Kudlien, "Medical Ethics and Popular Ethics," p. 102.)

46. This very topic of the doctor's moral responsibility (or lack thereof) is dramatized by the second-century-A.D. Roman writer, Apuleius, in his novel *Metamorphoses* (also known as *The Golden Ass*). Briefly, the story is told of a physician who is approached with a large sum of money for the sale of a lethal poison by a third party. This third party claims the poison is for a sick friend, who is described as suffering terribly from an incurable disease and wishes to quit life. Luckily, the physician guesses that this poison is intended for a murder plot of some sort. He substitutes for it a sleeping compound, thereby sparing the victim's life. Here, I think, Apuleius strongly hints at the vulnerability of the physician to witting or unwitting involvement in murder.

47. Some noteworthy alternative translations include Jones, trans., *Hippocrates*, vol. 1, p. 299: "Similarly I will not give to a woman a pessary to cause abortion"; John T. Noonan, "An Almost Absolute Value in History," in *The Morality of Abortion* (Cambridge, MA: University Press, 1970), p. 4: "Similarly I will not give to a woman an abortifacient pessary"; and Gordon, *Medicine Throughout Antiquity*, p. 417: "[A]nd in like manner I will not give to a woman a pessary to produce abortion." But John Chadwick and W. N. Mann, *The Medical Works of Hippocrates* (Oxford: Blackwell Scientific Publications, 1950), p. 9, join Edelstein as nonliteralists just here, translating: "Neither will I give a woman means to produce an abortion." So, too, are Charles Singer and E. Ashworth Underwood, who prefer: "[A]nd especially I will not aid a woman to procure abortion." (See Charles Singer and E. Ashworth Underwood, *A Short History of Medicine*, 2nd ed. [Oxford: University Press, 1962], p. 32.)

48. For example, the first-century-A.D. writer Scribonius Largus took the Hippocratic Oath to forbid abortion *simpliciter* (see chapter 8). So did his near contemporary, Soranus, who quotes the Oath as saying, "I will give to no one an abortive." Soranus, incidentally, disagreed with the Oath's categorical restriction (see chapter 6).

49. Liddell and Scott, *Greek–English Lexicon* (Cambridge, 1972), p. 487.

50. See chapter 6, pp. 123–24.

51. The Greek word *pessos* meant a "medicated plug of wool or lint to be introduced into the vagina, anus, etc., pessary," according to Liddell and Scott's *Greek–English Lexicon*, 9th ed., p. 1396. Among the few ancient authors who mention the pessary are the botanist, Theophrastus (fl. 340 B.C.), in his *History of Plants* 9.20.4. He cites a plant called birthwort (*Aristolochia rotunda*) as good "for the womb as a pessary: . . . in cases of prolapsed uterus it is used in water as a lotion." (See Arthur Hort, trans., *Inquiry into Plants*, Loeb Classical Library [Cambridge, MA: Harvard University Press], vol. 2, p. 319.) Another source is the medical writer, Celsus (fl. A.D. 25). In his *de Medicina* 5.21–22, he describes in detail various kinds of pessaries useful (a) for inducing menstruation; (b) "to mollify the womb"; (c) "against inflammations of the womb"; (d) to render the expulsion of an already dead fetus; (e) to control hysterical fits "owing to genital disease"; and (f) to promote conception. Oddly, no mention is made of the abortifacient pessary by these authors. But see Soranus's *Gynecology* 1.65, where several such recipes are provided. Cf. Dioscorides Medicus 1.106; 2.61.

52. Soranus does not mention death to the mother caused by a pessary. He does, however, warn that "one should choose those which are not too pungent, that they may not cause too great a sympathetic reaction and heat." (See *Soranus' Gynecology*, trans. Owsei Temkin (Baltimore, MD: Johns Hopkins University Press, 1956), p. 67.

53. The respect-for-human-life principle is discussed in detail in chapter 6.

54. William K. Frankena, "The Ethics of Respect for Life," in *Respect for Life: In Medicine, Philosophy, and the Law*, ed. Stephen Barker (Baltimore, MD: Johns Hopkins University Press, 1975), p. 38.

55. Kudlien, "Medical Ethics and Popular Ethics," pp. 109–10. Kudlien introduces the testimony of M. Nilsson, according to whom one need not search for Pythagorean influences to explain satisfactorily those ethical rules which were common to a religiously tinged stock of popular Greek beliefs. See Nilsson, *Geschichte der griechischen Religion*, 2nd ed. (n.p.:1961); München, vol. 2, p. 130.

56. DeVogel, *Pythagoras*, p. 241. Another objection that might be raised against Edelstein's contention that the Oath is of exclusively Pythagorean origin centers on a linguistic problem. The problem is that the Pythagoreans originally thrived in Dorian-speaking Greek communities on the more western Mediterranean shores of Italy. But since the oath is written in Ionic Greek—not in the Pythagorean-favored Doric dialect—this fact seems to further complicate Edelstein's thesis.

57. Liddell and Scott, *Greek–English Lexicon*, pp. 289, 303.

58. Jones, trans., *Hippocrates*, vol. 2, p. 259.

59. Hippocrates *Law* 1, trans. Jones, *Hippocrates*, vol. 2, p. 263.

60. Ibid., vol. 2, p. 265.

61. Compare the Hippocratic Oath's opposition to the practice of surgery discussed on pp. 86–90. *The Physician* thus contains another example of logical inconsistencies between The Oath and the Hippocratic Collection that point to multiple authorship. Additional inconsistencies regarding abortion and euthanasia will be treated in Part III.

62. On the topic of the development of the science of human anatomy in Greco-Roman times, see Ludwig Edelstein, "The History of Anatomy in Antiquity," in *Ancient Medicine*, pp. 247–301.

63. *The Physician* 1, trans. Jones, *Hippocrates*, vol. 2, pp. 311–13.

64. For one such attempt, see Edelstein, "The Professional Ethics of the Greek Physician," in *Ancient Medicine*, pp. 329ff.

65. *Precepts* 6, trans. Jones, *Hippocrates*, vol. 1, p. 319, emphases added. For a related passage on fee-setting that evidences a clear regard for the patient's welfare in relation to the hardship imposed by illness, see *Precepts* 4.

66. *Decorum* 5, trans. Jones, *Hippocrates*, vol. 2, p. 287.

67. *Decorum* 5, trans. Jones *Hippocrates*, vol. 2, , p. 295.

68. *Decorum* 14, trans. Jones, *Hippocrates*, vol. 2, p. 297.

69. *Decorum* 12, trans. Jones, *Hippocrates*, vol. 2, p. 295.

70. See the Oath, P6, p. 84, emphasis added.

71. This is not to say that the actual taking of craft-related oaths was rare, however, since they may have been kept secret through an oral tradition of instruction. Among Greek guilds, Marcus N. Tod singles out three of the more common types: (1) *religious guilds*, particularly those devoted to the Dionysiac art forms of music and drama; (2) *wholesale merchant association*s, devoted to religious, social, and commercial ends; and (3) *crafts guilds*, composed of workers of the same craft, industry, or trades such as launderers, tanners, doctors, cobblers. Of the last type, Tod states: "Their main function was religious and social rather than economic. . . ." He further states that, although these three types of guilds were numerous and very popular during both Greek and Roman times, there are few literary references to them throughout antiquity. See Marcus N. Tod, "Greek Clubs," in *OCD*, pp. 254–55, which contains a useful bibliography.

72. *Precepts* 6, trans. Jones, *Hippocrates*, vol. 1, p. 319.

PART III

ABORTION AND EUTHANASIA

6 The Problem of Abortion

They [midwives] cause miscarriages if they think them desirable.

—Socrates, as quoted by Plato

WE COME NOW to the third part of this journey into the origins of Western medical ethics. Having already investigated the social setting of ancient medicine as well as the rise of European medical ethics with Hippocrates and his successors, we are in the best position to explore the thinking of the ancients on abortion and euthanasia. Let us next see what the leading philosophers and physicians had to say about these topics. Let us also examine their related thoughts on infanticide and suicide. My final task will be to clarify the moral responsibility of the ancient physician in regard to his professional role as a potential abortionist or purveyor of euthanasia.

Among the specific questions to be pursued are these: What part did various philosophical attitudes toward death have in shaping the ethical perspectives of Pythagoras, Plato, Aristotle, and Seneca on the above issues? When did these philosophers, in particular, think that human life began and under what conditions, if any, did they allow that human life could be justifiably prevented or ended? Moreover, did members of the Greco-Roman medical and philosophical communities customarily acknowledge an inalienable right to life, or, on the other end of the spectrum, a right to die? Lastly, was suicide admitted to be a rational act in some instances, or was it almost always viewed as impulsive or blameworthy conduct?

Throughout Part III I shall test my earlier conjecture that many physicians who chose to ignore the teachings of the Hippocratic Oath on abortion and euthanasia (assuming they were familiar with some version of that document at all) did so in part because they were persuaded by powerful ethical arguments that directly opposed the Oath's restrictions against abortion and euthanasia. My contention is that some philosophical arguments, and the schools from which they issued, did contribute to the pluralistic sentiments of physicians and patients regarding the rightness or wrongness of abortion and euthanasia. The task that awaits us is to expose the premises of these philosophical arguments and then assess their individual strengths and weaknesses against the backdrop of Greek medicine and popular morals. In addition to the preceding quartet of philosophers, the medical writings of selected Hippocratic authors and the pioneer obstetrician and gynecologist, Soranus, will receive special attention.[1]

Finally, two qualifications must be placed on all that follows. First, I shall not delve at any great length into the complex subject of ancient law. I shall, however, comment on legal developments where this is helpful in setting the stage for my discussion of selected moral perspectives.

Second, it will be convenient at times to characterize various ancient moral positions as possessing *consequentialist* (teleological) or *nonconsequentialist* (deontological) tendencies. Roughly speaking, moral theories are classified as consequentialist if they equate right conduct with acts that cause the greatest balance of good over evil defined solely in terms of the consequences that the act in question produces. Nonconsequentialist theories, in contrast, insist that what finally determines the rightness or wrongness of an act has to do mainly with some criterion other than the consequences that a given act produces. One example of the former would be ethical hedonism: pleasure is the highest good, and right acts are those that produce the most pleasurable consequences for an individual in the long run. An example of the latter could be called Mosaic ethics: conforming to the divine imperatives of God is the highest good, and right acts are those which obey the Ten Commandments—regardless of the specific consequences which these acts may produce. Strictly speaking, however, such classificatory labels were foreign to the Greeks; in their moral theory, they generated what moral theorists today call uniquely eudaimonistic ethics.

As the words *eu daimon* (good spirit) literally imply, this kind of ethic involves creating a moral system that aims at making the moral agent a good spirit—one who acquires well-being. Moreover, contrary to some criticisms, eudaimonism does not necessarily entail ethical egoism. The latter states that only those actions that increase a given individual's total balance of good over evil are morally right and those alone. Yet acts of charity or benevolence were by no means a standard source of ridicule amongst the Greeks, for many were aware that the welfare of other citizens was linked to one's own welfare and to the well-being of the community. What is common to almost all of the Greek moral perspectives about to be examined, then, is this eudaimonist orientation, according to which to do good (*eu prattein*) is to fare well.[2] Hence, the moral agent as a whole, not his actions alone, is accorded the greatest attention in Greek ethical theories. In contrast, most modern and contemporary ethical theories have tended both (a) to shift the focus of attention from the agent to the praiseworthiness or blameworthiness of his act and (b) to downplay the notion that the virtuous person is more likely to be the happy person—in this earthly existence, at least. These differences in emphasis must be acknowledged at the outset since they are fundamental to comprehending Greek moral values.

PRELIMINARY CONSIDERATIONS

Not only abortion but also infanticide was widely practiced by the Greeks and Romans. In seeking to identify and understand the ancient philosophical arguments for and against these practices, it will be instructive to summarize some of the more interesting and historically important aspects of two practices that were entirely commonplace during most of antiquity. Lecky,[3] Westermarck,[4] and most recently Durant[5] have each written extensive social histories covering Greco-Roman attitudes and practices on these and many related topics from which all may profit.

The first observation I shall make is that the modern reader who approaches the ancient evidence on these topics for the first time almost faces a radical reorientation of values. One immediately confronts the fact that, with perhaps one known exception, parents throughout Greece and Rome had the legal right (though seldom the obligation) to kill their newly born children for virtually any reason.[6] It was not until the fourth century A.D. that Roman emperors began to enact measures that sought to protect the lives of free-born infants, at very least.[7] Notice, too, that in a social environment where infanticide is rife and rarely a matter of moral controversy among the general populace, the act of aborting a fetus (so long as the mother is not harmed) tends automatically to be viewed as well within the norm of the morally permissible.[8] In other words, since infanticide was judged morally acceptable under usual circumstances (i.e., when the parents consented, when the infant was still a newborn, etc.), then naturally the decision to carry out an abortion under similarly standard conditions (to be described below) could only with some difficulty be subject to condemnation from the pre-Christian moral perspective. In a sense, then, the whole subject of abortion for the pagans must be viewed as conceptually dependent on their logically prior reasonings about infanticide. For if infant life was expendable, why protest on moral grounds the killing of fetuses?

What's more, the contemporary reader is at first glance likely to locate the moral question of infanticide as an important branch of the central debate about euthanasia and the prospect of long-term, costly medical care for severely and irremediably defective newborns. But I suggest that a fresh conceptual orientation will need to be temporarily adopted in order to fully penetrate the logic of the pagan mind on this issue. For as will soon become evident, the reasons most often expressed by the Greeks and Romans for killing their newborns were by no means narrowly limited to modern considerations of what kind of hardship the infants would likely have to endure—given some defect or disease—were they allowed to live. In fact, ancient testimony strongly points to a diverse range of publicly admitted reasons for the justification of either infanticide or abortion. The typical reasons included: (1) the desire to preserve what some women viewed as their sexual, as opposed to their maternal, beauty;[9] (2) the desire to avoid the personal inconvenience and loss of freedom associated with caring for very young children;[10] (3) the desire to avoid poverty occasioned by the added material costs of child care;[11] (4) the related desire to limit competition for scarce resources by limiting the size of their community's population;[12] (5) the desire to have male offspring in greater proportion than female offspring based on perceived military and economic advantages;[13] (6) the desire to protect the woman from a life-threatening, difficult pregnancy;[14] (7) the desire to rid society of future citizens who, because they are born weak or defective, are considered to be a worthless burden to themselves or society;[15] (8) the desire to conceal adultery;[16] and (9) the desire to protect one's family or estate from a child of doubtful legitimacy.[17]

It is surely a mistake to imagine that the preceding nine reasons constitute an exhaustive list, or that the average citizens of either Greece or Rome constructed or consulted elaborate philosophical justifications for the above-mentioned deeds. When they acted, they did so partly out of habit and in accord with longstanding cultural approval, which they took for granted. Yet it is true, I would argue, that variants of these nine reasons, taken alone or in combination, are highly representative of the sorts of conscious motivations that led individual Greeks and Romans to perform acts of abortion or infanticide.

Nor can one absolutely say, in attempting to come to grips with the approach the ancients took on these matters of life and death, that reasons (5), (7), and (9) alone from the foregoing inventory constituted the usual sorts of justification for infanticide; while (1)–(4), (6), and (8) were standard justifications for abortion. To do so threatens to underestimate the complexity of the ancient social situation. It not only overlooks the likelihood of unique or mixed motivations for such deeds on the part of the moral agent, but it ignores completely that in a social environment where both abortion *and* infanticide are at very least legal, if not free of controversy, either act may in a given case serve to satisfy the motivation and final aim of the actor.

For example, a married couple may learn that the wife is pregnant. During the pregnancy they may entertain thoughts that they have enough children already and that an additional child will push them further into poverty, (3) above. If they vacillate during the pregnancy on whether or not to abort on account of their poverty, then (3) can still be legally accomplished by means of killing the infant shortly after it is born. There is good reason to believe, incidentally, that infanticide was more likely to result in tentative cases like the one under discussion if the newborn turned out to be a female, for a daughter usually required an expensive dowry to be paid upon her marriage. Also upon marriage, she became subject to the jurisdiction of another household or clan that had contributed nothing to her careful upbringing. Then, too, daughters were expected to do little in the way of outside productive labor that might enrich their family's income (not so, however, in the case of a son). And women in general performed no formal military duties in defense of their family or community.[18] Hence, there is little reason to doubt that throughout antiquity many more female than male children perished by infanticide. In Hellenistic Greece, the average family was quite small. It rarely contained more than one daughter. Thus it is fair to say that the comparative lack of value placed on female infants can be plausibly understood as the predictable outcome of an uncompromising and dominantly utilitarian appraisal of their worth.[19]

The preceding account of the social and legal setting in Greece and Rome has to this point been characterized in the broadest fashion. Again, my purpose is to provide only a general picture of relevant Greek and Roman popular thought and customs in preparation for introducing the philosophical literature which it is the main business of Part III to explore. Yet there remain three additional areas bearing on our topic that deserve some comment. These are: (1) contraception in antiquity; (2) methods of abortion and infanticide; and (3) the medical role of midwives.

Contraception

By the fifth century B.C., if not long before, the Greeks were generally aware of the causal connection between sexual intercourse and human pregnancy. In fact, embryology was a topic to which most of the sixth- and fifth-century pre-Socratic philosophers had directed at least a passing comment.[20] Yet it was not until the time of Aristotle and the Hippocratic authors of *On Semen* and *On the Development of the Child* that human embryology became a distinct biological science wedded to the search for nature's impersonal laws. Furthermore, though it is difficult to estimate how evenly distributed this embryological knowledge was among the general populace, it is certain that various sorts of contraceptive measures were known and used by the citizens of Greece and Rome.

These measures, however, were usually not reliable. If they worked at all, very often even their authors did not correctly understand why. Thus, Norman Himes, in his *Medical History of Contraception*, states that while Aristotle is the first Greek on record to mention a contraceptive formula—a formula involving the application of oil of cedar to the womb prior to intercourse—there is little reason to believe that he fully understood the causal principle behind this supposed remedy. "It is clear from the context that he regarded the quality of smoothness as the *modus operandi* of prevention; whereas we now know that oil has a contraceptive effect by reducing the motility of spermatozoa and by gumming up the external os."[21] In any case, Himes grants that Aristotle's formula might have worked on occasion. In addition, there were the more widely used mechanical devices, such as wool, salves, and resins. These, in the opinion of the physician and medical historian, Henry Sigerist, were probably somewhat more effective than the potion Aristotle mentions above when introduced into the vagina before intercourse.[22]

What would have constituted the ideal contraceptive device for both ancient and contemporary times, had it worked, was erroneously prescribed as follows by the Hippocratic author of *On the Nature of Women*: "If a woman does not wish to become pregnant, dissolve in water misy [a copper salt] as large as a bean and give it to her to drink, and for a year she will not become pregnant."[23]

Furthermore, the Roman poet and Epicurean philosopher, Lucretius (99–55 B.C.) declares at the end of the fourth book of his widely admired *On the Nature of Things* that the gods are definitely not responsible for human infertility and sterility. Instead, he says, natural causes are to blame. Hence, he mocks desperate childless couples for appealing to the gods and scolds husbands in particular for " . . . piling the raised altars with offerings, to make their wives pregnant with abundant seed. In vain they weary the divinity of the gods and the sacred lots."[24] Lucretius identifies the causes of infertility as including "too great thickness" or "undue fluidity and thinness" of the semen.[25] He also suggests that both diet and the modes of intercourse can improve or diminish one's chances of conception. For the consistency of semen is, he thinks, affected by certain foods; in addition, the quadruped position is said by Lucretius to promote conception. As for methods of contraception, he wrongly states that "effeminate motions" or gyrations on the part of women during intercourse help prevent conception. Lucretius thus concludes that " . . . for their own ends harlots are wont to move, in order not to conceive and lie in child-bed frequently, and at the same time to render Venus alone attractive to men. This method our wives have surely no need of [if conception is desired]."[26]

Lastly, the most accurate and impressive account of contraception in antiquity is rendered by the Greek physician of the Methodist school, Soranus (A.D. 98–138), universally credited as an early pioneer and founder of the medical specialties of gynecology and obstetrics (Fig. 7). More clearly than his contemporaries, he distinguished between contraceptives and abortifacients, saying, in part: "A contraceptive differs from an abortive, for the first does not let conception take place, while the latter destroys what has been conceived. Let us therefore call the one 'abortive' (*phthorion*) and the other 'contraceptive' (*atokion*)."[27]

Also, far in advance of his time, Soranus warned about the possible health risks involved in drinking alleged contraceptive potions of the sort cited above by the Hippocratic authors. He resisted superstition at every turn and discouraged the use of amulets (sometimes made in the form of genital organs), which were thought by the masses to influence the prevention or promotion of conception. According to Himes, Soranus also prescribed a host of ineffective contraceptive formulas among the 150 or so such prescriptions that he gave. But his main reliance was on the more rational mechanical techniques, such as vaginal plugs or pessaries, which used wool as a base mixed with oils or other gummy substances. As for his related views on the morality of abortion, which will be examined in the discussion below, Soranus observed: "It is much more advantageous not to conceive than to destroy the embryo. . . . "[28]

Given the results of our brief examination up to this point, I suspect that most Greeks and Romans would have shared Soranus's stated preference "not to conceive" rather than resort to abortion or infanticide. The Greeks and Romans were not a bloodthirsty people, and they were well aware of the risks and inconveniences attendant upon either remaining option.[29] But even so, universal ignorance of truly effective contraceptive measures would have rendered any such moral preferences entirely moot. As has been suggested, ancient medical science

Figure 7. Illustration (codex 1653) showing the fetus in utero, from a twelfth-century manuscript based on the writings of Soranus of Ephesus (A.D. 98–138), a Roman doctor who advocated contraception. Reprinted courtesy of The Royal Library, Copenhagen.

neither knew nor communicated any truly reliable contraceptive methods. It is generally agreed that the most effective and widely used method available was *coitus interruptus*. In addition, I am persuaded that the most our historical evidence entitles us to say is that the decidedly flawed contraceptive knowledge of antiquity was known to the more privileged segments of society, to be sure. But how widely dispersed these detailed formulae were among the uneducated and highly superstitious majority is hard to gauge. It is entirely possible that the masses experimented with an endlessly changing list of equally ineffective contraceptive techniques of every imaginable type and origin.

But if so, we must confront an additional important fact: limiting family size by whatever means was a widespread ancient practice. We possess several reliable reports, especially during the Hellenistic and Roman periods, of whole communities facing much lower population counts than their leaders and their own social critics deemed desirable from the standpoint of the national welfare. In Macedonian times, for example, Philip V was so worried about his country's depopulation that he created a law forbidding the willful limitation of the family by contraception, abortion, or infanticide. It is reported that in thirty years Philip's edict succeeded in raising the manpower of his nation by almost fifty percent.[30] Polybius, writing about 150 B.C., was well aware of the widespread practice of family limitation. He complained bitterly and wrote in alarming tones about the resulting depopulation:

> In our time the whole of Greece has been subject to a low birth rate and a general decrease of the population, owing to which cities have become deserted and the land has ceased to yield fruit. . . . For as men had fallen into such a state of luxury, avarice, and indolence that they did not wish to marry, or if they married, to rear the children born to them, or at most but one or two of them, so as to leave these in affluence and bring them up to waste their substance—the evil insensibly but rapidly grew. For in cases where, of one or two children, the one was carried off by war and the other by sickness, it was evident that the houses must have been left empty . . . and by small degrees cities became resourceless and empty.[31]

Can one fairly surmise from such testimony that the most common methods of voluntary family limitation in antiquity were abortion and infanticide, and not the relatively ineffective contraceptive measures of the sort outlined above? In my opinion, this is the only acceptable conclusion. Of the well-to-do families, Poseidippis (fl. 270 B.C.) writes: "Even a rich man always exposes a daughter."[32] Famine, sickness, poverty, and war, however great their toll, could not alone account for the reported facts. And, as we shall soon see, several Greek philosophers of the period condoned abortion or infanticide as morally justifiable practices for the control of the untoward social consequences of overpopulation. Is it not reasonable to think, therefore, that the public endorsements of philosophers may have influenced at least some segments of Greco-Roman society?

Methods of Abortion and Infanticide

Our investigation ought not to advance any further until we pause to define our two principal terms in this section. For our purposes, abortion shall be defined as the deliberate termination of pregnancy resulting in the intended death of the fetus prior to normal or spontaneous delivery.[33] Probably the most effective method, if not most popular, was to puncture the ovum by manual or other mechanical manipulation.[34] Another method, recommended by a Hippocratic author to a singer who unintentionally became pregnant, was to have the woman jump high into the air, kicking her heels repeatedly into her buttocks.[35] Embryotomy, the surgical cutting apart of the fetus, was also known to both the Greeks and Romans. But this was apparently a procedure of last resort. It was used by physicians primarily when the mother's life was threatened during delivery or when the fetus was thought to be dead in utero. Additionally, there were numerous recipes for abortifacient drugs taken orally or as pessaries (vaginal suppositories), which were touted by various medical writers. But most of these have since been shown by modern medical analysis to have had little effect.[36]

In contrast, the question of how to define infanticide in a way that conforms to ancient Greek and Roman thinking initially poses more of a problem. Straightforward infanticide, then as now, is commonly taken to mean the willful termination of the life of an infant. This definition may serve to capture standard cases in antiquity where the infant was actively killed by such common methods as smothering, strangling, drowning, crushing, and stabbing. But this definition fails to capture the subtleties involved in the allied and more passive methods vaguely called exposure or exposition.

Why? Because exposure sometimes involved merely acting to rid oneself of the burdens and liabilities of the infant, short of actively killing it. Hence, to say in antiquity that an infant had been exposed by its parents was not always the same as saying that the parents killed, or even intended to kill, their infant.

For example, a very common method of exposure in Greece and Rome was to carefully place the infant in an earthenware vessel and abandon it near a religious temple. The exposed infant was sometimes saved by some benevolent person wishing to adopt, or by someone hoping to profit by raising the child to serve as a slave or a prostitute.[37] Reflection on the latter possibility apparently inclined some parents to actively kill their unwanted infants rather than tempt fate to condemn such children to a wretched life of poverty or bondage at the hands of others. Thus, in one of the few characterizations of infanticide in Greco-Roman imaginative literature, the Roman playwright, Terence (ca. 190–159? B.C.) focuses on just such a concern. He portrays a husband and wife who are torn over what to do with their unwanted infant.[38]

> Terence represents Chermes as having, as a matter of course, charged his pregnant wife to have her child killed provided it was a girl. The mother, overcome by pity, shrank from doing so, and secretly gave it to an old woman *to*

expose it, in hopes that it might be preserved. Chermes, on hearing what had been done, reproached his wife for her womanly pity and told her she had been not only disobedient but irrational, for she was only consigning her daughter to the life of a prostitute.[39]

The moral and psychological significance of this distinction between infanticide, taken here to mean the active and certain termination of infant life, and exposure, taken here to mean passively subjecting the infant to the increased likelihood—but not always the certainty—of termination, cannot be overlooked. Psychologically, the uncertainty of the outcome of exposure in standard cases of abandonment, such as those described above, probably relieved some parents of their sense of moral responsibility for their deed. After all, whatever the outcome, it could be thought of as ultimately a matter now in the laps of the gods. Heaven could decide. Morally, it is quite possible that exposure was not popularly considered to be as blameworthy an act as outright infanticide. This was particularly so in regard to the infanticide of *healthy* infants, which custom, if not law, generally opposed. Thus, by the period of the Roman Empire, at least, the chances of healthy infants being rescued from abandonment were somewhat improved owing to the occasional intervention by the state.[40]

Midwives

No inquiry into Greco-Roman values and customs associated with the birth of new human life would be complete without some mention of the medical and social roles of midwives. It is probably true that most Greek and Roman women gave birth in a squatting position, perhaps sitting on a specially designed parturition chair. If medical services were rendered at all (and in most cases they were not thought to be needed), it was typically the midwife who attended. Socrates, himself the son of the midwife Phaenarete, is made to say at *Theaetetus* 149D that among the things midwives are known to do well is " . . . at an early stage to cause a miscarriage if they so decide."[41] Sigerist credits them with being able to diagnose early pregnancy better than any physician, and he speculates that midwives called in physicians during the birth process " . . . only in abnormal cases when something went wrong."[42]

It is not known with precision what, if any, the role of midwives may have been in association with acts of infanticide or exposure. But in the matter of procuring abortions, we have sufficient evidence to suggest that a good many midwives helped to provide these services for a fee. And this they did not only in cases of possible therapeutic abortion; i.e., those done to protect the mother's health—like the type to which Socrates may have been referring above. On this we also have the testimony of Soranus, who considered the subject of midwifery to be deserving of special comment. He emphatically demands of the ideal midwife that "she must not be greedy for money, lest she give an abortive wickedly for payment," a warning that would hardly have been necessary unless the temptation (to perform abortions) had been great in ancient Rome.[43]

Hence the moral implication of the role of midwives in ancient family life was this. Since midwives could detect pregnancy in the early stages, and could provide a woman with a relatively safe abortion, it was in principle possible for a woman, either married or unmarried, to secure an abortion without the knowledge or consent of her lover, her family, or her community. That this, in fact, sometimes occurred is well documented by certain Hellenistic legal prohibitions that presuppose such behavior.[44] A second moral implication here bears on the Hippocratic Oath. When the Oath-taker states, "I will not give a woman an abortive remedy," he is at once tacitly disassociating himself from the practices of many midwives with whom he does not agree, based on moral considerations predicated on at least some Pythagorean perspectives.[45] To these Pythagorean and other philosophical perspectives on abortion we now turn.

PHILOSOPHICAL PERSPECTIVES

The principal philosophers or schools of philosophy on which I have gathered ample evidence to permit a reliable identification and subsequent discussion of their respective stands on abortion or infanticide are just four in number: Pythagoreanism, Plato, Aristotle, and the Stoicism of Seneca. Whenever possible, I shall try to determine in each case the answers to two basic questions: First, at what point is the developing fetus taken to be a human being? Second, on what moral grounds is abortion approved or condemned? I shall limit the first question primarily to the metaphysical or early scientific considerations of when the preceding four authors judged the human embryo to be ensouled or animate. This was, after all, the characteristic form of that question among the ancients. In addition, I shall limit the second question primarily to the judgments of value placed on fetal or infant life. While some attention will eventually be paid to the more global question of what value was placed on adult human life per se, that is a broader issue which will be postponed until the remaining question of euthanasia is addressed in the next chapter.

Pythagoras

It will be recalled that Pythagoras (ca. 580–497 B.C.) placed the highest value on the soul. The earthly soul is said to be a temporarily fallen divinity, immortal in character, and the most essential and enduring part of each person's identity. In our discussion of Greek attitudes toward death in chapter 3, we saw that the Pythagoreans believed in what I termed *divine personal immortality*. We also saw that the soul is yoked to the alien and inferior human body (*soma*) for the sake of punishment, as in a tomb (*sema*). The personal salvation promised to humankind by the Pythagorean Brotherhood was that for the properly initiated at least, living on earth in accordance with the Pythagorean ethical virtues could render one's soul sufficiently pure in character to assure its speedy return at death to the heavenly station from which it originated. Again, the body alone is subject to decay: the soul, being divine, is deathless and is the object of highest worth from the Pythagorean perspective.

To these metaphysical and religious tenets the Pythagoreans added the dogma of the transmigration of souls. This stated that upon death, if one's soul was not sufficiently pure to return to its natural place among the gods in the heavens, then it would be required to inhabit fresh (newly born) bodies, of either human or animal form, until the requisite moral purity had been achieved. Thus, given the high value placed on the soul, it is little wonder that the Pythagoreans held it to be morally wrong to kill human or animal life. For while it is true that they downgraded the body and held the soul to be superior, they also held that it was divine law that decreed what kind of body, if any, a soul must occupy.

As we shall see in our upcoming discussion of euthanasia, Pythagoreans viewed it as abominable personally to take early leave from one's body (say, by suicide), or to assist or coerce any other living person or animal in doing so. To do so was both to mock the gods and soil one's soul with evil. This religious reasoning justifies at once, therefore, the Pythagorean observance of certain blood taboos, such as the abstention from eating meat. More importantly, it also justifies the judgment that it is morally wrong to cause a woman to have an abortion *if, in addition*, fetuses are believed to possess souls.

What, then, was the Pythagorean teaching on the question of the status of the fetus? As suggested in our preliminary discussion of abortion in connection with the Hippocratic Oath in chapter 5, the Pythagorean belief was that the fetus possessed a soul and was an animate being from the very moment of conception. Though the evidence for this claim cannot be traced directly to Pythagoras—since we possess nothing that he wrote—at least two pieces of evidence seem to justify this conclusion. The first is the testimony of Porphyry (A.D. 232/3–ca. 305), who, in his treatise on embryology, expressly attributes this position to the Pythagoreans.[46] The second is based on a Hellenistic account of the Pythagorean system of physiology compiled by Alexander Polyhistor (ca. 105 B.C.). On the latter account, the germ or seed is said to be a piece of brain containing hot vapors within it, and soul and sensation originate from this vapor at conception.[47] Similar views were also previously accepted by the Pythagorean Philolaus in the fourth century B.C., as reported by Diogenes Laertius.[48]

Thus, I see little reason to doubt the claim that the Pythagoreans unconditionally condemned abortion. As far as our evidence implies, fetal life was coequal in moral worth with adult human life, and this from the moment of conception. If so, this finding would appear at once to rule out the permissibility of therapeutic abortions for the Pythagoreans. For if the souls of both the fetus and the pregnant mother are divine, and if it is a decree laid by the gods upon mankind that the foreordained schedule of the arrival and departure of souls must never be tampered with by human beings, who, without contradiction, can claim that killing the fetus to save the mother's life is justified? Moreover, who would claim, granting the identical premises, that terminating the life of infants—for whatever reason—is on Pythagorean principles justified?

In addition, it is also worth noting that, on the above interpretation, not only human abortion and infanticide, but any effort to terminate the embryonic or new-born life of any species of animal would be subject to moral condemnation by the Pythagoreans. As Xenophanes, a contemporary of Pythagoras, mockingly re-counts: "They say that once a *puppy* was being whipped, Pythagoras, who was passing by, took pity on it, saying: 'Stop! Do not beat it! It is the soul of a friend; I recognize his voice.'"[49]

This concern for the lives of human as well as nonhuman creatures further illustrates a point that should not be skated over. That is, in talking about the concept of respect for life (also sometimes called the concept of sanctity or reverence for life), it is useful to distinguish between a *comprehensive* respect for life and a *noncomprehensive* respect for life.[50] The former covers all forms of life—vegetable, animal, and human. The latter is more representative of Western thinking: it is restricted to respect for life in the human form alone (whatever that designation is taken to be). In the case of the Pythagoreans, however, it is fair to say that their strong respect-for-life ethic approximated a more comprehensive scale than did any of the competing philosophical schools throughout antiquity.[51] Therefore, this ethic constituted a distinctive trait of Pythagorean moral and religious thinking—one that was sure to inform their equally nonconsequentialist stand against suicide and euthanasia.

Plato

The views of Plato on abortion and infanticide, like those of Aristotle, are predicated on considerations of a far more utilitarian and this-worldly sort than those associated with the Pythagoreans. (I am here using the word "utilitarian" in the broadest sense to mean the social consequences of an act or policy, not to be confused with the much later utilitarian school of philosophy associated with Bentham and Mill.) In a way, this is at first glance a bit puzzling in the case of Plato. As we have already seen, Plato believed in a version of *divine personal immortality*.[52] He also accepted the dogmas of the soul-body dualism and the transmigration of souls that had been associated with Orphic-Pythagorean thought. How, then, could he endorse both abortion and infanticide in his vision of the ideal state as set forth in his *Republic*?

The answer to a large extent lies in the fact that, unlike the Pythagoreans, Plato held that human life began at the moment of birth. This, at least, is the contention of Edelstein. While I have been unable to discover an explicit statement to this effect in Plato's dialogues, his mythical account of the soul's journey into successive human lives, known as the Myth of Er, does seem to imply this interpretation.[53] Moreover, that the successors of Plato at the Academy took this position is almost certain. Platonists and neo-Platonists alike denied the ensoulment of the fetus in utero. This they did on the grounds that the soul, being the special divine entity it is, had to enter the body from without (perhaps through the new-born's first breaths). Given this embryological theory, it is then possible to assert that aborting fetal life is an act falling in an altogether different category than kill-ing a human being, for the fetus remains a soulless creature.

What, then, are Plato's reasons for justifying abortion as he sets forth his blueprint for utopia in the *Republic*? In his organization of marriage and family life among his Guardian and Craftsmen classes, he accords the highest value to what he deems the good of the state. Ultimately, that highest value is identified as justice, the crowning virtue that emerges in the whole community when subordi-nate virtues are achieved in the right proportion among all the citizenry. If the state is to be the best, then its future citizens must not be allowed to live unless they can serve the productive interests of the state at some minimal level of compe-tence. In the main, it is on this policy that Plato attempts to justify abortion, in-fanticide, and euthanasia. For he does so, essentially, by tacitly appealing to the consequentialist principle that to permit these three acts in certain circumstances promotes the greatest long-term benefit for the entire community. Thus, in the final analysis, whatever rights or duties the individual may have to himself or to his family are subordinated by Plato to the higher duty to serve the state.

Specifically, Plato authorizes abortion as part of his eugenic program. This program entails the strictest regulation of marriage and mating, with the end in view of producing the most perfect human offspring possible for the alleged ben-efit of the entire state (*Republic* 5.459). Wishing to maximize the quality of the offspring of the Guardians in particular, he specifies that Guardians can legally mate only between the ages of twenty-five to fifty-five, and twenty to forty, for male and female partners, respectively. He prescribes these age ranges because he thinks they conform to the eugenic principle " . . . that children should be born from parents in the prime of life."[54] Then, in regard to abortion, Plato has Socra-tes state:

> As soon, however, as the men and the women have passed the age pre-scribed for producing children, we shall leave them free to form a connec-tion with whom they will. . . ; and all this only after we have exhorted them to see that no child, if any be conceived, shall be brought to light, or, if they cannot prevent its birth, to dispose of it on the understanding that no such child can be reared.[55]

It should also be observed that Plato's eugenic policy, when extended to cover the special case of fetuses conceived out of wedlock by women under the prescribed age of twenty, almost certainly entails the termination of these illicit pregnancies as well. For Plato held that offspring conceived by parents who were either too young or too old faced an unacceptably high risk of possessing inferior physical or mental attributes. This end—i.e., attaining the best bred and best ed-ucated Guardians possible—he thought morally justified these means.

So, too, Plato strongly implies that any fetuses conceived by lustful citizens who fall within his approved age ranges, but who, in addition, fail to secure the required legal and religious sanctions of the state (marriage), must thereby suffer abortion, even against the parents' will. Hence, all instances of bigamy, adultery, incest, and premarital sexual intercourse that produce offspring will be subject to abortion or infanticide.[56] In other words, illegitimate offspring were not to see the light of day. This suggests that Plato's legal sanctions for sexual incontinence or disobedience were grounded on eugenic principles, as well as on independent cal-culations of the overall good to be achieved by the anticipated deterrent value of these strict sanctions. For it is not hard to imagine that, in some of these illegal unions, offspring of a potentially high quality from the strictly genetic standpoint would result. Nonetheless, they are put to death by the state as a public warning to other like-minded citizens who would flirt with such folly.[57]

That Plato also favored infanticide for the purpose of securing the best pos-sible Guardian class, and that he specifically recommends getting rid of defective newborns judged to be below some minimal standard of fitness (which he does not specify in any detail), there can be little doubt. In a key passage he reveals that

> As soon as children are born, they will be taken in charge by officers ap-pointed for the purpose, who may be men or women or both, since offices are to be shared by both sexes. The children of the better parents they will carry to the crèche to be reared in the care of nurses living apart in a certain quarter of the city. Those of inferior parents and any children of the rest that are born defective will be hidden away, in some appropriate manner that must be kept secret.
>
> They must be, if the breed of our Guardians is to be kept pure.[58]

It is more difficult to determine, however, what additional reasons, if any, Plato supplied for the taking of infant life over and above the utilitarian reasons he advances for the taking of fetal life. On the heels of the passage just quoted, he supplies no new grounds. And I know of no other text where he does so in spe-cific reference to infanticide, even though we might well expect additional rea-sons, since he accords to the infant a higher moral status than he does to the fetus. But there are some hints of a possible reply, I think, in remarks that he makes at *Republic* 406 concerning the importance of living a productive life and the moral justification he advances there for euthanasia among the incurably sick or severely disabled adult population. Since it will be more convenient to explore this last matter a bit later on, it will suffice here to remark that there is an apparent weak-ness in Plato's ready endorsement of infanticide. This weakness stems from his inattention to taking into full account the possible divergent moral status of in-fants as compared with fetuses.

Aristotle

Arguing along utilitarian lines similar to Plato but emphasizing to an even greater extent the threat of overpopulation to the well-being of the state, Aristotle judges both abortion and infanticide to be morally justifiable. According to Aristotle, "if no restriction is imposed on the rate of reproduction, . . . poverty is the inevitable result; and poverty produces, in its turn, civic dissension and wrong-doing."[59] Aristotle, in other words, tacitly argues that since there is a causal link between overpopulation and occurrences of poverty or political revolution, and since these are social consequences that seriously threaten to reduce the overall balance of good and stability in the state, then the imposition of limits on family size is morally defensible. Such limits, he insists, must in any case be adjusted to allow for (1) infant mortality rates and (2) normally expected infertility rates among the married.[60]

Hence, it is fair to conclude further that, given the above reasoning, Aristotle would not have objected to couples resorting to contraceptive measures in order to achieve ideal population levels within the state. In fact, as we saw in a preceding section, Aristotle was well aware of such devices, and voiced absolutely no objection to their use.[61]

In this connection, his position on abortion and infanticide is a bit more complicated than the comparatively unqualified approval given it by Plato in the latter's morally eligible cases. In *Politics* 7.1335b.20, Aristotle states:

> The question arises whether children should always be reared or may sometimes be exposed to die. There should certainly be a law to prevent the rearing of deformed children. On the other hand, there should also be a law, in all states where the system of social habits is opposed to unrestricted increase, to prevent the exposure of children to death *merely* in order to keep the population down. The proper thing to do is to limit the size of each family, and if children are then conceived in excess of the limit so fixed, to have miscarriage induced *before sense and life have begun in the embryo*.[62]

First of all, in the prior case of infanticide, Aristotle deems this justifiable when and only when an infant is born deformed. The kind and degree of deformity he has in mind is nowhere specified. Thus, it would be misleading, I think, to attempt to associate Aristotle with a specific and perhaps overdetermined criterion on this matter. It must suffice to observe that he often stresses the importance of a sound bodily and mental constitution in his writings, as I suggested in a previous chapter. Also, he counts as life's chief nonmoral goods (i.e., qualities that contribute significantly to living the good life) both good birth (*eugenia*), which includes sound heredity, and health (*hygeia*), which includes freedom from disease and the full possession of bodily faculties.[63] Given that a deformed infant might well be judged to have little purchase on either or both of these valued attributes, one again observes Aristotle's concern for the supposed greater good of the whole community in his approval of infanticide. For a chronically sick, weak, or deformed child can, on utilitarian grounds, be judged of little worth either to himself or to the long-term productive interests of the well-ordered state.

But Aristotle's exact position on abortion is somewhat harder to interpret. In view of the preceding quotation, his position appears to depend almost entirely on when, according to his embryological and related metaphysical speculations, the human zygote was considered by him to have acquired "sense and life." In order to answer this question fully, it will be necessary to supplement what we have already learned concerning Aristotle's views on the human soul during our prior discussion of his concept of death.[64] We noted there that Aristotle regarded the soul to be inseparable from the body. He also taught that all living things, *zoa*, are single concrete entities comprised of soul and body. The soul he equated with the form of a given species. (Literally, soul [*psyche*] in Greek meant "life" or "vital principle;" it was then a word less closely associated with the religious connotations it tends to have now in English.[65]) In addition, Aristotle taught that non-living or inanimate things are soulless (*apsychon*). Hence, the possession of a soul made all the difference in Aristotle's system in regard to whether an entity of a given kind was to be sorted into the living (literally besouled [*emsychos*]) or non-living categories.[66] Observing this, David Ross has written:

> Aristotle is helped here by the fact that the natural expression in Greek for a living thing is *empsychon soma*, "besouled body," where "besouled" evidently stands for the attribute that distinguishes living from other bodies, the power (at the least) of self-nourishment with or without the powers that mark off the higher living things from the lower. Soul, then, is the form or actuality of a living thing [whereas body is its potentiality].[67]

In reference to Aristotle's view on the status of the human zygote in his theory of the ascending scale of being, it is further necessary to ask: What, in the broadest terms, distinguishes higher living things from lower? Briefly put, his answer is that all living things are possessed of souls, and of souls there are three basic kinds. These are, in ascending order of worth: (1) the nutritive soul; (2) the sensitive soul; and (3) the rational soul. These three forms of soul constitute a series with a definite order, such that each type presupposes all that come before it in this order, without being strictly implied by them.

Hence, the minimal soul ascribable to all living things is the nutritive soul. The human zygote, or conceptus, is in Aristotle's view at very least besouled in the nutritive sense, for it is capable of nourishment and growth. So, too, all plant life is in this sense "alive." But plants, unlike persons, are limited to this nutritive level of existence.

Higher up the scale of being are creatures to whom the sensitive soul is properly ascribable. All animals are, at very least, besouled in virtue of their capacity to touch, and so they feel pleasure and pain, and also desire.[68]

Finally, there is the rational soul, which is ascribable to man alone of all earthly creatures. I conclude that, for Aristotle, to be a human being in the fullest sense means to possess the capacity for reason, contemplation, and rational choice. If there is to be talk about degrees of *human* existence, for Aristotle, such talk must ultimately be referred to various stages of growth, development, and eventual decay based on the preceding account of his psychology.

In regard to his theories of human embryology and psychology, Aristotle's position on the morality or immorality of abortion now may be properly assessed. It will be recalled that he condemns infanticide " . . . *merely* in order to keep the population down." He then says that the proper or right thing to do is to secure an abortion only if a given family has exceeded its fixed quota of children. It is significant, I think, that he does not cite any other immediate reasons than population control as grounds for abortion. Thus such possible grounds, common enough in his time, as the desire to preserve feminine beauty, avoid personal inconvenience, conceal adultery, etc., he does not even mention. Hence, I am inclined to think that he considered these motives to be morally ineligible.

At any rate, though Aristotle justifies abortion in the lone case mentioned, he does so by adding a strict condition, which, if it is not met, renders the deed morally objectionable. That condition is, in Aristotle's own words, " . . . to have miscarriage induced before sense (*aisthesis*) and life (*to zen*) have begun in the embryo." We are now in a position to see that, by life, Aristotle was referring minimally to a living thing possessing the nutritive soul. This, as I have suggested, is the status of the human zygote at and shortly after conception.[69] Sometime later—Aristotle nowhere says how long but perhaps in a month or so—the developing fetus is informed by the sensitive soul ascribable to all animal life. Aristotle remains curiously silent as to the precise moment in utero when the fetus acquires the rational soul, though this was usually conjectured to occur a bit later on during the second trimester of pregnancy.

Let us suppose, as did his followers in antiquity, that some point between the fortieth and ninetieth day of gestation marked the cut-off date during which induced abortion (for the lone eligible reason of family limitation) became morally wrong. This is the case supposedly because abortion then involved the destruction of a fetus endowed with the animal capacity to feel pain. In other words, abortion was then wrong because it involved the destruction of sentient *and* potential human life. If we suppose this, we come at once to a dilemma, noted in Aristotle's *History of Animals*:

> In the case of male children the first movement usually occurs on the right-hand side of the womb and about the fortieth day, but if the child be a female then on the left-hand side and about the ninetieth day. However, we must by no means assume this to be an accurate statement of fact, for there are many exceptions. . . . And, in short, these and all such-like phenomena are usually subject to differences that may be summed up as differences of degree.
>
> About this same period [forty days for the male, ninety days for the female] the embryo begins to resolve into distinct parts, it having hitherto consisted of a fleshlike substance without distinction of parts.[70]

Now if one is willing to assume, as did some of his followers, that Aristotle is here implying that the fetus acquires the sensitive soul at forty and at ninety days in the case of the male and female embryo, *respectively*, then how did the moral agent in the relevant case proceed? For it was impossible in antiquity to know in advance the sex of the unborn with any precision, as Aristotle here admits.

There is the additional problem, which Aristotle also acknowledges, that not all women can know within forty days that they are truly pregnant. If so, is it always too late to justifiably abort after forty days (waiving here the added difficulty of ascertaining the exact date of conception)? It would appear so. For again, if one waited until, say, the sixtieth day after suspected conception, and if to one's surprise the fetus was identifiable as male, then on Aristotle's view one has acted improperly. Therefore, it is safe to infer that the most conscientious thing a married couple ought to do, according to Aristotle, is to adopt birth control methods of some sort in cases where the family quota of offspring has already been reached. If these devices failed, as they commonly did in his day, then abortion in the eligible case becomes morally acceptable only if both of the following conditions are met: (1) the date of conception can be reasonably determined and (2) the woman realizes that she is pregnant and aborts *prior to the fortieth day* of gestation. From this I conclude that Aristotle's moral position regarding abortion is fairly clear: He gives it limited approval on utilitarian grounds. But practical difficulties of an epistemological nature concerning the dilemma of accurately pinpointing the date of acquisition by the human embryo of the relevant sensitive soul effectively cast Aristotle's moral stand on abortion into a sea of confusion. For if one assumes, for the sake of argument, that it is, in fact, morally justifiable to abort during some favored period of time (t_1), and not at a successive time (t_2), but there is no reliable way to verify whether one is aborting within the favored time period, then practical problems in ethical decision making result.

Therefore, as to Aristotle's views on abortion, I see no natural solution to this dilemma. Indeed, it is probable that he himself was aware of these epistemological difficulties. But even though he made an attempt, he apparently found no fully satisfactory solution to them.[71]

Seneca

The Roman Stoic, Seneca (4 B.C.–A.D. 65), conveniently aids our initial approach to the Stoic perspective on abortion and also serves to anticipate his own position on euthanasia (to be discussed later on). In one telling passage, he states:

> Just as the mother's womb holds us for ten months, not in preparation for itself, but for the region to which we seem to be discharged *when we are capable of drawing breath* and surviving in the open, so in the span extending from infancy to old age, we are ripening for another birth. . . . The day which you dread as the end is your birth into eternity.[72]

In actuality, Seneca felt that the best state of affairs was never to have been born in the first place.[73] This did not mean that he had no regard at all for human life. Rather, he shared a sentiment common to many Stoics and Epicureans who lived during the Hellenistic and Roman periods. This somewhat nihilistic sentiment stemmed in large measure from the growing feeling that the satisfactions of human existence are ordinarily too short and too few. Life holds many apparent pleasures, to be sure, but they seldom abide owing to their frail and transitory nature. Even those things that, on the Stoic view, men and women ought to prize most of all are extremely hard won and always subject to loss: peace of mind (*apatheia*), above all else; personal and communal well-being; a sense of at-oneness with God and Nature; and, to a lesser extent, personal health.

The means to spiritual peace of mind, which the wise man or woman alone could hope to sustain but which all might experience to some degree if they lived life in the right manner, was constituted by the four cardinal virtues. These four virtues were identified by the Stoics as: (1) wisdom (knowing what is truly good and bad); (2) courage (knowing what to truly fear and what not to fear); (3) justice (knowing how to give everyone what properly belongs to him); and (4) self-control (knowing what impressions to assent to and what passions to moderate or ignore). These virtues, and their supposed benefits, were also quite representative of the eudaimonist ethical perspective, according to which to live virtuously promotes the well-being of the whole person—both his body and soul, his commerce and relations with others, and his sense of unity with the greater universe of which he is but a small part.

Returning to Seneca's preceding quotation, it is evident from his words that he associates being born with the initial capacity of the individual to draw breath. This turns out to be an important observation. For, according to later Stoic physics and psychology, (a) the soul is a corporeal thing and (b) its essence—and indeed the defining attribute of being a member of the human species—is the possession of the vital breath (*pneuma*).[74] As pantheists, the central Stoic teaching in this connection was that each person's soul is a tiny, fiery piece of the greater world-soul, which is God. Hence, on the Stoic perspective, birth marks the start of human life in virtue of the manifest capacity of the newborn to draw breath.[75] (The fetus is ontologically akin to a mere plant: it possesses a *physis*, a nature, but not yet a *psyche*, a soul.)

Breath or *pneuma* was also said to be fed by exhalations from the blood. It was taken to be diffused throughout the entire unified soul (though the heart was its principal seat) owing to the interpenetration of breath-currents throughout the body. Human death, therefore, is signaled by the absence of breathing. It is occasioned by the loss of *pneuma*, which, in the Stoic view, was causally linked to the final cessation of cardiopulmonary functions. The dominant Stoic teaching about the dead, then, involved a variant of *natural personal dissolution*: the deceased's *pneuma* reunites in death with the larger *pneuma* of the world-soul, extinguishing thereby any trace of personal individuality.

Given this orientation, it comes as little surprise to learn that generally the Stoics were not adamantly opposed to abortion. After all, the fetus was not counted as a human being in either the biological or moral sense. Here a useful contemporary distinction may be introduced. One may talk about humanhood (or personhood) in two senses: (1) in the *biological* sense, designating the essential properties a being must have to count as a member of the species *homo sapiens*, and (2) in the *moral* sense, designating the properties a being must have in order to be counted a member of the moral community entitled to certain rights, duties, and related legal or moral protections—such as, for example, the rule against homicide.[76] Roughly, many of the Stoics of Seneca's period believed that the human soul, following birth, continued to expand its powers until around the age of fourteen, when it acquired the full capacity of rationality.

Fundamentally, the Stoics held that justice only extended to rational beings. In addition, only rational beings could be the bearers of rights. Therefore, only those fourteen or older were considered mature enough to possess rights protecting them against homicide (among other things). So while personhood in the biological sense was acquired at birth, personhood in the moral sense was acquired only at the point of young adulthood in the normal individual. The fetus, though not totally worthless, is entitled to our moral concern mainly insofar as nature intends fetuses to become rational beings in the usual scheme of things. Thus, since one generally ought to follow the designs of nature, it would be wrong to adopt a frivolous attitude toward the act of abortion.

However, even though children are not persons in the moral sense, and fetuses even less so, the Stoics felt it was appropriate (a duty) for parents to have a certain kind of attachment to their children—namely, the kind of attachment that will encourage parents to raise their children to be as rational and disciplined as possible. But all things that are appropriate—all duties—admit of exceptions, according to Stoicism. Thus it is generally a duty to preserve one's own or another's (e.g., a child's) life. Yet the Stoics did not judge life to be a good. In contrast, the natural order of things, and acting in accordance with the perceived natural order, was a good. So if one realizes that another's existence no longer contributes to the natural order of things, reason requires that one ought to terminate that life. But, as I shall emphasize in the next chapter when examining the Stoic position on suicide, this imperative leads to serious difficulties. At best, the Stoic could claim to know the natural order (fate) only in rough outline, not in sufficient detail to determine precisely what role the life any given individual plays in the larger scheme of things. Therefore, deciding whether to commit infanticide, say, could be extremely anguishing for the conscientious Stoic. Abortion posed less of a moral ordeal since, *inter alia*, the fetus possessed no real moral status to begin with. Since the fetus was not a member of the moral community, to abort violated no rule against homicide. True, Roman custom did stipulate that in the case of a married woman, her husband's prior consent to abortion was legally necessary.[77] But that the Stoics attached this legal requirement to their moral theory is most doubtful.

The favorite argument of the Stoics in support of abortion was based on an analogy. They held that the fetus is merely part of the mother's body, analogous to the fruit of a tree. Therefore, technically she may do with the fetus as she pleases until such time as it becomes ripe and falls down.[78] That point was said to occur at birth, when personhood in the biological sense, as suggested above, was in actuality deemed to begin.

Thereafter, in the absence of overriding reasons that would require an independent moral justification, the Stoics regarded the newborn as a future member of the moral and legal community (though not a bona fide member). As such, the newborn was usually treated as if he had the *prima facie* right to life. Again, all things being equal, the newborn ought to be nurtured and preserved. Hence, the life of an infant must not be arbitrarily terminated on the Stoic view. To be terminated, there must be a good, overriding reason for doing so. In contrast, almost any reason was admissible for the justification of abortion.

The main reason that was considered by the Stoics morally sufficient to warrant infanticide was that the newborn was found to be defective. About this Seneca is emphatic. He writes: "We destroy monstrous births, and we also drown our children if they are born weakly and unnaturally formed." He adds the justification that it is an act of reason thus to separate what is useless from what is sound.[79]

In my view, the full force of Seneca's argument is predicated on at least two aspects of Stoic ethics and physics. The first has to do with the eudaimonist emphasis on the importance of cultivating the required virtues in order to live well. Since, as I have suggested, the four cardinal virtues were said to be necessary to a life worth living, and since a malformed baby was, on account of its physical or mental defects, subject to being judged incapable of attaining the required virtues, to terminate the life of such defective newborns was seen as an "act of reason" from the Stoic perspective.

Second, this interpretation seems *a fortiori* all the more convincing in view of the Stoic teaching that whatever happens in this existence happens in accordance with Divine Providence. Hence, there are no accidents and no chance events. Therefore, if a person feels regret over the workings of Nature—including the fact that some newborns are pathetically defective and are, in accordance with Divine Reason, allegedly better off dead—then this regret must be overcome by recalling that whatever happens is for the best. As Seneca himself taught, it is through human reason and its capacity to appreciate the harmony of the universe that individuals may soothe their sometimes aching spirits. For it is comforting knowledge that " . . . Divine Providence extends even to the smallest details of life."[80] If so, it is arguable from the Stoic perspective that to terminate a malformed infant is, in fact, to exercise a duty in accordance with God. For God (Nature) may be said to ordain infanticide as an act of human reason in conformity with divine justice on those occasions when we correctly grasp the difference between what is useless and what is sound.

However, this Stoic position raises a definite criteriological problem concerning just how to tell when an infant is sufficiently defective to be judged useless. It also ignores the related difficulty of determining exactly in reference to whom the infant's life should be judged useful or useless. Therefore, these difficulties cast serious doubt on the soundness of Seneca's position on infanticide. The position on abortion is equally flawed: one can plausibly pressure the tenuous Stoic claim that the relationship of a pregnant woman to her fetus is merely analogous to that of a tree to its unripened fruit.[81] Persons and trees are such vastly different forms of life that it is only with incredible effort that this analogy can be made to stick. For these reasons, the above Stoic arguments in support of abortion and infanticide are fraught with serious difficulties.

SUMMARY

To summarize our findings on the moral positions adopted by Pythagoras, Plato, Aristotle, and Seneca on the question of abortion and infanticide, Pythagoras alone was opposed to both of these measures. For the Pythagoreans, human life was said to begin at conception. It was a duty to God not to injure human or other sentient life. For bodily life, into which divine souls had descended as a punishment, possessed derivative value as the temporary residence in which souls could be purified by choosing to live wisely. Hence, to terminate either fetal or infant life was wrong because it deprived the victim of the immediate opportunity to at least attempt to live an embodied, earthly life in such a way as to win for his soul both the admiration and divine invitation of the gods. For this reason, the Pythagoreans also likely would have taken a dim view of contraception, though there is no evidence that it was formally condemned.

As for Plato, he was an advocate of both abortion and infanticide in the *Republic*. He saw in these biomedical measures the opportunity to promote the best possible offspring. Therefore, on utilitarian grounds predicated on his understanding of eugenic principles, he prescribed abortion and infanticide in specific circumstances that he judged to be useful to the overall quality of life in his utopia. These circumstances included the endorsement of infanticide for defective newborns or those born of parents considered past their prime for childbearing and the endorsement of abortion in cases of adultery, premarital sex, or other unauthorized sexual unions that bore fruit. Although Plato does not address the question of contraception per se, he probably would have encouraged it for those couples that had exceeded his prescribed age for childbearing but were still sexually active. Since Platonists held that human life did not begin until birth, neither abortion nor contraception was considered to be morally objectionable.

As we saw, Aristotle, like Plato, also endorsed both abortion and infanticide on utilitarian grounds. But he put the start of actual human life at some point in utero when the fetus is informed by the rational soul, after first receiving at conception the nutritive and then, not long after, the sensitive souls. In *Politics,* Aristotle emphasized population control as a way to reduce poverty and civil unrest. But his argument in favor of infanticide was restricted to cases of defective infants alone. I argued that Aristotle's argument is ultimately grounded on his vision of the minimal good life and his implied judgment that highly defective newborns were better off dead in view of their permanent deficiencies, not to mention their possible drain on the resources of the well-functioning community. Furthermore, Aristotle considered abortion morally justifiable for population control purposes alone only when the fetus is incapable of sensation. But, as I argued, at what point an individual fetus acquires a sensitive soul is very difficult to say with precision, using Aristotle's embryological guidelines. Therefore, the practical application of his moral theory on abortion appears flawed. I conjecture, in addition, that Aristotle might have ideally preferred contraception over abortion in the eligible case. If such measures had been effective (which they were not in his day), they would have limited population without raising the serious epistemological and practical problems of the sort described.

In contrast with Aristotle, the later Stoics considered human life in the biological sense to begin at birth with the child's first breath. It was not until the individual reached young adulthood (around the age of fourteen) that he became a person in the moral sense, with the full protection of the moral rule against homicide. But, like Aristotle, Seneca and the other Stoics prescribed infanticide for defective newborns alone on moral, if not religious, grounds. The defective newborn was taken to be so bereft of the opportunity to acquire the virtues necessary in order to live with some semblance of tranquility that it was considered an act of reason to acknowledge their unfitness by actively hastening their death. In addition, the Stoic position on abortion was more permissive than Aristotle's. The Stoics definitely opposed the Pythagorean perspective, which unconditionally protected fetal life. Their liberal approval of abortion even exceeded Plato's position in the *Republic*; unlike the Stoics, Plato would have at least required the prior consent of the state. But the Stoics likened the fetus to the fruit of the tree before it was ripe and had descended. Strictly speaking, the fetus possessed no moral worth of its own (since it had neither a *psyche* nor rationality) and was ontologically akin to a mere plant. From this analogy, the Stoics argued that women had the discretionary right to abort at their own option. In so doing, they chose to ignore the critical disanalogies to which their argument was also vulnerable.

But just as at life's beginning the human community faces questions of moral import, so too at life's end. To this latter group of questions we now turn in examining various ancient moral arguments for and against euthanasia.

Discussion Questions

1. Were infanticide and abortion both legal in Greece and Rome? Were these practices widely considered morally acceptable?
2. How effective were ancient methods of contraception? Was abortion the only means of limiting family size?

3. What was the likely role of midwives in caring for expectant mothers? In procuring abortions?
4. What philosophical school opposed both infanticide and abortion? Why?
5. The Stoic Seneca supported a woman's right to an abortion by comparing her fetus to a body part. Is this analogy valid?
6. Review the nine common reasons cited that sometimes drove women in antiquity to abortion or infanticide. Do any of these motivations persist today? If so, which ones?
7. In Rome, was it legal for a married woman to secure an abortion without her husband's prior consent?

NOTES

1. It appears certain that Galen wrote no commentary on the Hippocratic Oath, and he nowhere mentions the Oath by name. What his personal views were on abortion, infanticide, or euthanasia is highly conjectural. But since he much admired Aristotle's ethical theories, it is possible that he followed Aristotle pretty closely on these matters, too. Norman E. Himes reports that one ". . . Dr. Moissides of Athens informs me that he has searched the works of Galen and has been able to find no discussion of contraception." (See Norman E. Himes, *Medical History of Contraception* [Baltimore, MD: Williams and Wilkins, Co., 1936], p. 75.) Similarly, I am unaware of any direct evidence of Galen's views on abortion.

2. Typical of such a commitment to the relation between doing good and faring well is Plato at *Republic* 10.621d. There is an instructive discussion of eudaimonism in Vernon J. Bourke, *History of Ethics*, 2 vols. (New York: Image Books, 1970), vol. 1, chaps. 1–3. See also Alasdair MacIntyre, *A Short History of Ethics* (New York: Macmillan, 1976), chaps. 7–8, for a useful comparison of ancient eudaimonism and contemporary moral theory.

3. William E. Lecky, *History of European Morals: From Augustus to Charlemagne*, 2 vols. (London: Longmans, Green, and Co., 1905); see especially vol. 2, pp. 19ff.

4. Edward A. Westermarck, *The Origin and Development of the Moral Ideas,* 2 vols. (London: Macmillan, 1906–8); see especially vol. 1, pp. 393–413 (chap. 18, "The Killing of Parents, Sick Persons, Children–Feticide").

5. Will Durant, *The Story of Civilization,* 10 vols. (New York: Simon and Schuster, 1939), vols. 2 and 3.

6. The exception here was the Greek city of Thebes. It is conjectured that the Pythagorean, Philolaus, who was known to have advocated a strict respect-for-human-life ethic, lived in Thebes and succeeded in influencing that city's legislation, which, according to legend, barred both infanticide and suicide. The principal evidence for such laws is to be found in Aelian's *Varia Historiae* 2.7, cited by William Lecky, *European Morals*, vol. 2, p. 26. Yet there is reason to believe that the Theban law referred only to healthy, not deformed, infants. The crime was punishable by death in any case.

7. In A.D. 318, the Christian emperor, Constantine, falling under the influence of the Judeo-Christian respect-for-human-life ethic, declared the act of fathers slaying their sons and daughters at any age a crime. According to William L. Langer, "Infanticide: A Historical Survey," *History of Childhood Quarterly, The Journal of Psychohistory* 1 (1974): 355, Constantine never explicitly forbade infanticide by name, though pre-

sumably he meant to include it. But infanticide was made a crime punishable by death toward the end of the fourth century by the emperors Valentinian, Valens, and Gratian. All this must be understood in the context of ancient Roman legal powers, extending back to the early Roman republic, which gave the *paterfamilias* the legal power (*patria potestas*) of life and death over members of his household, especially his children and slaves. Similar laws or customs were ascribed to Greek fathers during the Archaic period. William Langer, commenting on infanticide and the laws of the late Roman Empire, notes that even the Christian emperors were somewhat ambivalent. For example, they did nothing to abolish exposure (a passive form of infanticide) or the sale of exposed children (by those who rescued such children) as slaves. In fact, it was not until the time of Justinian in A.D. 529 that the subjection of foundlings to slavery was outlawed. (See Langer, "Infanticide," p. 363, note 8.)

8. This is not to imply that there were *no* voices to be heard during pagan times in opposition to abortion or infanticide. Among those writers from the Roman period who described the widespread practice of abortion with disapproval were Ovid (*De nuce* 22–23); Seneca (*Ad Helviam* 16); *Favorinus* (quoted by Aulus Gellius in his *Noctes Atticae* 12.1); and Juvenal (*Sat.* 6.592). At Athens during the golden age, both custom and law provided that on or before the *tenth day* of its new life, the infant was formally accepted into his family in a religious ritual around the hearth, receiving presents from well-wishers and a name. Parents who thereafter exposed such children to die were punished by the state. (See Durant, *Civilization*, vol. 2, pp. 287–88 and Westermarck, *Moral Ideas*, vol. 1, p. 410.) In Hellenistic times, the Jewish philosopher Philo Judaeus (ca. 30 B.C.–A.D. 45) denounced the exposure of children on religious grounds, calling it murder. Early Christian writers like Tertullian (ca. A.D. 160–ca. 240), an active proponent of the Judeo-Christian respect-for-human-life religious ethic, condemned as morally wrong not only infanticide but also abortion. For he construed the developing fetus as a human life, declaring, "He also is a man who is about to be one. Even every fruit already exists in its seed" (Tertullian *Apologeticus* 9).

9. This was particularly a motive of some upper class Hellenistic and Roman women. "Seneca thinks Helvia worthy of special praise because she has never destroyed her expected child within her womb 'after the fashion of many other women, whose attractions are to be found in their beauty alone,'" states Westermarck, *Moral Ideas*, vol. 1, p. 416. He quotes Seneca from *Ad Helviam* 16. See also Durant, *Civilization*, vol. 1, p. 567.

10. Writing on infanticide in antiquity, William Langer suggests that "modern humanitarian sentiment makes it difficult to recapture the relatively detached attitude of the parents toward their offspring. Babies were looked upon as the unavoidable result of normal sex relations, often as an undesirable burden rather than as a blessing." (See Langer, "Infanticide," p. 355.) While this may be *part* of the story, I think Langer may mislead his readers into thinking that little warmth or compassion was commonly felt and expressed by Greek and Roman parents toward their young. This is, of course, an unwarranted inference. Once parents decided to keep their newborn (a decision customarily made within a day or two of its birth), they were standardly raised with a great deal of indulgence and affection.

11. This was no doubt a recurring motive for both abortion and infanticide. William Lecky states that "Quintilian [fl. A.D. 60] speaks in a tone of apology, if not justification, of the exposition of the children *of destitute parents* (*Declamationes* 306) and even Plutarch speaks of it without censure (*De Amor. Prolis.*)." (See Lecky, *European Morals*, vol. 2, p. 28, note 1, emphases added.)

12. The Greeks felt the pressures of population growth more than the Romans. The Greek city-state was comparatively small, and the mainland provided proportionately little arable land. Rome was expanding its territories and was in need of citizens for soldiering and colonization. Hesiod, Plato, Aristotle, and Polybius, among others, discussed various aspects of the population problem. Hesiod, Xenocrates, and Lycurgus were partisans of the one-child family, Himes claims, and, as we shall soon see, Plato and Aristotle favored a stationary population. (See Himes, *Contraception*, p. 79, and M. Moissides, "Le Malthusianisme dans l'Antiquite Greque," *Janus* 36 (1932): 169–79, cited by Norman Himes.

13. See female infanticide, p. 118.

14. Therapeutic abortion was practiced by the ancients as is clear from the testimony of Soranus. See p. 174.

15. It is well known that the Spartans practiced eugenics. The newborn was subjected both to (1) the father's right to kill any of his defective offspring, as well as (2) the state's right to inspect and kill babies that appeared too weak. According to Durant, ". . . any child that appeared defective [to the Spartan council of inspectors] was thrown from a cliff of Mt. Taygetus, to die on the jagged rocks below." (See Durant, *Civilization*, vol. 2, p. 81.) Infanticide was also practiced at Athens, though it was not a legal obligation, nor did the state engage in inspection or eugenics per se. None of this must obscure the fact that healthy infants were killed throughout Greece and Rome; though public opinion was mixed on the morality of this, it was tolerated.

16. During Hellenistic times, abortion was punishable by the law only if a husband's consent was not first secured by his wife. One motive for a wife not securing it was her desire to conceal her adultery. Hence, it was also punishable if a married woman got an abortion at the instigation of her seducer. (See Durant, *Civilization*, vol. 2, p. 567.) Eduard Westermarck states that in Rome abortion " . . . was prohibited by Septimius Severus (ca. A.D. 145–211) and Antoninus, but the prohibition seems to have referred only to those married women who, by procuring abortion, defrauded their husbands of children." (See Westermack, *Moral Ideas*, vol. 1, p. 415.)

17. The Roman satirist Juvenal (fl. A.D. 80) speaks to this when he instructs a husband "rejoice; give her the potion . . . for were she to bear the child you might find yourself the father of an Ethiopian." (Juvenal *Satires* 5.141, cited by Durant, *Civilization*, vol. 3, p. 364.)

18. The main exception here is the Spartan women, who did receive some military training.

19. This judgment of a female child's worth was naturally linked to emergent social customs and institutional expectations. The revolutionary character of Plato's reforms for women in Greek society, whereby they are made full-fledged rulers, soldiers, and artisans in his ideally conceived state may be understood in part as a bold rejection of the normally low status accorded women in classical Greek society. Though he does endorse infanticide on eugenic grounds in his *Republic*, Plato does not favor the preservation of the male child over the female child—as did his countrymen at large. Hence, Plato's advocacy of equality between the sexes extends to his policies on infant care and selection. (Plato *Republic* 445b–466d passim.)

20. For a complete discussion of their contributions, see Joseph Needham, *A History of Embryology*, 2nd rev. ed. (New York: Abelard-Schuman, 1959), pp. 27–31.

21. Himes, *Contraception*, p. 80. See Aristotle, *History of Animals* 4.583a.

22. Sigerist, *History of Medicine*, vol. 2, p. 230. Norman E. Himes devotes an entire chapter to "The History of the Condom or Sheath." In it he concludes that such devices

were known in antiquity, at least by Imperial Roman times, " . . . though we know nothing of the extent of such use. In the absence of more positive knowledge, we must assume that it was not in common use." (See Himes, *Contraception*, chap. 8, p. 188.)

23. Littré, *Oeuvres*, vol. 7, p. 415, cited by Himes, *Contraception*, p. 81. This unusual contraceptive formula is, in fact, given again in the Hippocratic Collection at Littré, *Oeuvres*, vol. 8, p. 171.

24. Lucretius, *On the Nature of Things*, trans. H. A. I. Munro (London: Bell, 1913), pp. 165–66, cited by Himes, *Contraception*, p. 83.

25. Ibid., p. 166.

26. Ibid., p. 167.

27. *Soranus's Gynecology*, trans. Temkin, p. 62.

28. Ibid., p. 63.

29. See my remarks on this matter in note 10.

30. Durant, *Civilization*, vol. 2, p. 568.

31. Polybius *Histories* 36.17, trans. W. R. Paton, cited by Durant, *Civilization*, vol. 2, p. 568.

32. Durant, *Civilization*, vol. 2, p. 567.

33. This definition purposely does not conform in every detail to the latest lexical definition now in use by contemporary physicians. One variant of the latter standardly includes what laymen often call miscarriages. Hence, nowadays abortion is defined in medical parlance as "termination of pregnancy, *spontaneously* or by induction, prior to viability. Thereafter termination of pregnancy is called delivery," according to André E. Helleger, "Abortion: Medical Aspects," in *EB*, vol. 1, pp. 2–3. The definition I am using, however, captures the central sense in which the term was usually employed in the ancient medical literature, especially when moral appraisals were offered.

34. Sigerist, *History of Medicine*, vol. 2, p. 230. In general, see R. Hähnel, "Der künstliche Abortus in Alterum," *Archiv für Geschichte der Medizin* 29 (1936): 224ff.

35. Littré, *Oeuvres*, vol. 8, p. 610, cited by Sigerist, *History of Medicine*, vol. 2, p. 230.

36. Ibid.

37. Durant, *Civilization*, vol. 2, p. 287, and vol. 3, p. 365. See also Westermarck, *Moral Ideas,* vol. 1, p. 40, and Lecky, *European Morals*, vol. 2, p. 28.

38. Terence *Heauton-timorumenos*, Act III, Scene 5, cited by Lecky, *European Morals*, vol. 2, p. 28, note 1.

39. Ibid., emphases added. Another similar literary example occurs in Apuleius, *Metamorphosis* 10. It, too, involves a mother's pity for her female infant that her husband commanded her to kill.

40. Will Durant states, "Sometimes, in the first century, girls or illegitimate children were exposed, usually at the base of the Columna Lactaria—so named because the state provided wet nurses to feed and save the infants found there." (See Durant, *Civilization*, vol. 3, p. 364.) Even so, it is true that more often than not exposed infants throughout antiquity died.

41. *Collected Dialogues*, trans. F. M. Cornford, p. 854.

42. Sigerist, *History of Medicine*, vol. 2, p. 232.

43. Soranus, *Gynecology*, trans. Temkin, p. xl.

44. See note 16.

45. Notice that *unlike* the Oath's prohibition against surgery in its very next paragraph (see P5, p. 84), in the case of abortion the Oath-taker does not say that he "will withdraw

in favor of such men [or women] as are engaged in this work." This strongly implies that the Oath's prohibition against abortion is absolute. Moreover, it is not intended to protect the holiness of the physician *alone*. It is intended to protect the patient and the fetus from moral wrongdoing as well. Moreover, Durant states that by the time of the Roman Empire, women were engaged in medicine not only as midwives but as doctors. Though he may exaggerate their numbers, he claims: "There were many women physicians; some of them wrote manuals of abortion, which were popular among great ladies and prostitutes." (See Durant, *Civilization*, vol. 3, p. 313.)

46. Prophyry *Pros Garaun.* See Edelstein, "Hippocratic Oath," p. 19, note 42.

47. Edelstein, "Hippocratic Oath," p.19. Edelstein also notes that the ascetic rigor engendered in the Pythagorean way of life, scientific beliefs aside, militated against abortion. For example, extramarital relations were banned, and coitus, even in matrimony, was only considered honorable if it aimed at producing children.

48. Diogenes Laertius *De vitis* 8.28–29.

49. Ibid., 8.36, cited by John M. Robinson, trans., *Early Greek Philosophy,* p. 61, emphasis added.

50. Frankena, "Respect for Life," p. 25.

51. This observation adds some support to the ancient tradition that ascribes to Pythagoras possible travels to the East, perhaps as far as Babylonia, between the time he left Samos and before he settled in Croton, on the east coast of southern Italy, around 530 B.C. But Herodotus is surely mistaken in ascribing to the Egyptians (*Histories* 2.123) a belief in the transmigration of souls, and further implying that the Pythagoreans (though he does not name them) borrowed that doctrine from Egypt. In any case, there is no evidence that the Pythagoreans ascribed souls to vegetative life or regarded it as sinful to take such life. This is why, strictly speaking, they do not fully qualify as embracing a *comprehensive* respect-for-life ethic, though they come close.

52. See chapter 3.

53. At *Republic* 10.621b–c, Er states that after the souls whom he observed in the afterworld had suffered their punishments and rewards and had selected their next earthly, soon-to-be-embodied lives, each drank from the River of Forgetfulness. He states: "When they had fallen asleep, at midnight there was thunder and an earthquake, and in a moment they were carried up . . . *to their birth* . . . " (See *Republic*, trans. Cornford, p. 359, emphases added.)

54. *Republic* 5.461, trans. Cornford, p. 161.

55. Ibid.

56. The relevant passage on which I base this claim is *Republic* 5.461a–c.

57. For a somewhat less restrictive and seemingly more humane set of regulations bearing on matters relating to population control and the abortion option, see Plato *Laws* 5.740d. There, Plato does not say that he endorses abortion or infanticide in order to control populations in excess of 5,040—a number he deemed ideal for the state. In fact, he refers to setting up colonies abroad from the mother country as "the last resort." Hence, it is conceivable that in his old age, Plato drew back a bit from the position he advocates at *Republic* 5.462. Plato's handling of adulterous citizens is also greatly toned down at *Laws* 6.784–5 and 8.841ff.

58. *Republic* 5.460ff., trans. Cornford, p. 160.

59. Aristotle *Politics* 7.1265b.10ff., trans. Ernest Barker, *The Politics of Aristotle* (Oxford: Oxford University Press, 1946).

60. Aristotle *Politics* 7.1265b.5ff.

61. See p. 119. The ideal size of a city-state, according to Aristotle, was 10,000.
62. Aristotle *Politics,* trans. Barker, emphases added. The Greek of the final sentence reads, in part: " . . . *tei aisthesei kai to zen estai.*"
63. See Aristotle *Nicomachean Ethics* 1.8 and *Rhetoric* 1.5.
64. See chapter 3, pp. 60–62.
65. Another word in Greek meaning life was *bios.* This word referred not to biological life per se, but rather to an individual's personal experiences as in "the course of life." (See Liddell and Scott, *Greek–English Lexicon,* p. 130.) The word *zoa* in Greek also meant life, but especially life in the sense of what we would now call biological subsistence (ibid., p. 297). Hence, when to this list is added a third Greek word, *psyche,* meaning in our day the "life of the spirit" or "mind," but capable of meaning in Aristotle's day life *simpliciter,* it becomes imperative that the concept of life Aristotle intended in his writing on abortion be specified. Minimally, he means that the human fetus ought not be aborted if it possesses life (*zen*) at such a level that it has the sensitive capacity (*aisthesis*) to feel pleasure or pain. This latter capacity is found in almost all animals and in higher forms of life, according to Aristotle.
66. Significantly, the verb *empsychoo* in Greek meant "to animate." The Latin word *anima* was associated with the Greek word for soul (*psyche*), and was often used to contrast the body. Also, *anima* originally denoted the sign of life: breath. (See Liddell and Scott, *Greek–English Lexicon,* p. 798.) It is directly from this Latin word *anima,* not the Greek *psyche,* that we get the animate-inanimate distinction in English. This is a distinction standardly made between things that are alive and capable of self-movement, and those that are not. Aristotle, moreover, held that plants moved in the minimal sense of undergoing generation, growth, and decay. Plants did not, however, possess locomotion, as did most (but not all) animals.
67. David Ross, *Aristotle* (New York: Harper and Row, 1974), p. 134, and, for a more detailed account of Aristotle's psychology, pp. 129–42.
68. The relevant passages are: *De Anima* 414a.2–4; 415a.3–6; 435a.12. Aristotle has it that as an outgrowth of the sensitive soul there occurs in most animals, on the cognitive side, imagination (of which memory is a further development); and, on the appetitive side, the capacity for movement (locomotion).
69. Aristotle elsewhere states: "What is called *effluxion* is a destruction of the embryo within the first week, while *abortion* occurs up to the fortieth day." (Aristotle *Historia Animalium* 8.3.583a.10ff, emphases added.) His switch from "effluxion" to "abortion" in this passage cannot have been arbitrary, it seems to me. "Effluxion" probably signals the conceptus possessing the nutritive soul alone. See D. W. Thompson, trans., *The Works of Aristotle,* eds. J. A. Smith and W. D. Ross, 11 vols. (Oxford: Clarendon Press, 1910), vol. 4, p. 583.
70. *Historia Animalium* 8.3.583b, in Thompson, trans. *The Works of Aristotle,* vol. 4, p. 583. By "distinct parts," Aristotle means the presence of heterogeneous organs, such as hands, eyes, heart, etc.; by "fleshlike substance," he means homogeneous constituents, such as tissue, blood, and bones. In his embryological theory, Aristotle embraced a theory of epigenesis, according to which the individual organism develops by structural elaboration of the unstructured zygote rather than by a simple enlarging of a preformed entity.
71. According to Crawley, "Foeticide," in *ERE,* vol. 6, p. 56. Aristotle's followers grappled with this issue, attempting to bring certainty and consistency to his teachings on abortion. "His followers distinguished between the male and female embryo in the

date of animation. The male was regarded as being forty days after conception, the female eighty days [sic]. Later the moment of animation was fixed for both sexes at the fortieth day. The Roman jurists adopted the latter view. The general distinction between the animate and the inanimate foetus was clearly held by Canon and Roman law alike, and lasted to modern times. It was applied by Augustine thus: 'The body is created before the soul. The embryo before it is endowed with a soul *and is informatus*, as its destruction by human agency is to be punished with a fine. The embryo *formatus* is endowed with a soul; it is an animate being: its destruction is murder, and is to be punished with death.'" (See Augustine *Questiones in Exodum* 80; *Questiones Veteris et Novi Testamenti* 23, cited by Crawley.) Variants of this distinction endured in Roman Catholic theology until A.D. 1869, at which time Pope Pius IX formally eliminated the distinction between an animated and unanimated fetus. He further decreed that all fetuses should be considered ensouled from conception and that therefore *any* abortion was equivalent to murder.

72. Seneca *Consolation to Marcia* 24.4, trans. M. Hadas, cited by Choron, *Death and Western Thought*, p. 69, emphases added.

73. Seneca Consolation to Marcia 22.3.

74. As a major Hellenistic philosophical movement, Stoicism flourished for well over five centuries. It originated in the fourth century B.C. with its founder, Zeno of Citium (ca. 336–264 B.C.) and counted among its many adherents the Roman Emperor Marcus Aurelius, who ruled from A.D. 161 to 180. Traditionally, Stoic thought is divided into three main periods during which there occurred significant changes in doctrine. Roughly, these periods are early (336–186 B.C.); middle (185–5 B.C.); and late (4 B.C.–A.D. 200). Seneca belongs to the last of these periods. Yet, he was influenced by the Middle Stoics, Panaetius and Posidonius, with whose views on the development of the human soul I here associate him. Seneca wrote no treatise on human embryology. My account of his theory of human personhood is thus necessarily speculative. I am indebted to Michael Frede, Princeton University, for clarifying some of the details of Stoic moral psychology. An unusually concise and useful treatment of the Stoics can be found in F. H. Sandbach, *The Stoics* (New York: W. W. Norton, 1975).

75. *Stoicorum Veterum Fragmenta* 2, cited by Edelstein, "Hippocratic Oath," p. 18, note 42. For a useful description and analysis of Stoic psychology, see R. D. Hicks, *Stoic and Epicurean* (New York: Russell and Russell, 1962), pp. 60–63. Concurrent with these Stoic doctrines, it may be observed that Roman law and custom distinguished sharply between abortion and infanticide in the following way: The unborn child was not said to be *homo* (a human being), nor was it even an *infans* (infant). Rather, it was said to be a *spes animantis* ("the prospect of a living being"). (See Crawley, "Foeticide," in *ERE*, vol. 6, p. 56.)

76. This useful distinction between the *moral* and *biological* (or what she calls the "genetic") sense of the term "human" has been pointed out by Mary Anne Warren. See her "On the Moral and Legal Status of Abortion," *The Monist* 57 (1973): 43–61. In general, unless I indicate otherwise or the context clearly demands the biological sense, it is personhood in the *moral* sense with which this investigation is most concerned.

77. See note 7, and Crawley, "Foeticide," in *ERE*, vol. 6, p. 56, who has it that the father *alone* could legally order an abortion in Rome.

78. Spangenberg, "Verbrechen der Abtreibung der Leibesfrucht," in *Neue Archiv des Criminalrechts*, vol. 2, pp. 22ff., cited by Crawley, "Foeticide," in *ERE*, vol. 6, p. 56

and Westermarck, *Moral Ideas*, vol.1, p. 415. The modern reader recognizes in this Stoic defense of the discretionary right of a woman to seek an abortion the paradigm of contemporary arguments of a similar sort. In particular, there is the contemporary, proabortion argument that asserts a woman's putative property rights over her body, likens the fetus to any one of her organs, and concludes that the discretionary right of a woman to have her appendix removed extends, by analogy, to her right to abort or not. Criticisms against these and other contemporary variants of Stoic and related ancient positions for and against abortion are readily available. For specific criticisms of the property rights argument, see Joseph Margolis, *Negativities: The Limits of Life* (Columbus, OH: Charles E. Merrill Publishing Co., 1976), chap. 3, pp. 45ff., and Joel Feinberg, *Matters of Life and Death*, ed. Tom Regan (New York: Random House, 1980), pp. 203–5.

79. Seneca *De ira* 1.15.
80. Hicks, *Stoic and Epicurean*, p. 26.
81. Some commentators are fond of quoting Seneca's *Consolation to Helvia*, his mother, in which (at 16.3) he praises her for not crushing " . . . the hope of children that were being nurtured in your body," as if Seneca were opposed to abortion. This, however, misses the point. The Stoics never argued that women ought to abort, only that it was their *discretionary right* to do so. In other words, she has neither the strict duty to bear, nor the obligation to abort her child. Hence, although her choice is sovereign in respect to the fate of the fetus, this does not bar the moral community from criticizing some women as thoughtless or frivolous in their exercise of this right. It is in this tradition that Seneca praises his mother. For he personally holds in contempt women whose " . . . only recommendation lies in their beauty," and who therefore regard pregnancy " . . . as if an unseemly burden," as he says in that same passage. (See Seneca, *Moral Essays*, trans. John W. Basore [London: William Heinemann, 1932], vol. 2, pp. 471–73.)

7 The Problem of Euthanasia

*By happy dispensation all travel to an end
which sets free from woe.*

—PINDAR

PRELIMINARY CONSIDERATIONS

Suicide and Language

In our prior examination of attitudes toward death, I argued that the Greek concept of euthanasia (a) referred to a manner of dying; (b) literally translated meant an easy or good death; and (c) logically entailed no one particular theory about what happened to the dead. This account must now be expanded in two important ways.

First, the modern reader, accustomed to restricting the current English versions of this concept to discussions of mercifully ending the life of a hopelessly suffering or defective patient, must appreciate that the Greek use of the term was broader in scope. The Greeks sometimes employed the term to describe *the spiritual state* of the dying person at the impending approach of death. Hence, euthanasia was a term far broader in scope than contemporary English usage normally allows: its meaning was not anchored in medical contexts alone, though some of these contexts were also covered by it.

Second, for the Greeks euthanasia did not necessarily imply a means or method of causing or hastening death. However, when quick-acting and relatively painless drugs such as hemlock were first developed by the Greeks in the fifth century B.C., which allowed the individual to quit life in an efficient and bloodless manner, the linguistic result was that these forms of suicide were sometimes described as instances of euthanasia. But, even then, this ascription primarily involved a favorable appraisal of the subject's state of mind, not the means by which death came. Hence, on the whole there were no rigidly followed rules that fixed the application of the term euthanasia to contexts involving terminal illness or suicide alone, even though these situations could be properly referred to in selected cases.

Having thus recognized at the outset the decidedly broader scope that the concept of euthanasia enjoyed among the Greeks in comparison with the narrower contemporary English usage of this term, I propose to investigate one small piece of this Greek concept that comes closest to, and, in fact, originally included, what is often meant today by euthanasia. I am referring to the notion of *voluntary* euthanasia. This is characteristically defined to mean that with the prior consent of the patient, either the patient or someone else may bring about a relatively quick and painless death to one who is judged on medical grounds to be the victim of an untreatable, painful terminal illness or disability. This limited definition of the term in question admittedly involves only one of the several eligible senses in which that term may be used in our own historical epoch.[1] But, despite this limitation, it does succeed in capturing two relevantly allied meanings that wed it to its older Greek ancestor: namely, (1) voluntary euthanasia normally connotes a genuine human concern for the psychological state of mind of the suffering patient for whom life has apparently become an intolerable burden and (2) it crucially links the moral appraisal of the conduct of the patient (and those supplying his medical services) to the precondition that the patient is free to make a reasoned decision regarding the option to hasten or not hasten his own death.

To clarify further, (2) attests to the fact that the Greeks did not admit involuntary euthanasia as part of their general concept of euthanasia at all. If someone's life was terminated without his consent, normally this was *prima facie* a case of homicide. Such cases did not qualify as euthanasia principally because for adults, at least, it was popularly held that those who involuntarily died at the hands of others did not die well. Typically, they were not thought to have experienced good deaths. Just the opposite: if murdered, their souls were held to be restless, rancorous, and bent on revenge against their assailants.[2]

The obvious exception to all this was, of course, infanticide. But here the victim of infanticide was treated as a special case: a widely held Hellenistic view claimed that the infant was not really a human being until he was first fed.[3] Nor was pagan religion obsessed about the disposition of the deceased infant's soul, as Christianity would later be. Hence, since infants were usually killed before they were fed, popular moral condemnation did not normally attach to this deed. As for those infants who *were* fed, though they were later involuntarily killed as an act of mercy or prudence owing to their chronic and painful ill-health, their deaths were customarily deemed tragic and pitiable. Such deaths were not, in the Greek mind, standardly considered good or easy deaths either for the victims or the parents. At best, they were regarded as necessary. Perhaps reflecting this fact, popular Greco-Roman sentiment tended to resist the killing of *nondefective*, healthy infants, even though Roman law did not prohibit this practice until the fourth century A.D., as we have already noted. Therefore, infanticide, which is by its very nature involuntary since the infant lacks the verbal skills by which to give or withhold consent, was not customarily included in the Greek concept of euthanasia.

Also, (1) cannot be overemphasized. When talking about voluntary euthanasia, the current tendency is to freight the concept heavily with its moral, appraising sense. But doing so misses the dominant ancient connotation of this term, which *primarily* involved a psychological appraisal, and only secondarily a moral one. To illustrate this subtle difference, I suspect that the pivotal ancient question regarding euthanasia in its broadest sense was, typically: Did the subject voluntarily meet death with peace of mind and minimal pain? In contrast, the looming contemporary question involving euthanasia tends to be: Is euthanasia under any conditions morally justifiable?[4] Moreover, I do not think it is correct to infer from this that the Greeks were oblivious to the moral challenge voluntary euthanasia represented. They did not ignore the task of trying to furnish a coherent ethical defense of the practice. In fact, after we explore what some of the Greek and Roman philosophers had to say about the general question of the morality of suicide, I think quite the opposite impression will be left. At any rate, I do contend that the term's ability to confer or withhold a favorable appraisal of the apparent state of the subject's mind during his final conscious days and hours marked its primary linguistic function. Despite this emphasis, however, it is doubtless true that such a psychological appraisal was not readily separable from the allied moral appraisal of whether the subject evinced sound thinking, on moral or other grounds, for choosing to withdraw from life. Hence, the Greek *euthanasia* was indeed capable of bearing two senses, both psychological and moral, and surely in everyday discourse these two senses were sometimes mingled together.

As to the related notion of suicide—by which I here mean, in a rough and preliminary way, those forms of conduct in which the individual intentionally kills himself—the Greeks and Romans were generally sympathetic provided that the deed was done *for the right sorts of reasons*. Just what these reasons amounted to from the vantage point of some of the leading philosophical schools is a question that awaits our further treatment. Presently, it is worth noting that of all the ancient cultures it is in the Greek culture of the fifth and fourth centuries B.C. that suicide is first represented as a *mode of dying* instead of as an act of killing, which, historically, was its prior sense.[5] Why this is so can only be conjectured. But the philologist David Daube plausibly suggests that in the case of suicide, " . . . the most conspicuous thing for the onlooker is that a man kills himself: it is this arresting deed that the earliest words notice. That he dies in a certain fashion is a more subjective feature, a feature concerning him alone, to which attention is paid only at a later, more reflective stage."[6] It was especially due to the flowering of Greek philosophy and, I would add, to the peculiar emphasis of eudaimonist ethics, which tended to link isolated appraisals of acts of personal conduct to more general appraisals of the moral agent's whole way of life—from birth to approaching death—that likely fostered this higher reflective stage with respect to acts of suicide. For a person's life was viewed as a whole; and hence his birth, life, and death were open to moral as well as aesthetic evaluations based on considerations of proportion, measure, and order. To end life at the right time, then, approached an *aesthetic* challenge for some.

Furthermore, a second factor may have been the introduction and perfected use of hemlock. As a matter of fact, this agreeable potion reportedly did contribute to an increase in the suicide rate in antiquity.[7] Daube states:

> Its role in the human carrying out of capital sentences is familiar from the story of Socrates; and it may well have been a factor in the creation of such myths as that of a utopian island whose inhabitants, when the desirable maximum span of life is reached, take their leave by lying down on a plant that produces eternal sleep.
>
> It would also make for a linguistic turn toward a more passive concept of suicide—as a mode of dying rather than killing. When a man falls upon his sword, the external violence, *the killing*, is incomparably more impressive than when he takes a drink that brings about a slow ebbing away of his life—*a dying*.[8]

One can add to this the additional point that insofar as what we now call voluntary euthanasia was construed by the Greeks and Romans as one possible type of suicide, the phrase bears a definite family resemblance to the Latin expression for suicide, *mors voluntaria*, which also stressed the voluntary nature of such dying. In contrast, our English word "suicide"—literally, "self-killing"—lays stress on the peculiar fact that one's self is the object of one's killing. In this, the English language has lost touch with many of the most characteristic Greek and Roman expressions for suicide, which tended to emphasize suicide as a mode of death, and so decidedly downplayed the novel and sometimes violent side of self-killing. It is precisely this sort of linguistic legacy, incidentally, that in my view lends support to the claims of Joseph Margolis that, given the culturally variable character of the ascription of suicide, there can be no truly value-neutral concept of suicide. What is allowed or disallowed linguistically is always colored by some specific partisan perspective that is adopted (consciously or unconsciously) by the individual observer.[9]

Indeed, even within a single culture one may discover a rich and variable repertoire of expressions that refer to suicide. This is especially evident among the Greeks, whose historians, playwrights, and philosophers coined many such expressions. To sample just a few of these, Daube records Xenophon's *haireo thanaton* (to seize death); Euripides' *aporregnymi bion* (to break off life); Plato's *hekonein haidou* (to go voluntarily to Hades); Aristotle's *biazesthai heauton* (to flee living); and the Stoic's *eulogos exagoge* (sensible removal).[10] Surprisingly, the first noun phrase for suicide does not regularly appear in Greek until the first century B.C. It was *autocheiria*, "an act with one's own hand," or "own-handedness." Somewhat later, in the second century A.D., *autoktonia*, "self-killing," became standard.[11] But by that time the concept of suicide as *a way of dying*, rather than as a peculiar form of killing, was thoroughly embedded in Greco-Roman thought. Hence, such thinking regularly tended to overlook the literalness of these later noun phrases.

We must turn now to briefly consider two remaining points: First, the types of suicide recognized by the Greeks. And, second, the typical methods by which this act was carried out. Following that, we shall examine some of the leading philosophical schools to discover whether they would have supported or opposed that form of suicide we call voluntary euthanasia, and which the Greeks, too, would have thought of in that way.

Types and Methods

It is possible to distinguish at least eight recurring types of suicide that were recognized as such during the Greco-Roman period.[12] What distinguishes these from each other is primarily a variable estimate of the supposed motives of the subject for taking leave from this world. My purpose here is to suggest where in this constellation of ancient specimen cases having to do with self-murder the concept of voluntary euthanasia likely would have belonged.

It must be added that I shall limit my account to noncompulsory instances of suicide. It is true that the ancients sometimes forced people to take fatal poisons in capital executions. It is also true that they occasionally recognized cases of suicide that were thought to be linked to some sort of mental health disorder.[13] But the former case is of little concern to us here, since suicide by direct coercion precludes the relevant sort of moral appraisal of the praiseworthiness or blameworthiness of the agent's conduct. That is, one would surely not be inclined to praise or blame the conduct of one who had no other real choice but to imbibe a fatal poison; the question even may be legitimately raised as to whether this is, properly speaking, an instance of suicide at all. Similarly those individuals who, on account of some form of illness or disability, are judged to have lost control of their senses and conduct are thereby also rendered ineligible subjects of moral appraisal. In antiquity, as now, it was presumed that individuals so qualified were in some sense acting involuntarily.[14] But it is suicide in the Latin sense of a voluntary death (*mors voluntaria*) that deserves our utmost attention here, for we are preparing to analyze ancient philosophical arguments for and against noncompulsory instances of this deed. And these arguments ultimately presuppose some capacity for reason and choice on the part of the individual.

Resuming our main task, at least eight types of noncompulsory suicide, distinguishable primarily by their presumed leading motives, are discernible in Greek and Roman literature. These may be conveniently divided into two somewhat arbitrary groups. First, *heroic suicide*, characterized by the subject's desire to escape present or impending shame and dishonor; or the noble wish to devote one's life to one's country; or to slay oneself in order to relieve excessive grief. Second, *nonheroic suicide*, which, by degrees only, tended as a group not to be as inspiring to the ancients, perhaps partly because they were perceived to be on the whole more egoistically motivated or because they were thought to occur regularly in less glorious circumstances.

To the first (heroic) group belong four recurring cases motivated by: (1) the desire to escape shame and dishonor, as in the case of Ajax, who, after realizing that he had slaughtered his own camp's herds in a fit of madness, fell on his sword;[15] (2) the desire to demonstrate total self-devotion to one's country, as in the case of the last Athenian king, Kodras, who, after learning from the oracle at Delphi that the only way his country would not be captured by the Spartans was for him to die at their hands, arranged in that manner for his own self-sacrifice;[16] (3) the desire to end unrelieved grief over the death of a loved one, as in the sad tale of King Aegeus, who, owing to his receipt of the false signal that his son, Theseus, had perished, threw himself into the sea that today bears his name;[17] and (4) the desire to atone for the death one has accidentally caused to another person, as in the case of Adrastos, who, having inadvertently killed the son of Croesus, begs Croesus to arrange for his own death in recompense.[18]

To the second (nonheroic) group belong four additional types of suicide motivated by: (5) the desire to end personal grief owing to persistent and degrading poverty, which was explicitly recognized in the writing of Theogonis as sufficient cause to quit life;[19] (6) the desire to be reunited in death with a deceased loved one or companion, as in the case of Paris's beloved Oenone, who, owing to her intense longing and sorrow, threw herself on his funeral pyre;[20] (7) the desire to quit life owing to the sheer sense of how boring, pointless, and futile it may appear, a motive that, significantly, is often redescribed as a form of madness, since most bystanders are not so powerfully in agreement, and one that may have been at work in the mass suicides of the maidens of Miletos[21]; and, finally, (8) the desire to escape a relentlessly painful illness or infirmity, usually thought to be incurable in nature, and usually (though not always) associated with the approach of old age. This last type of suicide, which we may call voluntary euthanasia, is illustrated in the case of the elderly citizens of Ceos, who, once they had passed age sixty, were in the habit of taking leave from life by drinking hemlock.[22] Also, there is the case of Titus Aristo, who, not untypically by the period of the Roman Empire, carefully reasoned that he would end his life if his physicians reported that his insufferable illness was definitely beyond their means to cure.[23]

In sum, it is to this second group of nonheroic suicides that voluntary euthanasia in most cases belonged. The last illustration of the suffering patient, Aristo, and our preceding observations about the possession of lethal drugs by the ancient physician point to the unique opportunity of the doctor to declare his patient untreatable and, if so requested, supply to him the appropriate "cup of death." Since, especially by the late Hellenistic and Roman Imperial periods, almost all of the older religious stigmas attached to suicide had lost their force and since, excepting the cases of slaves and soldiers, civil penalties against suicide were practically unknown throughout both Greece and Rome, there was little to constrain an individual bent on quitting life from acting on his resolve.[24] The methods chosen are readily imaginable. They included, besides the ever-popular hem-

lock, self-immolation, jumping from high places, drowning, self-starvation, hanging, and running oneself through by the sword or dagger. Moreover, of these foregoing methods starvation alone would qualify in modern times as *passive* voluntary euthanasia, wherein the subject's death is brought about by *omitting* those
elements necessary to the support of biological life. The others would qualify as
active forms of euthanasia, wherein death occurs as the more immediate result of
committing a fatal act of some sort.[25]

All this prompts one to ask: On what moral grounds did some of the leading ancient philosophers support or oppose voluntary euthanasia (either active or
passive) in the sense we have characterized it above? In particular, what position
did the Pythagoreans, Plato, Aristotle, and the Stoic Seneca take on this issue, and
what bearing, if any, did their attitude toward death likely have on their moral or
religious reasoning in regard to suicide or euthanasia?

PHILOSOPHICAL PERSPECTIVES

Pythagoras

It is not necessary to re-examine here the tenets of Pythagoras already discussed
in the preceding chapter concerning the doctrines of (a) *divine personal immortality* of the soul; (b) transmigration of souls upon death; (c) earthly life as penal
servitude marked by the fallen soul's entombment in the body; and (d) earthly life
as an opportunity to purify the soul through the proper study of philosophy and
mathematics, so that one day the soul might be liberated and return to its origins
in heaven. Instead, let us focus on the fact that the Pythagorean opposition to all
forms of suicide, including euthanasia, ultimately rests on a religious principle
from which this moral teaching is derived. In our discussion of abortion, I alluded
to the Pythagorean religious principle that it is a direct violation of an individual's
higher duty to God to behave in such a way as to prematurely end his or another's
life. In the *Phaedo*, this principle appears to be linked by Socrates to the teachings of the fifth-century-B.C. Pythagorean Philolaus:

> The allegory which the mystics tell us—that we men are put in a sort of
> guard post, from which one must not release oneself or run away—seems
> to me to be a high doctrine *with difficult implications*. All the same, Cebes,
> I believe that this much is true: that the gods are our keepers, and we men
> are one of their possessions.[26]

The religious character of the absolute Pythagorean rejection of suicide is
readily discernible. The entire argument presupposes these crucial premises: (1)
God exists; (2) man's highest moral duty is always to obey the commands of God;
and (3) one of these divine commands unconditionally bars the individual from
taking early leave from his embodied, earthly existence. Therefore, if any one of

these three premises is, in turn, successfully undermined by the religious skeptic, the Pythagorean position against suicide at once collapses. Perhaps it is, in part, Plato's awareness of the inherent frailty of this religiously endowed argument that led him to make Socrates acknowledge the "difficult implications" of this perspective. For it is a perspective founded ultimately on mysticism and faith—not reason and dialectic—which Plato and Socrates both preferred, notwithstanding their own admitted religious tendencies.

Before leaving the Pythagoreans, I would like to make three related points having to do with my earlier claim that theirs was a philosophy imbued with the respect-for-human-life ethic. First, the word "life" is, as already noted, ambiguous.[27] One can have respect for: (a) each individual human life; (b) the life of the human species taken as a whole; (c) the life of one's lineage; and (d) the life of one's tribe, nation, or race. William Frankena is right in saying that it is primarily concern for (a), the individual's life, that is of central concern in bioethical discussions of euthanasia and abortion.[28] He is equally right, I think, in observing that, in speaking of the individual, we can speak of his bodily or physical life; and, in addition, we can speak of his mental or spiritual life. In the Pythagorean view, it is the *spiritual* life that has the highest value, owing to its divine religious character. Therefore, if bodily life has value, as it certainly does for the Pythagoreans, it is wholly parasitic on the value it receives from being the temporary residence of the divine soul. Even so, in our ordinary conversations about the value of human life, it is really *bodily* life that, for all intents and purposes, is minimally at issue. For it is most clearly life of this physical sort that is prevented or terminated in acts of abortion, infanticide, suicide, euthanasia, and the like.[29]

Second, to this must be added the distinction between respect for human life in the biological, physical sense just defined (*zoa*), and respect for the career and personality of the individual (*bios*). These two senses are by no means equivalent, as witnessed by the fact that one could assert without contradiction that, although Jones possessed life in the first sense, he was entirely devoid of life in the second sense following his unfortunate automobile accident. Hence, the alleged sanctity of human biological life, and the sanctity of human personality, bear at most a loose logical relation. If so, this implies, against the Pythagorean position, that one can fairly claim to be a partisan of the respect-for-human-life ethic, in the primary sense (a) taken above and still legitimately admit overriding conditions for the moral justification of euthanasia.

Third, it is revealing that throughout human history there have been few partisans who, without any qualification at all, have endorsed the respect-for-human-life ethic in and of itself. For if one were such a partisan, then one would have to be willing to assert that human bodily life has absolute value per se simply because it is human life. That claim would be taken as a basic, unappealable first principle. Yet even the Pythagoreans did not choose to make this basic claim; nor, incidentally, did the Christians of later antiquity.[30] For both groups found little satisfaction in such a bold, tautologous, and empty-sounding secular principle. And so, although from vastly different religious traditions, Pythagoreans and Christians alike made the value of human bodily life at least partly, if not totally, conditional on the higher and antecedent principle that God valued man. Therefore, it remains true that the Pythagoreans were partisans of the respect-for- human-life ethic. But, even for them, it is questionable whether human life was taken to be intrinsically valuable per se. Its value, though genuine and of binding importance for their medical ethics, was a *derivative* value resting ultimately on religious, not moral, considerations.

Plato

If one assumes that the opposition to suicide voiced by Socrates in the above-quoted *Phaedo* passage (see p. 153) mirrors the actual sentiments of Plato, and if one further considers the discussion of euthanasia for the incurably sick in passages from *Republic* and *Laws*, one senses an evolution taking place in Plato's thinking on this subject. It seems to me that the absolute opposition toward suicide voiced at *Phaedo* 62bff. is significantly softened at *Republic* 3.405ff. This is done in such a way as to furnish a moral argument in favor of rational suicide among the incurably ill. Moreover, at *Laws* 11.873cff., which was probably written when Plato was an old man himself approaching death, it appears that a decidedly intermediate position between the two earlier accounts is struck. The account finally given in the *Laws* both moderates and seeks to incorporate salient features of Plato's earlier antithetical positions.

Of the three relevant passages, scholars have devoted more attention to the *Phaedo* than to the other two combined. This is certainly understandable. The *Phaedo*, together with the *Apology* and *Crito*, includes the earliest sustained treatment of the timeless moral and legal questions associated with death and dying ever to have been bequeathed by antiquity to the modern era. A fair amount of attention has thus been paid to the problem of attempting to unravel which views in the trilogy were owned by the historical Socrates, and which by his student and admirer, Plato. I shall not stop here, however, to enter into that particular debate, but I shall venture to express my sympathy for those commentators who have linked the historical Socrates with the comparatively agnostic view toward death expressed by the figure of Socrates in the *Apology*. There, at *Apology* 40Cff., the following alternatives are advanced:

> Death is one of two things. *Either* it is annihilation, and the dead have no consciousness of anything, *or*, as we are told, it is really a change—a migration of the soul from this place to another. Now, if there is no consciousness but only a dreamless sleep, death must be a marvelous gain. . . . If, on the other hand, death is a removal from here to some other place, and if what we are told is true, that all the dead are there, what greater blessing could there be than this, gentlemen?[31]

Significantly, although Socrates does not here claim to know which account of being dead is correct, he does claim that in either case death is nothing to fear.

What's more, this was an original insight, the importance of which was not lost on the Epicureans and Stoics who followed in the Socratic tradition of debunking the terrors of the afterworld.

If we recast Socrates' preceding disjunction into the terminology suggested in chapter 3 of this book, his position comes close to saying that at death one faces either the prospect of (1) *natural personal dissolution* or (2) a variant of *chthonic personal immortality*. (The latter he strives to dress up in order to emphasize the potential for pleasantries even in Hades!) The above digression into the question of what happens when one dies is settled in the *Phaedo*. For there Socrates is made to embrace the second disjunct: the soul is immortal. Moreover, the immortality it possesses is depicted not with Homeric, chthonic imagery, but rather with the Orphic-Pythagorean imagery associated with *divine personal immortality*. Furthermore, life itself is now described as a preparation for death. The true philosopher does not recoil with fear at the thought of his own death but anticipates it with longing. For death, the separation of the soul from the body, at last affords him the ultimate opportunity to behold universal knowledge in its purest splendor, unencumbered by the mere appearances and base distractions with which he had formerly been afflicted while embodied on earth.

All this brings us to a central puzzle regarding the moral acceptability of suicide in the *Phaedo*; namely, if it is conceded for discussion's sake that the above account in the *Phaedo* represents a true picture of the afterworld, is it not then natural to ask why philosophers at least—after their souls have been sufficiently purified—ought not take early leave from their inferior bodies by suiciding? To this question Socrates unequivocally replies (*Phaedo* 62Cff.): "No man has the right to take his own life, but he must wait until God sends some necessity upon him, as he has now sent to me."[32] Socrates' reasoning here also appears to be grounded on religious premises. It bears a faint resemblance to the Pythagorean metaphor (see p. 153) of the soul being required to serve a faithful guard duty for and in the body as a form of penance from which " . . . one must not release oneself or run away."

But on closer inspection, Socrates' argument is not quite the same as the Pythagoreans'. First of all, it is conjectural whether Socrates or Plato embraced the Orphic-Pythagorean view that embodied life is a penal servitude for past sins. It was not central to Socrates' teaching, nor was it central to Plato's, that human life was a form of punishment. Instead, both men acknowledged the mixed character of human existence, and both emphasized the value of living a reflective philosophical life in order to successfully meet the challenges of this middling, earthly plane. Second, the Pythagoreans, emphasizing the penance constituted by human life as a duty placed on man by the gods, argued that humans therefore had no right to end their penance by committing suicide.

This is not, however, the content of the full argument developed by Socrates at *Phaedo* 62b–cff. Rather, Socrates is made to rest his case against suicide on the analogy that " . . . the gods are our keepers, and we men are one of their possessions." Moreover, he suggests that the gods are very good masters and that, as their mere possessions or chattel, it would be morally wrong for individuals to take flight from their rightful and benevolent masters through an act of suicide, barring some divine necessity or compulsion (*ananke*). Such a compulsion would presumably need to be an *external* one, like Socrates' predicament of facing capital punishment via poisoning. Hence, quitting life out of a sense of boredom, out of personal fear, out of a desire to escape earthly struggles, or out of thoughtlessly succumbing to destructive internal impulses would in no case pass muster morally. Therefore, the philosopher who is motivated to commit suicide by the desire to win immediate universal knowledge (and in so doing escape the earthly struggles of inquiry) would be violating his higher duty to the gods. The true philosopher finds life to be a "rehearsal" for death only in a special sense. By living in a reflective manner so as to carefully prepare his immortal soul for its eventual release from the body due to natural causes, he may succeed in conditioning his real self—his soul—for its most inspiring and satisfying odyssey. He does not, like a greedy guest, rush uninvited to death's banquet; nor like a disobedient slave does he willfully desert his benevolent keeper (Fig. 8). Such is the negative picture of suicide presented in the *Phaedo*.

Figure 8. Detail, artist's reconstruction of Tholos, originally designed by Polycleitas the Younger, at the Temple of Asclepius at Epidaurus (ca. 360 B.C.). Patients for whom no cure could be found by scientifically minded Hippocratic physicians were free to seek palliative comfort, if not actual cure, in the over two hundred temples of the physician-god Asclepius. Incantations, purifications, and dream therapy were commonly used there. Reprinted by permission of Harry N. Abrams, Inc., New York.

The *Republic*, however, appears to all but ignore these religious constraints against suicide. In the *Republic*, Socrates is made to advance the argument that *rational suicide* is not only possible but morally warranted in at least two related cases. The whole issue of whether suicide can cogently be said to be rational is a hotly debated one in our own time. By ascribing such a position to *Republic* 3.405ff., I here mean that Socrates talks as if sound reasons do, in fact, morally justify suicide in cases of (1) incurably debilitating disease, or (2) incurably debilitating disablement. If so, for our purposes Plato may be said to support *voluntary* euthanasia for adults in the *Republic*. By extension, *involuntary* euthanasia may also here be understood to be justified on similar grounds for incurably defective younger children. This latter inference would then further serve to illuminate Plato's qualified support of infanticide for defective newborns—a position of his found to be somewhat flawed in our earlier discussion.[33]

What, then, are his grounds for supporting euthanasia? They appear to be primarily utilitarian, not religious, in nature. Speaking in admiring tones of the legendary physician-god, Asclepius, whom he compares favorably over contemporary practitioners like Herodicus, who practice bad medicine by coddling and nursing their hopeless patients (and themselves) to a lingering and painful death, Socrates asks:

> Shall we say, then, that Asclepius recognized this [folly] and revealed the art of medicine for the benefit of people of sound constitution who normally led a healthy life, but had contracted some definite ailment? He would rid them of their disorders by means of drugs or the knife and tell them to go on living as usual, so as not to impair their usefulness as citizens. But where the body was diseased through and through, he would not try, by nicely calculated evaluations and doses, to prolong a miserable existence and let his patient beget children who were likely to be as sickly as himself. Treatment, he thought, would be wasted on a man who could not live in his ordinary round of duties and was consequently *useless to himself and to society*.[34]

The gist of Plato's position, in effect, is this: In his ideal society, he envisions the welfare of the state as a whole to hold a higher worth than the welfare of any one individual. Duties to the state here override duties to self and to family. In fact, religious duties, one recalls, are in Plato's utopian scheme finally invented and orchestrated to serve the purposes of the state as "convenient fictions." His aim in so doing is to further influence the masses so that they make whatever personal sacrifices are deemed necessary in order to ensure the full productivity and strength of the community. Hence, Plato's support of euthanasia in the *Republic* drops the religious underpinnings and analogies found in the *Phaedo*. Dropped, too, is an explicit eschatological argument attempting to allay natural human fears of the unknown that are associated with death. Substituted in their place is the more immediate specter of living out a tormented existence. This last prospect, made possible by a person's jealously guarded option and allegedly selfish insistence on surviving as a sickly, parasitic, unproductive citizen, is vigorously ridiculed as morally blameworthy behavior.[35]

It follows that hopelessly sick individuals are, to a very real extent, expendable from the moral point of view, according to Plato's *Republic*. Thus it is safe to infer that in the case of older children and adults, he approved of *voluntary* euthanasia on utilitarian grounds as an eligible form of rational suicide in the aforementioned instances. Whether he also approved *involuntary* euthanasia in the case of adults remains an open question that he does not speak to explicitly in the *Republic*. It would be unfair, however, to convict him of this on his silence. But that he approved involuntary euthanasia in the case of infants there can be no doubt. Though Plato acknowledged infants as human beings, he regarded their continued existence, if incurably sick or defective, as an unreasonable liability too great for the state to endure. Unlike the Pythagoreans, who in other ways informed much of Plato's thinking, their respect-for-human-life ethic was one moral principle he did not care to own in their absolute terms.

Yet, oddly enough, in Plato's last major work, *The Laws*, which, like his earlier *Republic* shares the goal of imagining an ideal commonwealth in which to live, Plato condemns suicide as morally wrong in all but four cases. He further prescribes legal penalties according to which the bodies of suicides must be (a) buried alone apart from all others; (b) buried "in disgrace" in deserted places that have no name, somewhere on the outskirts of the state; and (c) buried without any headstone or marker. Doubtless these sanctions reflect, in part, some of the traditional religious stigmas associated with blood pollution, and specifically pollution by self-murder, still current in some of the city-states of Plato's own day.[36] More important for us, however, is the observation that of the four excusing conditions Plato lists as *not* deserving of moral blame, the second explicitly excuses individuals, like Socrates in the *Phaedo*, who take their lives in obedience to a legal order from the state. No less important, the first and third excusing conditions could apply to those cases of the incurably ill or disabled, like Plato refers to in the *Republic*, who are deemed morally justified for electing voluntary euthanasia. (The remaining fourth condition excuses those who slay themselves in order to atone for "some irremediable disgrace" with which they cannot live.)[37]

The one remaining motivation for suicide that was the most prevalent in antiquity, and, I dare say, remains so in our own day, is described in the *Laws* in condemnatory terms as follows: It is the case of one who " . . . imposes this unjust judgment on himself in a spirit of slothful and abject cowardice."[38] In other words, it is the case that covers all those (including the pseudo-philosopher), who, acting from the mere motives of boredom, sloth, fatigue, or simple rejection, take it upon themselves to impulsively quit life. This is most clearly the kind of suicide opposed by Socrates in the *Phaedo*. It is also the kind that Plato studiously avoids endorsing in the *Republic*. Yet the case of voluntary euthanasia, which Plato does endorse there on moral grounds of a utilitarian sort, is also specifically excused (if not endorsed) in *The Laws*. In unmistakable language to that effect in condition three, alluded to above, Plato's proposed punitive legislation does *not* apply to those whose hand is " . . . forced by the pressure of some excruciating and unavoidable misfortune."[39] For such are the misfortunes of incurable injury or disease, to be sure.

Hence, there is little doubt in my mind that in his old age Plato sought to harmonize in some condensed fashion his earlier thoughts on the topics of suicide and euthanasia as found in the *Phaedo* and *Republic*. But whether or not he struck a morally defensible compromise in his *Laws* is left, characteristically, for his readers to decide.

Aristotle

One who disagreed with Plato's stand in support of euthanasia was his student and former colleague at the Academy, Aristotle. Aristotle did not devote so much of his attention to the problem of suicide as did Plato. But what he contributes to the discussion in two key passages from his *Nicomachean Ethics* is concise and to the point. These two passages show his unqualified opposition to suicide and, in particular, his opposition to the proposition that it is morally acceptable for a person suffering from an incurable disease or disability to quit life.[40]

Aristotle's opposition to suicide is expressed in one of these two passages in the context of his broader examination of the question of whether a person can be properly said to treat himself unjustly.

> . . . one class of just acts are those acts in accordance with any virtue which are prescribed by the law; e.g., the law does not expressly permit suicide, and what it does not expressly permit it forbids. Again, when a man in violation of the law harms another (otherwise than in retaliation) voluntarily, he acts unjustly, and a voluntary agent is one who knows both the person he is affecting by his action, and the instrument he is using; and he who through anger voluntarily stabs himself does this contrary to the right rule of life, and this the law does not allow; therefore, he is acting unjustly. But toward whom? Surely toward the state, not toward himself. For he suffers voluntarily, but no one is voluntarily treated unjustly. This is also the reason why the state punishes; a certain loss of civil rights attaches to the man who destroys himself, on the ground that he is treating the state unjustly.[41]

The point is that the person who suicides is blameworthy not just because he has seen fit to mortally injure himself (which in itself is deplorable as being " . . . contrary to the right rule of life", i.e., unnatural). Most of all, the person who suicides is blameworthy because his act violates his duty to the state to remain a productive, contributing citizen so long as he possibly may.

This raises two questions: First, is Aristotle really intending to include here the incurably ill, who by their disabilities may already be unable to render useful service to the state? Second, what, in any case, is the logic behind punishing the *successful* suicide with "a certain loss of civil rights"? Let us pursue these questions in turn.

It will be recalled from our earlier examination of Aristotle's attitude toward death that he squarely labels death " . . . the most terrible of all things; for it is the end, and nothing is thought to be any longer either good or bad for the dead."[42] Moreover, in his writings on courage, he defines the brave man as " . . . fearless in the face of noble death" [i.e., death in battle], and fearless as well in " . . . all emergencies that involve death." The admirable courage of the brave man confronted by the personal prospect of death or disease stems almost entirely from his sense of what is honorable conduct and what is base, says Aristotle. This rests, ultimately, on his intellectual ability to find the mean relative to himself between the opposing vices of cowardice and rashness. He may grasp some notion of this mean by observing the conduct of the prudent man who has mastered the right moral rules by which ends are achieved. Moreover, psychologically even the courageous person, according to Aristotle, is not invulnerable to fear at all times: there are some things deserving of fear. For example, " . . . things terrible even beyond human strength."[43] Yet, in general, even such things as these (and certainly impending death and some forms of painful disease would qualify) are only feared by the brave person " . . . from the right motive, in the right way, and at the right time. . . ."[44]

It is fair to inquire how the virtuous person ought, in Aristotle's view, to conduct himself if faced with a terminal, debilitating disease that saps his powers to exercise the minimal duties of citizenship. Would such a person be excused from moral censure if he killed himself? The answer is no. On this Aristotle appears to be unequivocal: "But to die to escape from poverty or love *or anything that is painful* is not the mark of a brave man, but rather of a coward; for it is softness to fly from what is troublesome, and such a man endures death not because it is noble but to fly from evil."[45]

Thus, I conclude that Aristotle did not approve of the individual who quit life on account of the infirmities of illness. I further conclude that Edelstein, who attempts to argue that Aristotle's opposition to suicide did not really involve moral censure but only amounted to a plea for more backbone, is just wrong about this.[46] Furthermore, our evidence suggests that euthanasia was blameworthy for Aristotle not simply because it deprived the state prematurely of one of its own, but because such an act typically constituted an excessive degree of rashness or cowardice. This was especially true of the subject who ended life out of excessive anger or grief at his helpless suffering or who acted deficiently by not meeting his predicament with the requisite courage called for in order to face nobly the trial of his affliction.

Second, as to the logic of calling for civil penalties involving the loss of rights for the successful suicide, surely some sense can be made of this. In the context of the city-state, Aristotle is particularly intent on condemning the act of suicide, not simply the actor. Although he does not specify what this loss of rights involves, I conjecture that he has in mind special prohibitions concerning the burial of suicides similar to those prohibitions mentioned by Plato in the *Laws*. For example, it is known that in Aristotle's day the hand of the suicide was sometimes severed and buried separately from the remaining corpse. Moreover, the institution of nameless graves and the prospect of inglorious and isolated burials far from the hallowed burial grounds of the community's honored dead may have served a double purpose as a warning to the living who were considering suicide or euthanasia.

A final question: Since, as I have argued, Aristotle opposed both suicide and euthanasia on moral grounds without any apparent exception, can he be identified as a partisan of the respect-for-human-life ethic in either its basic or derived sense?[47] I think not. For we saw that to be a partisan of the respect-for-life ethic, one must either accept as basic the proposition that human bodily life has absolute value per se just because it is human life. Or one must accept a similar proposition that would also confer absolute value to human life even though that value derives from prior principles. In either case, Aristotle fails to qualify. It is true that he opposes suicide. But his moral justification of infanticide for defective newborns on utilitarian grounds disqualifies him from further serious consideration. For is it not self-contradictory to assert, on the one hand, that all human bodily life has absolute value just because it is human and, on the other hand, that some human lives should be terminated just because they are judged to be defective? Such a position would appear inconsistent. It represents, at any rate, a peculiar departure from our ordinary way of talking about respecting the lives of our fellow human beings.

Seneca

We have seen that the Stoics viewed death as nothing to fear. In the main, they taught a version of *natural personal dissolution* according to which the tiny fiery pneuma dwelling within each person dispersed at the moment of death to reunite with the world-soul Pneuma of God.[48] Thus, there were no punishments awaiting the deceased's ghost in the netherworld, for there were no ghosts. Individuality and personality effectively ceased with death. Death was viewed as the natural and inevitable resolution of human life itself. Hence, only the fool would attempt to oppose death; the wise man would arrange to meet it head on if he could, timing his exit from this world with the aplomb of a thoughtful dinner guest who seeks to avoid boring or detaining his hosts. Hence, the wise man withdraws from life's banquet in just the right way, under just the right conditions.[49]

This raises two important questions: First, did the Stoics hold that suicide, and particularly euthanasia, was a rational act? Second, did they hold that each person possessed what amounts to a moral right to end his own life? I shall argue that the writings of Seneca suggest affirmative answers to both of these queries. But, as we shall see, they do so only by insisting on some very strict qualifications that were quite characteristic of the Stoic perspective on suicide and euthanasia.

In general, the Stoics were not the first philosophical school to approve of suicide. We have already seen that Plato approved of it in a limited way, especially for the incurably ill who suffered their fate under compulsion (by external necessity, as it were). Moreover, representatives of two minor Socratic schools, the Cynics and the Cyrenaics, at various times also looked favorably upon suicide.[50] What distinguished the Stoics, however, was that they were mightily inspired by the moral example of Socrates' courageous death. Following Socrates, they viewed philosophy not only as the art of right living, but also as the art of dying well. Very likely, learning to die nobly became one of the central problems in Stoic ethics, partly because the Stoics came to view the act of dying as an important test of a person's moral strength and stature.[51] Thus it is little wonder that the Stoic founder, Zeno, committed suicide in his old age prompted by the agonizing pain of a foot injury; his successor, Cleanthenes, suicided after developing a boil in his mouth; Seneca himself slashed his wrists at around age sixty-eight after it appeared certain that his former student, Nero, would otherwise order him executed on the dubious charge of treason.[52]

This last mention of the circumstances of Seneca's death, in particular, highlights a crucial Stoic idea concerning suicide: To have the capacity to willfully depart from life was viewed as the greatest boon to mankind; it constituted a real choice that epitomized moral freedom. In the following passage, Seneca expresses this central idea. He also tacitly rebukes thinkers like Pythagoras and Aristotle who opposed suicide, and demonstrates his sympathy for voluntary euthanasia on account of the cruelties of disease.

> You can find men who have gone so far as to profess wisdom and yet maintain that one should not offer violence to one's own life, and hold it accursed for a man to be the means of his own destruction; we should wait, say they, for the end decreed by nature. But one who says this does not see that he is shutting off *the path to freedom. The best thing* which eternal law ever ordained was that it allowed to us one entrance into life, but many exits. *Must I await the cruelty either of disease or of man*, when I can depart through the midst of torture, and shake off my troubles? *This is the one reason why we cannot complain of life*: it keeps no one against his will. Humanity is well situated, because no man is unhappy except by his own fault. Live, if you so desire; if not, you may return to the place whence you came. You have often been cupped in order to relieve headaches. You have had veins cut for the purpose of reducing your weight. If you would pierce your heart, a gaping wound is not necessary; a lancet will open the way *to that great freedom*, and tranquillity can be purchased at the cost of a pin-prick.
>
> What, then, is it which makes us lazy and sluggish? None of us reflects that some day he must depart from this house of life; just so old tenants are kept from moving by fondness for a particular place and by custom, even in spite of ill-treatment. Would you be free from the restraint of your body? Live in it as if you were about to leave it. Keep thinking of the fact that some day you will be deprived of this tenure; then you will be more brave against the necessity of departing.[53]

Yet it would be a mistake to infer from the above quotation that (a) the Stoics placed no limit on the eligible reasons for suicide or that (b) they thought suicide was permissible without serious prior reflection.

As for (a), the only category of situations provisionally eligible was that which required of the individual intolerable or unworthy endurance. Ultimately, it was for the individual to decide whether his present circumstances truly met this requirement. Owing to the myriad of conditions that could sincerely be considered unendurable, a great variety of circumstances became in practice eligible for the Stoic act of suicide. Seneca, for example, argues that merely the anticipation of a considerable disturbance in one's conduct and peace of mind constituted a sufficient reason for committing suicide.[54] But he tempers this statement with the admonition that no philosopher should rush to suicide simply in order to escape ordinary forms of human suffering. Suicide is most clearly warranted, according to Seneca, only when it represents choosing " . . . an easier mode of death instead of a more painful one, thus avoiding a freak of destiny and the cruelty of man."[55] In general, vice and human folly must be met by other means than by suicide. Death furnishes no real deliverance from them, since it makes the bad no better, as Edward Zeller has aptly remarked.[56]

According to one ancient authority, just five cases were normally admitted by the Stoics to warrant suicide: (1) if one's death could render a real service to others; (2) if by suiciding one could avoid being forced to commit an unlawful deed; and (3) if one were impoverished, (4) chronically ill, or (5) no longer in possession of a sound mind. All of these cases are also approved by Seneca. Therefore, it is fair to conclude that the Stoics *did* recognize the moral right to take one's own life. But this right was not in principle unlimited: some, not all, situations morally justified suicide. And one of these situations, as we have seen, was to be the victim of incurable or chronic disease.

In regard to (b), no act of suicide is considered praiseworthy by Seneca unless it is preceded by careful reflection. To Lucilius he writes:

Whichever of these ideas you ponder, you will strengthen your mind for the endurance alike of death and of life. For we need to be warned and strengthened in both directions—not to love or to hate life overmuch; even when reason advises us to make an end of it, the impulse is not to be adopted without reflection or at headlong speed. The brave and wise man should not beat a hasty retreat from life; he should make a becoming exit. And above all, he should avoid the weakness which has taken possession of so many—the lust for death. For just as there is an unreflecting tendency of the mind towards other things, so, my dear Lucilius, there is an unreflecting tendency towards death; this often seizes upon the noblest and most spirited men, as well as upon the craven and the abject.[57]

Furthermore, this emphasis on reflection is suggested by the favorite Stoic phrase to denote suicide, which, as we saw above, was "sensible" or "reasonable removal" (*eulogos exagoge*). This phrase implies that any defensible act of suicide must, in fact, manifest a rational character on the Stoic view. But, if so, what was the logic behind so-called rational forms of suicide, according to the Stoics?

Two key elements of their thinking converge to provide an answer. The first is the claim that life and death are themselves matters of indifference (morally neither good nor bad) to the wise person. The second is the claim that the reflective individual must await some evidence from destiny (God) based on an internal signal that the time to die is now. I shall discuss the second of these two claims, suggesting a serious difficulty that arises.[58]

Since life and death are for the Stoics indifferent in the sense specified above, the decision of whether or not one ought to suicide really turns on an individual's own preferences. The individual must somehow gauge whether he is living his life in accordance with nature—which was the Stoic ideal. His reason alone has the capacity to determine this, and man alone of all earthly creatures was said by the Stoics to be possessed of this divine faculty. But how could one tell whether the time for removal from life was at hand? How could one tell whether the personal conditions thought to be essential for the preservation of the Stoic way of life were irretrievably beyond reach?

By the period of the Roman Empire, later Stoics, like Seneca, began to think it was possible that the soul survives the body at death. Seneca occasionally wavered on the traditional Stoic view of death as natural personal dissolution to permit a poetic vision of divine personal immortality of the sort Plato sponsored.[59] But either under the traditional or the late Stoic concept of death, the task of the Stoic partisan reasoning about his own possible suicide remained approximately the same. A.W. Mair has plausibly characterized this task as a modified extension of Socrates' claim in the *Phaedo* that suicide was only admissible when some compelling constraint or force of circumstances (such as his own impending execution) made death unopposable. But Socrates had spoken of this compelling constraint (*ananke*) in the sense of an *external compulsion* found in one's environment. Later Stoics, including Seneca, tended to reinterpret the nature of this compulsion to mean that an *inner compulsion* need only be present. The trick was then to try to introspectively read off from one's own life situation whether any suicidal impulses one may be experiencing are, in fact, an omen from God that the time to leave life is at hand.[60]

This approach, of course, marks a decisive departure from Socrates' original sentiments opposing suicide in the *Phaedo*. Some would call it a sweeping rationalization for almost all varieties of suicide, reasoned or hasty, noble or base. My own opinion is that such a conceptual maneuver does indeed appear so broad as to invite conflating cases of putatively reasoned suicide, resembling the five admissible cases discussed above, with cases of merely impulsive, cowardly suicide, of the sort Seneca and his predecessors totally disowned.

Hence, the most serious flaw I have discovered in the decision procedure behind late Stoic efforts to characterize *some* forms of suicide as rational acts amounts basically to this. Any effort put forward by an individual to interpret his own life situation as one truly qualifying for suicide in accordance with the above Stoic ideals is an effort that can never be *objectively certified* as morally defensible. What's more, owing to possible self-deception, a person may misinterpret his situation and quit life for trivial reasons. A given act of suicide may, in fact, be morally defensible—at least relative to the Stoic perspective. But the final decision to commit suicide, though a limited right of every individual according to the Stoics, admits of rather few certifiably warrantable instances. Significantly, one of these instances is that of the very sick, suffering patient. But even such an unfortunate person is obliged, in the Stoic view, to weigh his plight with the greatest care, lest he quit life too soon.[61]

SUMMARY

To summarize the various positions adopted by Pythagoras, Plato, Aristotle, and Seneca on the question of suicide and euthanasia, the Pythagoreans were clearly opposed to both of these measures. Their opposition is unconditional in both cases. It was shown to rest directly on the respect-for-human-life ethic, which is itself a moral principle derived from their logically prior religious principle that God values each embodied soul. Therefore, bodily life must not be prematurely ended, nor, as we saw earlier, prevented. At bottom, then, suicide and euthanasia are blameworthy because each embodied human soul is ordered by the gods to complete its natural lifespan: to desert one's station is tantamount to violating divine law. In a word, it is a sin, as Philolaus implies.

Plato, on the other hand, decisively sought to moderate the unconditional opposition of the Pythagoreans against suicide and euthanasia, even though he shared much of their vision of death as divine personal immortality. In the *Phaedo*, Plato opposes suicide on what would have to be characterized as religious grounds. Yet even in the *Phaedo* his opposition is not unconditional. That is, if environmental constraints make imminent death irreversible, one may perhaps take early leave when no other course appears open; but that opportunity rarely occurs, despite efforts by the later Stoics to broadly reinterpret this passage. In contrast, in the *Republic* Plato softens his view against suicide. This he does by approving voluntary euthanasia for the incurably ill or disabled on what amounts to utilitarian grounds. Plato also approves involuntary euthanasia in the form of infanticide for defective newborns. In both instances, he links and subordinates the value of the individual to the individual's ability to perform his functions well for the state. The chronically sick and defective are seen as useless both to themselves and to society. In *Laws*, Plato combines his earlier positions in the *Phaedo* and *Republic* with the added suggestion that the suicide who leaves life merely to escape his lawful duties brings shame upon himself and his community. The resulting blood pollution in this last case of cowardly self-murder is reprehensible. To demonstrate both religious offense and civil outrage against the suicide, an ignominious burial is required. Plato nowhere embraces the respect-for-life ethic as we have defined it here, else his stands favoring abortion and euthanasia would never be admitted.

As for Aristotle, he unconditionally stood opposed to both suicide and euthanasia. In the case of suicide, he thought it blameworthy not because the subject wronged himself but because he wronged his community by violating his duty to live a productive life. Unlike Socrates in the *Phaedo*, Aristotle's argument is not predicated on religious considerations but rather on social considerations having to do with the proper way in which citizens should hold themselves accountable to the state. Furthermore, Aristotle offers little encouragement to proponents favoring voluntary euthanasia, since he argues that death must be met bravely by the virtuous person, no matter what. As the Stoics were to suggest later on (but with an altogether different twist), Aristotle felt that dying courageously—by not willfully giving into death—constituted a significant moral test. At any rate, despite his opposition to suicide and euthanasia on moral and political grounds, it would be overhasty to characterize Aristotle as a partisan of the respect-for- life ethic. For he did approve what we would characterize as involuntary euthanasia for defective newborns. He also approved abortion, though this he restricted to fetuses thought to be incapable of sensation. In either case he furnished utilitarian grounds that no absolute proponent of the respect-for-life ethic could accept.[62]

As our principal representative of the Stoic school, Seneca, like almost all partisans of the Stoic tradition before and after him, found favor with both suicide and euthanasia. But although he held that suicide could be characterized as a rational act, and although he thought that each person had a limited right to quit life, there were at least two necessary conditions that the justified would-be suicide had to meet. First, the antecedent circumstances of the subject's proposed act must fall roughly into at least one of those five specified categories already examined, which included, as we saw, being victimized by chronic or incurable disease. Second, the subject must duly reflect on his present circumstances, weighing the pros and cons with regard to himself and others. He must thereby try to ensure that his proposed act does not amount to little more than an impulsive, ill-timed wish to escape life's legitimate duties, from which the virtuous person does not lightly flee through death's door. Therefore, Seneca's endorsement of suicide and euthanasia, though sympathetic, is not unconditional. Though he is no proponent of the so-called respect-for-human-life ethic, that he did in the ordinary sense respect the lives of others, especially his friends, relatives, and countrymen, few would seriously deny.

Discussion Questions

1. Did any Greek philosophers count acts of infanticide as morally equivalent to acts of abortion or euthanasia? Why?
2. Did the Greeks and Romans generally oppose suicide? Which philosophers condemned suicide and why?

3. Distinguish between heroic and nonheroic forms of suicide. To which class does euthanasia belong?

4. On what moral grounds did Pythagoras, Plato, Aristotle, and Seneca support or oppose voluntary euthanasia?

5. Define the respect-for-human-life principle. How has this principle impacted the contemporary moral debate concerning abortion, infanticide, suicide, and euthanasia?

6. What were Aristotle's views on abortion? On suicide? Do you agree with him?

NOTES

1. For example, euthanasia is now also standardly qualified as *involuntary* euthanasia, evidenced by the absence of the patient's consent to quit life, and *active* versus *passive* euthanasia, discussed above, p. 153. Sissela Bok provides a straightforward account of euthanasia in its various modern senses in "Death and Dying: Euthanasia and Sustaining Life," in *EB*, vol. 1, pp. 268–77.

2. See chapter 3, p. 58, particularly points (2) and (3).

3. Philo attributed this view to the Hellenistic masses (*hoi polloi*). Philo *Vit. Mos.* 1.11, cited by Immanuel Jakobovits, *Jewish Medical Ethics* (New York: Bloch Publishing Co., 1976), p. 174, note 51.

4. This shift in emphasis is supported by examples of more recent uses of the term in the last century or so, as recorded by the *Oxford English Dictionary*, 12 vols. (Oxford: Clarendon Press, 1961), vol. 3, p. 325, in regard to the English word *euthanasia*.

5. David Daube, "The Linguistics of Suicide," *Philosophy and Public Affairs* 1 (1972): 391.

6. Ibid.

7. See Rudolf Hirzel's classic "Der Selbstmord," *Archiv für Religionswissenschaft* 2, (1980), p. 243, for which I thank Truman Eddy for his kind assistance. See also Aristophanes *The Frogs* 116ff., wherein he alludes to the advantages of hemlock over other methods as an aid to suicide; and Theophrastus *History of Plants* 9.16.8, wherein he remarks on the powerful and incurable effects of poisons produced from hemlock and poppy.

8. Daube, "Linguistics of Suicide," p. 393. Daube gives Diodorus Siculus 2.57.5 as one ancient source of the myth to which his quote refers.

9. See Joseph Margolis, *Negativities*, chap. 2, pp. 23–35 ("Suicide"), which is also reprinted in Tom L. Beauchamp and Seymour Perlin, *Ethical Issues in Death and Dying* (New Jersey: Prentice Hall, 1978), pp. 92–97.

10. Daube, "Linguistics of Suicide," pp. 399–400, 406. Daube gives as sources for these Greek expressions: Xenophon *Hellenica* 6.2.36; Euripides *Iphigenia in Tauris* 974; Plato *Phaedo* 68a; Aristotle *Nichomachean Ethics* 9.4.8.1166b; Diogenes Laertius *Lives* 7.130 (on Zeno).

11. Daube, "Linguistics of Suicide," p. 403. Daube offers the anthropological theory that, regarding the evolution of any native language in a given culture, "The emergence of the noun betokens a decisive advance in abstraction, systematization, institutionalization" (p. 397). If so, the regular appearance of Greek nouns to refer to suicide suggests a trend toward wider acceptance or at least reflection concerning the practice.

12. I have benefitted from the literary and historical evidence amassed in A. W. Mair, "Suicide," in *ERE*, vol. 12, pp. 26–33.

13. The prevalent social attitudes of antiquity, however, tended to construe suicidal behavior, which nowadays is widely classified as symptomatic of a medical problem, as alternatively symptomatic of moral problems or general problems of living. This observation suggests the normative character of the ascription of illness, particularly mental illness—a topic I shall not treat here. For more on mental disorders in antiquity, see George Rosen, "History in the Study of Suicide," *Psychological Medicine* 1 (1971), p. 272. In general, see Margolis, *Negativities*, chaps. 7–8.

14. This statement stands despite my remarks in note 13, for the ancients did, in fact, recognize as involuntary (and hence blameless) *some* instances of supposed mental disorder. But they counted such instances far fewer in number. See Hippocrates *Epidemics* 7.89, cited by Rosen, "Suicide," p. 272, as one example.

15. Homer *Odyssey* 11.548 and Sophocles *Ajax*.

16. Lycurgus *c. Leokrat* 84ff., cited by Mair, "Suicide," in *ERE*, vol. 12, p. 27.

17. Plutarch *Theseus* 12.

18. Herodotus *History* 1.45.

19. Theogonis 173ff., cited by Mair, "Suicide," in *ERE*, vol. 12, p. 27.

20. Ovid *Her.* 5, cited by Mair, "Suicide," in *ERE*, vol. 12, p. 29.

21. Plutarch *Mulierum Virtutes* 249b-4, cited by Mair, "Suicide," in *ERE*, vol. 12, p. 29.

22. Strabo 10.486, cited by Mair, "Suicide," in *ERE*, vol. 12, p. 29.

23. Pliny (the younger) *Epistle* 1.22. See also Diogenes Laertius *Lives* 7.130; and Pliny *Epistle* 3.7 for related illustrations.

24. Mair, "Suicide," in *ERE*, vol. 12, pp. 30–31, 34.

25. The first recorded theoretical discussion of *active euthanasia* occurred in Thomas More's *Utopia*, first published in 1516, although the term "euthanasia" had not yet been explicitly coined. In its modern sense, the term first appeared around 1870, according to W. Bruce Fye, "Active Euthanasia: An Historical Survey of Its Conceptual Origins and Introduction into Medical Thought," *Bulletin of the History of Medicine* 52 (1979): 492–94 passim.

26. *Phaedo* 62b–c, trans. Hugh Tredennick, *Collected Dialogues*, p. 45, emphases added. In an interesting article, J. C. G. Strachan suggests that—contrary to J. Burnet and R. Hackforth, among others—this allegory, its body-guardpost imagery, and its accompanying rationale opposing suicide, may not have belonged either to Philolaus (as was assumed even in later antiquity) or to the fifth-century-B.C. Pythagoreans of Plato's day. The thrust of his argument, though far from conclusive, turns on (a) emphasizing the hiatus and possible ambiguity in the text between the introduction of Philolaus' name at 61dff., and the introduction of the allegory at 62b, which bears no explicit attribution to Philolaus; (b) establishing the far firmer association of the allegory at 62b with Orphic, not Pythagorean, religious teachings by the fifth-century-B.C. period in question; and (c) underscoring the subsequent confusion of sorting out the true ownership of the allegory at 62b, which was occasioned by the eventual acceptance of the body-prison doctrine by the Pythagoreans toward the end of the fourth century B.C. (a confusion that also allegedly misled Cicero in his *De Senectute* 20 and modern scholars who followed). Strachan has, I think, succeeded in undermining any *unqualified* ascription of this passage to Philolaus. But he is surely fanciful in suggesting that perhaps " . . . Plato was unwittingly responsible for the adoption of this particular piece of Orphism by the Pythagorean school." (See J. C. G. Strachan, "Who *Did* Forbid Suicide at *Phaedo* 62B?" *Classical Quarterly* 20 [1970]: 216–20.) For more on this controversy, see J. Burnet, *Plato's Phaedo* (Oxford: Clarendon Press, 1911), pp. 22ff.; R. Hackforth, *Plato's Phaedo* (In-

dianapolis, IN: Bobbs-Merrill, 1960), p. 38; and R. S. Black, *Plato's Phaedo* (Indianapolis, IN: Bobbs-Merrill), pp. 195ff., cited by Strachan.

27. See chapter 6, note 65.

28. Frankena, "Respect for Life," pp. 25–26.

29. Ibid., p. 26.

30. Ibid., pp. 38–42.

31. Hugh Tredennick, trans., *Collected Dialogues*, p. 25, emphases added.

32. *Phaedo* 62c–4, trans. Benjamin Jowett, *Republic and Other Works* (New York: Doubleday), n. d.

33. See chapter 6, pp. 128–29.

34. Plato *Republic* 3.407d., trans. Francis Cornford, *Republic of Plato* (Oxford: Oxford University Press, 1973), p. 97, emphases added.

35. Such, in fact, is the precise picture we get of the infamous gymnastic master and trainer, Herodicus. Socrates describes Herodicus in unflattering terms. He is one who, after losing his health " . . . combined training and doctoring in such a way as to become a plague to himself first and foremost and to many others after him . . . by lingering out his death. He had a mortal disease, and he spent all his life at its beck and call, with no hope of cure. . . . Every departure from his fixed regimen was a torment; and his skill only enabled him to reach old age in a prolonged death struggle." (Plato *Republic* 3.406b–c., trans. Cornford, *Republic of Plato*, p. 96.) Cf. William A. Heidel, *Hippocratic Medicine: Its Spirit and Method* (New York: Columbia University Press, 1941), p. 123.

36. See Mair, "Suicide," in *ERE*, vol. 12, pp. 30–31, and Herbert J. Rose, "Disposal of the Dead," in *OCD*, pp. 314–15.

37. *Laws* 873c–e, trans. Trevor J. Saunders, *The Laws* (New York: Penguin Books, 1976), p. 391. Note that this fourth condition is not, as qualified in the text, equivalent to what I classify as a form of heroic suicide. For to be heroically characterized, the subject and others must regard his disgraceful deed as genuinely accidental and unintended. In contrast, the fourth condition in *Laws* simply excuses the subject who has " . . . fallen into some irremediable disgrace he cannot live with." The tragic element of not intending to cause such disgrace is missing, or, at least, not required by Plato. Cf. pp. 151–52.

38. *Laws*, trans. Saunders, *The Laws,* p. 391.

39. Ibid.

40. Edelstein, "Hippocratic Oath," p. 17, note 36. Edelstein contends that under the onslaught of the later Stoic attack on their views, sometime after Aristotle died, his disciples deserted his teachings against self-murder.

41. *Nicomachean Ethics* 5.10, trans. W. D. Ross, *Basic Works*, pp. 1020–21.

42. For Aristotle's full quotation on death and courage, see chapter 3, pp. 50–51.

43. *Nicomachean Ethics* 3.1115b.7, trans. Ross, *Basic Works*, p. 975.

44. Ibid., 3.1115b.18, trans. Ross, *Basic Works*, p. 976.

45. Ibid., 3.1116a.12–15, trans. Ross, *Basic Works*, p. 977, emphases added.

46. Edelstein, "Hippocratic Oath," p. 17. Edelstein tries very hard to downplay Aristotle's moral censure of suicide. If so, was this done in order to protect his own theory concerning the exclusive Pythagorean origins of the Hippocratic Oath? See chapter 5.

47. This distinction is discussed on pp. 154–55.

48. See pp. 134–35. There is some evidence that the late Stoic Seneca occasionally flirted with a version of *divine personal immortality*. But he admits that on this score philosophers of old (referring to Plato) promised more than they could deliver, and doesn't

seem to take the notion of personal immortality seriously. Such a notion is not, at any rate, central to Stoic teaching, and I am convinced that Jacques Choron exaggerates Seneca's dependence on this perspective. (See Choron, *Death and Western Thought*, p. 69.) Cf. Seneca *Epistles* 24, 102.

49. The metaphor of life as a banquet, at which only the greedy guest overstays his visit, was a favorite of Seneca's.

50. The Cynics based the right to suicide on the prior right to be able to separate oneself from one's community at any time. They advocated an *unlimited* right to commit suicide, therefore, which the Stoics refused to grant. (See Hirzel, "Der Selbstmord," pp. 279ff.) As for the Cyrenaics, it is true that *only some* of them endorsed suicide on moral grounds. Theodoros opposed it unconditionally. But Hegesias argued the case for rational suicide so eloquently that a rash of suicides occurred in Alexandria, and Ptolemy II ordered him banished from Egypt in consequence. (See Diogenes Laertius *Lives* 2.86; and Cicero, *Tusc.* 1.34.) The Epicureans were officially opposed to suicide since the wise man neither seeks death as a refuge nor declines life—fearing nothing. Even so, the Roman Lucretius broke with Epicurus on this issue. He granted suicide limited warrant for those to whom life had grown distasteful. It appears, moreover, that many late Epicureans sided with Lucretius, who himself is reported to have committed suicide. For more on the Epicureans and suicide, see Jacques Choron, *Suicide* (New York: Charles Scribner's Sons, 1972), pp. 112–15.

51. On death as a test of moral strength, see Seneca *Epistle* 70.17–19.

52. Tacitus (*Annals* 15.64) sympathetically records the manner of Seneca's death, which showed much bravery. It involved the initial supply of a poison by Seneca's physician, which did not act as speedily as hoped for.

53. Seneca *Epistle* 70.14–18. *Seneca: Ad Lucilium Epistulae Morales*, trans. Richard M. Gummere, 3 vols. (Cambridge, MA: Harvard University Press, 1962), vol. 2, p. 65, emphases added. Critics of the Stoic position in support of suicide have long observed an inherent contradiction in the Stoic perspective. On the one hand, Stoics claim that the wise person must resign himself to the course of destiny by making his will conform to what must happen anyway. On the other hand, they allow that when a person is placed in circumstances calling for intolerable or unworthy endurance, this resignation can justifiably warrant active resistance. As Edward Zeller has challenged: Is it " . . . consistent with unconditional resignation to the course of the world, to evade by personal interposition, what destiny with its unalterable laws has decreed for us?" There appears to be no clear way out of this dilemma for the Stoics, though I must waive that controversy here. (See Edward Zeller, *The Stoics, Epicureans and Sceptics* [New York: Russell and Russell, Inc., 1962], p. 339.)

54. Seneca *Epistle* 70.

55. Zeller, *Stoics*, p. 337. See *Epistles* 58.36 and 70.11.

56. Zeller, *Stoics*, p. 336.

57. Seneca *Epistle* 24.24–26, trans. Gummere, *Seneca,* vol. 1, p. 181.

58. The first claim is critically discussed by Zeller, *Stoics*, pp. 338–39.

59. Seneca *Epistle* 65 and 102. See also note 48.

60. Mair, "Suicide," in *ERE*, vol. 12, p. 31. The passage in question from *Phaedo* 62C was also treated on pp. 155–56. Mair credits the later Stoics Panaitios (ca. 140 B.C.) And Posidonios (ca. 130–146 B.C.) for modifying Socrates' emphasis on *external* compulsions, which force suicide, to *internal* compulsions, such as inner, overmastering impulses of ambiguous origin. Cf. Seneca *Epistle* 102.23. In any case, note that one re-

sult of such a reinterpretation meant that a Stoic could be said to have chosen suicide on religious grounds, if he took his internal impulses to end life as the divine decree of heaven.

61. Seneca himself wrote that he once considered ending his life as a young man on account of an annoying illness (catarrh) that caused him to become dangerously thin. But discovering that his prognosis was not terminal, he endured and overcame his sickness with the help, he says, of philosophy and friends. He gives as his primary reason for not killing himself at the time his profound love for his father, and the grief his suicide would cause the old man. (See Seneca *Epistle* 78.)

62. The question, however, can be raised as to whether Aristotle could be plausibly said to be a proponent of the respect-for-human-life ethic at least *prima facie*, in W. D. Ross's sense. This is certainly conceivable, though one will search in vain for textual evidence in Aristotle to satisfy such an approximate reinterpretation. Even so, the point remains that the concept of respect for human life admits of at least two possible forms: (1) the absolute form, which states that it is *always* wrong to end or prevent a human life or (2) the nonabsolute form, which states that it is *not always* or finally wrong to prevent or shorten a human life, since other overriding considerations may still make it right in certain instances. I have focused on the first form, as this is the most useful expression of the principle in relation to my analysis of the origins of the Hippocratic Oath, particularly its absolutely formulated prohibitions against abortion and euthanasia. See W. D. Ross, *The Right and the Good* (Oxford: Clarendon Press, 1930), pp. 19ff., and Frankena, "Respect for Life," pp. 32–33.

8 The Physician's Moral Responsibility

No physician, insofar as he is a physician,
considers his own good in what he prescribes, but
the good of his patient; for the true physician is
also a ruler having the human body as a subject,
and is not a money-maker.

—PLATO

WHAT SENSE OF MORAL RESPONSIBILITY did the ancient physicians characteristically possess when granting or denying their patients' requests for abortive remedies or lethal poisons? This is the question we are now prepared to explore. The term "responsibility" is an exceedingly rich one containing several different meanings. I intend to focus on what H. L. A. Hart has called "role responsibility." What duties or institutional constraints are borne by an individual in virtue of his or her working role in a given society?[1] Our purpose here is not to reconstruct an ancient scale by which to praise or blame the conduct of the pre-Christian physician. Rather, our purpose is to comprehend the moral force of some of the relevant craft and related institutional values that may have influenced the typical Greek and Roman doctor's conduct when his medical assistance was sought by patients seeking to prevent or end life.

I shall argue that the dominant medical ethical values expressed by the Hippocratic Collection as a whole do not unequivocally oppose the collaboration of physicians in abortion or voluntary euthanasia. In fact, that body of authoritative medical writings furnished no unified ideological opposition to such practices. I shall further suggest that this absence of opposition by the Hippocratics and most other pre-Christian medical sects can be partly understood as the result of a pluralistic philosophical climate in which no philosophical school succeeded in persuading the educated public that abortion and voluntary euthanasia were morally wrong. In fact, as we have seen, philosophers themselves were split on these issues: almost all but the Pythagoreans furnished some grounds for abortion, and most eventually defended euthanasia as well.

Let us turn at once to some of the more pertinent evidence from the Hippocratic Collection that fails to oppose or, in some instances, condones abortion or euthanasia.

ABORTION

As for abortion, in the Hippocratic treatise *On the Development of the Child* there exists a passage in which the author admits, in a very casual and non-defensive manner, to having helped a young dancer abort her unwanted child in the earliest stages of pregnancy. The method appears crude: ". . . I thereupon told her to jump in such a way that the heels touched the buttocks; she had now jumped seven times when the semen fell to the ground with a plop. And when the woman saw this, she stared at it and exclaimed."[2]

The second-century-A.D. Greek gynecologist Soranus observed this apparent contradiction regarding abortion in the Hippocratic Collection. For the Oath had stated: "I will not give to a woman an abortive remedy." Soranus's comments imply that in Roman times there existed at least two schools of thought among physicians on the question of abortion. The first group, inspired by the Oath and perhaps early Christian teaching, refused to aid in abortion for any reason. According to Soranus, this group held that " . . . the specific task of medicine [is] to guard and preserve what has been engendered by nature."[3] The second group, which was the larger of the two and the one to which Soranus belonged, held that abortion was indicated whenever the mother's life was at serious risk. Abortion for the purposes of preserving youthful beauty or to conceal adultery, however, was explicitly condemned by Soranus. Moreover, as we saw above, Soranus preferred contraception to abortion because it constituted a safer remedy for the mother than destroying her fetus, and he labored to invent many contraceptive devices to that end.[4]

Then there is the interesting testimony of the first-century-A.D. Roman physician, Scribonius Largus. Scribonius was a keen admirer of Hippocrates, whom he called "the founder of our profession."[5] Along with the first-century Roman writer Erotian, Scribonius is our earliest known source to mention the Hippocratic Oath; happily, we possess Scribonius's comments on some of its teachings, notably on abortion.

In the preface of his book *On Remedies*, Scribonius observes that the Hippocratic Oath forbids abortion. He sees in this prohibition a lesson to all in humanity. He writes: " . . . [Hippocrates] has gone a long way toward preparing the minds of learners for the love of humanity. For he who considers it a crime to injure future life still in doubt, how much more criminal must he then judge it to harm a full grown human being."[6] Here Scribonius does not explicitly state that he is himself opposed to abortion. But these admiring remarks, plus his cosmo-

politan philosophy of medical humanism, according to which "medicine promises her aid in equal measure to all who seek her help . . . and professes never to
injure anyone," implicitly sets him apart from those pagan physicians who routinely administered abortions for virtually any reason.[7] Very possibly Scribonius
stands ideologically allied with Soranus, who, as we saw, criticized the unrestrained cooperation of physicians in abortion. In fact, Scribonius's preceding remarks suggest that he may have regarded the fetus as having some measure of
moral worth. If so, then like the author of the Hippocratic Oath, Scribonius, too,
may have been morally opposed to abortion.

It is far more certain that many ancient physicians, and I suspect most, consented to aiding women in abortion for a variety of reasons. While the Hippocratic
Oath opposed even therapeutic abortions designed to spare the mother's imperiled life (since its prohibition against abortion was unconditional), physicians
were free to dissent, and many did so, Soranus among them.

Yet, the comparatively small circle of physicians who were in complete
sympathy with the Oath must have faced occasionally a serious ethical dilemma
while ministering to the needs of expectant mothers. For, as Oswei Temkin has
rightly emphasized, on the one hand the Oath-taker pledges to keep his patients
free " . . . from harm and injustice" (P3, p. 84). On the other hand, abortion is prohibited, even for therapeutic reasons.[8] Therefore, when the prognosis indicated
that the mother would be harmed or killed owing to the frailty of her health or to
the expected complications of an abnormal delivery, adherents of the Oath must
have faced a serious conflict of duty.[9] To be sure, the duty to obey the Oath's prohibition against abortion could clash logically (and emotionally) with the correl-
ative duty to keep the patient from harm. Significantly, this particular dilemma
found no solution from within the profession of medicine for over two thousand
years. For it was not until the late nineteenth century that *safe* Caesarean section
procedures and related techniques for reducing hemorrhaging and infection were
invented.[10]

It is also relevant to note that the Hippocratic author of *Development of the
Child*, quoted above, apparently declined to be bound by the Oath (if, indeed, he
knew of it at all). For his young dancer is a single girl, though possibly also a
slave. By aborting early on she rids herself, through her doctor's cooperation, of
any inconvenience that an unwanted pregnancy would have represented in her
role as a musical performer. Therefore, the Hippocratic physician in this instance
instructs his client on how to terminate her suspected pregnancy for reasons of a
non-life-threatening sort. He may well have belonged to a third group of physicians, perhaps the largest, who were willing to grant abortions for almost any
reason at all.[11] Yet Soranus, who, like many of his fellow practitioners, ignored the Oath on the matter of abortion, would have nonetheless found this particular girl's motives for abortion morally unacceptable. So, too, her doctor's
complicity.

Hence, we are again reminded of the freedom enjoyed by members of the
medical craft throughout most of antiquity: physicians could ply their trade as

they saw fit, subject only to the laws of the land, almost none of which barred abortion or, for that matter, voluntary euthanasia. We are also in a position to confirm that the Hippocratic teaching on abortion is by no means cut and dried, despite popular misconceptions to the contrary.

EUTHANASIA

What, then, of the Hippocratic teaching on euthanasia? Did the majority of the Hippocratic authors and their disciples advocate or oppose voluntary euthanasia? On what grounds?

The straightforward way to approach this question is to observe that the Hippocratic authors advocated not even beginning medical treatment in cases where patients were known to be suffering from incurable illnesses. In the Hippocratic treatise *The Art*, the art of medicine (*techne iatrike*) is defined as follows: "In general terms, it is [1] to do away with the sufferings of the sick, [2] to lessen the violence of their diseases, and [3] to refuse to treat those who are over-mastered by their diseases, realizing that in such cases medicine is powerless."[12] The last part of this statement may strike some readers as evidence of a hideously stern and uncaring attitude on the part of the Greek physician. The logic behind such an attitude, however, is not complicated. It rests on at least two motivations, one of which may be described as humanitarian, the other prudential.

First, as the author of the treatise eloquently proceeds to argue, every art or craft has its own limitations and proper ends. It is madness, he says, not to accept the fact that some diseases are by their very nature beyond the physician's power to arrest. If so, it is a dictate of reason that no thoughtful physician ought to initiate treatment when he determines in advance that a particular patient now soliciting his healing services is well beyond medical hope. To treat an incurable patient, therefore, is tantamount to willfully drawing out his suffering and raising false hopes: such a practice is unethical and smacks of bad medicine, for nature in such cases cannot be intelligently opposed.

Second, it is true that the Hippocratic physician, like his Egyptian counterpart, made extensive use of medical forecasting in order to determine rationally which patients to treat and which to leave alone. But prognostication was also useful as a prudent tool by which the doctor could simultaneously protect his own reputation by not attempting therapy on hopeless incurables whose final demise under his care might be bad for business. So this concern for reputation constituted a second motivation that was grounded primarily on economic and not simply moral or humanitarian constraints. The Hippocratic author of the treatise *Prognostic*, for example, unabashedly links the value of this art to remaining blameless in the eyes of others:

> Now to restore every patient to health is impossible. To do so indeed would have been better even than forecasting the future. But as a matter of fact

men do die, some owing to the severity of the disease before they summon the physician, others expiring immediately after calling him in. . . . It is necessary, therefore, to learn the natures of such diseases, . . . and to learn how to forecast them. For in this way you will justly win respect and be an able physician. For the longer time you plan to meet each emergency, the greater your power to save those who have a chance of recovery, while you will be blameless if you learn and declare beforehand those who will die and those who will get better.[13]

Furthermore, if the patient was thought to be hopeless, the Hippocratic physician was not inclined to inform him directly, unless perhaps he pleaded to be told. Instead it was customary for the physician to inform a third party, who might, in turn, break the bad news as gently as possible to his sick friend or loved one.[14] Moreover, if requested to supply a lethal poison, the ancient physician was not legally barred from doing so; many apparently chose to accommodate their patients' pleas for euthanasia in just this way. Hence, the patient was not necessarily doomed to be totally abandoned by the medical community in his last days and hours.[15] If a physician declined to treat him, the patient could at least be made as comfortable as possible, or seek palliative or alternative care at a nearby Asclepian temple. He could also quit life altogether with the aid of fast-acting drugs sold by the willing practitioner. That such pharmaceutical assistance was often motivated by the physician's sincere compassion for his patient's unbearable suffering, I do not personally doubt.[16] If so, a decision "not to treat" cannot justifiably be ascribed merely to the ancient physician's selfish concern to protect his business reputation as a gifted healer. At least an equally important part of the story is that, on ethical grounds, many physicians sought to avoid raising false hopes or to avoid irresponsibly prolonging their patient's agony by staging costly mock treatments.

Therefore, although the Hippocratic Collection is not stocked with imperatives commanding doctors to assist consenting patients to end their tortured lives, with the notable exception of the Oath not a single Hippocratic writer voices opposition to voluntary euthanasia. Granted, this does not constitute an endorsement. But it does represent a significant fact that squares with the known medical practices of those times during which the cooperation of physicians in aiding acts of suicide among the very sick was widespread.[17] It is also a fact that further casts doubt on any popular acceptance of the Hippocratic Oath by ancient medical doctors as a whole, including those several medical writers whom we lump together under the name "Hippocrates."

So far, we have discovered that it was not generally considered morally wrong inside or outside the craft of medicine for the Hippocratic physician of the fifth and later centuries to aid in the practices of abortion or voluntary euthanasia. That is, the physician was not normally vulnerable to moral condemnation for engaging in these practices, given his vocational role as a craftsman belonging to a largely itinerant, totally unlicensed and unregulated working class that specialized in the various healing arts. In fact, we have seen that the Greek physician could practice medicine pretty much as he saw fit under the social conditions of the Hellenic and Hellenistic periods, subject only to those general legal constraints that applied to all citizens.

"DO NO HARM"

Yet, in attempting to further delineate the role responsibility of the Greek and later Roman physicians in regard to abortion and euthanasia, it is pertinent to ask whether evidence from the Hippocratic Collection supports the positive claim that it was considered by the Hippocratics and their followers to be the physician's moral duty to aid in patient-requested abortion or euthanasia. Alternatively put, it is pertinent to ask whether the physician was usually liable to blame or to charges that he had violated his professional responsibilities if he declined to perform these services. The answer to these questions is no. To support my contention, I shall re-examine one additional piece of much debated evidence from the Hippocratic texts.[18] The evidence, which is sometimes touted as excluding abortion or euthanasia, is, in fact, *neutral* on this question of there being positive moral duties to abort or to assist in voluntary euthanasia.

The evidence in question comes from *Epidemics* I. It constitutes one of the best known maxims of Greek medical literature, and it appears below, as it seldom does elsewhere, in its wider context:

> Declare the past, diagnose the present, foretell the future; practice these acts. *As to diseases, make a habit of two things—to help or at least do no harm.* The art has three factors, the disease, the patient, the physician. The physician is the servant of the art. The patient must cooperate with the physician in combating the disease.[19]

It is not hard to imagine that in the case of a woman seeking abortion, if her physician refused assistance and she thereafter undertook to independently terminate her pregnancy by her own methods, the woman thus greatly increased her own personal risks. For the average citizen, then as now, did not possess sufficient medical knowledge of her own to minimize possible damage to herself (Fig. 9). Therefore, the doctor's refusal to abort might in some cases be fairly viewed as a contributing factor leading to a desperate patient's personal decision to take matters into her own hands, thereby very possibly doing lasting harm to herself.

These sorts of considerations make it overhasty to tag the preceding passage as one that clearly forbids physicians to help patients abort. In fact, if a particular physician did not, on philosophical grounds, conceive of the fetus as a sentient creature, nor even as a human being, then the imperative "not to harm"

Figure 9. Interior medallion of a cup by the Brygos Painter, ca. 490–480 B.C. "First, do no harm . . ." has always been a paradoxical imperative. Some short-term harm is frequently involved in rendering a cure, as in this man vomiting to rid his body of excess, offending humors. Promising experimental therapies may also harm until refined or refuted. Reprinted by permission of Martin von Wagner Museum, Wurtzburg University, Germany. (Photo: K. Oehrlein)

could thereby be understood to have no moral force in cases of abortion. And, indeed, with the exception of the implied respect-for-human-life ethic engendered in the Hippocratic Oath, the remaining Hippocratic writings take no reasoned stand whatever on the specific question of whether the fetus is a human being whose right to exist must never be challenged by the mother, the physician, or the community.

Also the preceding passage deals with the physician's duties to his patient in arresting his *patient's* disease. If, therefore, the physician determined that his patient's pregnancy was threatening to harm her own life (given her present constitutional state), is it not then conceivable that the full context of this imperative could be rightly interpreted to justify abortion for therapeutic purposes? This cannot be ruled out. Even so, the passage in question admittedly does not succeed in clearly establishing any positive duty that physicians ought to perform abortions on request. At best, it remains neutral on that question, subject only to the partisan philosophical ideology of the attending physician.

But what about voluntary euthanasia? Don't the words " . . . at least do no harm," unequivocally condemn that practice? Probably not. For if the patient is judged to be suffering from a terminal disease, and if he is presently in great agony and is begging for death, it is far from obvious that to furnish the patient with a lethal poison in such cases is to do harm in the required sense. At least there is no reason to think it incredible that such assistance on the part of a physician might have been construed by many citizens as a kindness. This remains an open question: it would be a gross oversimplification to stereotype all pre-Christian Greek or Roman physicians as personally favoring voluntary euthanasia. What *can* be legitimately claimed, however, is that a considerable number did. And they did so partly owing to their own partisan philosophical perspectives on the question of euthanasia—perspectives that were doubtlessly influenced to some extent by the flourishing philosophical schools of their time.

In any case, the passage under consideration from *Epidemics* I appears neutral on this issue. My analysis suggests that the passage neither entails nor excludes the ascription of positive duties on the part of the Greco-Roman physician to supply patients requesting drugs for voluntary euthanasia or, for that matter, abortion.

SUMMARY

Since there is no clear ascription of such positive duties involving abortion or euthanasia throughout the Hippocratic Collection, and since the Hippocratic Oath unequivocally opposes these two practices, where does this leave us?

I have argued in chapter 5 that the Hippocratic Oath represents a small and largely ignored reform movement within the ranks of fifth- and fourth-century-B.C. medical practitioners. This implies that its contemporary moral force was quite limited. The Oath's prohibitions, then, were morally binding only on proportionately few of those craftsmen who practiced ancient medicine. Most physicians were not even aware of the Oath's existence. Those who were chose to adopt or ignore whatever provisions of it they felt they could stomach, based on their professional experiences, philosophical ideologies, and individual consciences. Thus, all things considered, the following characterization comes closest to capturing the fairest picture of the average Greek doctor's moral situation with regard to abortion and voluntary euthanasia. Given his vocational role *qua* physician, the Hippocratic healer of the fifth and fourth centuries was never morally bound by positive duties to assist in abortion or voluntary euthanasia on request. He could, of course, assist in these practices without much risk of moral disapprobation from either inside or outside the ranks of his craft, if he so chose. Therefore, he possessed what may be described as a *discretionary* professional right to assist in abortion or voluntary euthanasia: he was not obliged *qua* physician either to take part or to refrain from such services. It was entirely up to his own judgment and moral sense of things.

If so, was there not also a discernible symmetry in the ancient doctor-patient relationship, especially in regard to the options of abortion and euthanasia? For, depending on the moral or religious perspectives of a given patient, is it not true that—legally, if not morally—almost all patients felt that they were similarly possessed of a parallel discretionary right to seek or decline these controversial medical services, according only as their individual consciences dictated?

This, I submit, was for a long time the case. It was not really until the Western world fell under the influence of Christianity in the last two centuries of the Roman Empire that the moral duties of the ancient physician became decisively redefined. When this occurred, his discretionary rights regarding abortion and euthanasia (and those also of his patients) were at first publicly condemned and then socially pressured.[20] From the early Christian perspective, the Hippocratic Oath, more than any other medical ethical work of the pagan period, contained much to be admired—though it, too, was recast to include the new deity.

For example, the earliest known Christian version of the pagan Oath, probably written some time before the third century A.D., was entitled: "From the Oath According to Hippocrates Insofar as a Christian May Swear It." Translated from the Greek, the first several lines of this Christianized version read:

> Blessed be God the Father of Our Lord Jesus Christ, who is blessed for ever and ever; I lie not. I will bring no stain upon the learning of the medical art. Neither will I give poison to anybody though asked to do so, nor will I suggest such a plan. Similarly, I will not give treatment to cause abortion. . . .[21]

Surely this basic acceptance of the Hippocratic Oath was due in no small measure to the Oath's implied respect-for-human-life ethic. For this was an ethic accorded high favor among the celebrants of this latest of the great mystery religions, just as it had won the favor of a comparatively smaller circle of religiously inspired Greek physicians many centuries earlier.

Discussion Questions

1. Does the entire Hippocratic Collection consistently oppose the participation of physicians in acts of abortion? What about euthanasia? Explain.
2. What is meant by the "role responsibility" of an individual working in a particular job? In your opinion, who or what determines the parameters of this responsibility?
3. What were Soranus's views on whether the physician should assist in abortion? Was abortion ever justified in his view?
4. Is Scribonius Largus's philosophy of medical humanism consistent with the ethical values of the Hippocratic Oath?

5. In spite of the Hippocratic Oath, did Greek and Roman doctors perform abortion for almost any reason? What about infanticide? Euthanasia? How do you account for this?

6. Did the Hippocratic imperative, "[F]irst do no harm," argue for or against the Hippocratic doctors assisting in voluntary euthanasia? Discuss the various ways this notion can be understood.

NOTES

1. H. L. A. Hart, *Punishment and Responsibility* (Oxford: Oxford University Press, 1968), pp. 211–30. Such role responsibilities can be classified into two types of duties: (a) moral duties and (b) legal duties. I shall mainly deal with the former.

2. Hippocrates, *On Intercourse and Pregnancy*, trans. Tage Ellinger (New York: Henry Schuman, Inc., 1952), and Littré, *Oeuvres*, vol.13, p. 490.

3. *Soranus' Gynecology*, trans. Temkin, p. 63.

4. See chapter 6, pp. 120–21.

5. Scribonius Largus, *Compositiones*, ed. Georg Helmreich (Leipzig: Teubner, 1887), p. 2. Scribonius and Erotian took Hippocrates to be the true author of the Oath.

6. Ibid.

7. Ibid. Scribonius Largus's concept of humaneness (*humanitas*), which was a central idea in his medical philosophy, meant more than simply affecting a friendly disposition. It involved what he called a " . . . proficiency and benevolence toward all men without regard to race, creed, or color." Though there is no evidence that he was a Christian convert, he may have been tinged by Christian or Stoic notions of the universal brotherhood of man. At any rate, Scribonius was aware that his philosophy of medical humanism went considerably beyond the moral scope of the Hippocratic writings on ethics and etiquette.

His use of the word *humanitas* corresponded, at the time he wrote, with the then dominant meaning of the Greek word *philanthropia* (the love of mankind). Yet it is not likely that the Hippocratic Oath was consciously animated by *philanthropia* at the time it was written; that sentiment was not native to Greek thinking in pagan times. Even so, I must concur with Ludwig Edelstein's judgment that the Oath nonetheless " . . . assumes full significance and dignity [from the modern point of view] only if interpreted in the way in which it was understood by Scribonius and those who came after him." (See Ludwig Edelstein, "The Professional Ethics of the Greek Physician," in *Ancient Medicine*, p. 374.)

8. Oswei Temkin, "The Idea of Respect for Life in the History of Medicine," in *Respect for Life*, pp. 10–11.

9. But to what degree did pagan followers of the Oath feel this conflict of duty? If they were devoutly religious, as presumably many were, is it not likely that they saw the irresistible will of heaven in the tragic loss of the mother's life during childbirth? Indeed, have not some modern partisans of the Hippocratic Oath's stand on abortion traditionally found solace in a similar theological conviction, i.e., that the regrettable loss of the mother, or fetus, or both, is God's will?

It will be recalled that the ancients did not construe the question of abortion (therapeutic or otherwise) in the now familiar language of competing moral rights. For example, weighing the putative right to life of the fetus versus that of the mother, community, etc. The claim that moral rights exist is mainly a modern one.

10. The Caesarean section is one of the oldest surgical procedures. It was almost always fatal to women throughout antiquity and the Middle Ages. Legend had it that Julius Caesar was born in this fashion, which is most doubtful. The operation is named for a branch of the ancient Roman family of the Julii, whose cognomen, Caesar (cf. *cadere*, "to cut"), originated from a birth by this means, according to Pliny. "Caesarean Section,"in *Encyclopaedia Britannica* (London: Encyclopaedia Britannica Inc., 1971), vol. 4, p. 577. Zeus performed a version of the Caesarean when he rescued his still unborn son, the infant Dionysus, from the womb of his mortal lover, Semele, who had suffered a tragic and sudden death. Fortunately for mankind, Dionysus flourished.

11. One religious consideration related to the pre-Christian acceptability of physicians supplying abortifacients was this. By Hellenistic times, it was not widely believed that the ghosts of terminated fetuses sought revenge against their living offenders, if indeed that was ever a serious constraint. There is evidence suggesting that, in earlier times, some types of ghosts were thought to "walk" or to be restless, but few sought revenge against the living for their misery. It is true that Plato records the souls of some suicides suffering penance in the afterworld (*Republic* 10.615c). But the absence in pagan thought of anything like the Christian doctrine of Original Sin, which eventually was thought to damn the souls of fetuses whose lives were ended without baptism, must have lessened the religious anxieties of the pagans in regard to abortion. (See Mair, "Suicide," in *ERE*, vol 12, pp. 30–31.)

12. *The Art* 3, trans. Jones, *Hippocrates*, vol. 2, p. 193.

13. *Prognostic* 1, trans. Jones, *Hippocrates*, vol. 2, pp. 7–8. Other relevant passages in the Hippocratic Collection that show a marked concern for professional reputation include *Precepts* 9 and *Decorum* 11, 17.

14. Hippocrates, *Pyorrhetic* 2, cited by Littré, *Oeuvres*, vol. 6, pp. 4–6. See Danielle Gourevitch, "Suicide among the Sick in Classical Antiquity," *Bulletin of the History of Medicine* 43 (1969): 501–18. One must beware of inferring from this discussion that the Hippocratics regularly shunned difficult cases. For evidence to the contrary, see *On Joints* 69; *Ancient Medicine* 9; and *Precepts* 7.

15. In an interesting paper, Ludwig Edelstein has argued that the role of religious or temple medicine for the terminally ill, by the fifth century B.C. and for centuries later, was roughly this. Those patients declared untreatable often sought refuge and alternative therapies of a supernatural sort under the auspices of the temple priests of Asclepius (see Fig. 5). The Hippocratic physicians did not customarily prescribe such religious therapies themselves, it is true, but they studiously left that option open. Hence, those of their patients declared untreatable were not, in fact, deserted by all representatives of the medical community: the religious segment was a last resort, providing comfort and solace, if not lasting cures, to the suffering multitude. (See Ludwig Edelstein, "Greek Medicine in Its Relation to Religion and Magic," in *Ancient Medicine*, pp. 205–46.)

16. Could another factor in the physician's motivation have been his financial gain through the sale of lethal drugs? This possibility cannot be dismissed. As suggested in chapter 1, most physicians had to work for a living; some had trouble making ends meet. But as Apuleius's *Metamorphoses* implies, it is entirely unwarranted and even slanderous to depict the ancient physician as an unseemly poison-peddler who practices only for

the sake of his purse. For more on Apuleius, see chapter 5, note 46. Plato's ideal physician functions *qua* to serve others, and only in a subsidiary capacity does he function as a wage-earner (*Republic* 1.341cff.). In general, see Fridolf Kudlien, "Medicine as a 'Liberal Art' and the Question of the Physician's Income,"*Journal of the History of Medicine* 31, no. 4 (1976): 448–59.

17. Gourevitch, "Suicide among the Sick," pp. 508ff.

18. The passage about to be discussed (construed *primum non nocere* in Latin texts) is also examined in chapter 5, in a somewhat different context.

19. *Epidemics* 1.11., trans. Jones, *Hippocrates*, vol. 1, p. 165, emphases added.

20. Abortion was formally condemned in the West by the Church as early as A.D. 305 by the Council of Elvira meeting on the Iberian Peninsula (canon 52); later it was condemned in the East within a decade by the Council of Ancyra in A.D. 314 (canon 21). (See J. T. Noonan, "An Almost Absolute Value," in *Morality of Abortion*, p. 14.) Severe penalties were imposed, including excommunication for women who aborted in order to conceal adultery. For further developments during the early Christian period, see Noonan, pp. 11–18 *passim*. As for euthanasia, Darrell Amundsen has observed that while the early Christian tradition held it to be a sin for the physician to terminate life using active euthanasia, " . . . it laid no stress, apparently, on the positive correlate that would require the physician actively to prolong life." (See Amundsen, "The Physician's Obligation to Prolong Life," p. 27.) The Christian position was based largely on the principle that God alone gives life and man ought not interfere with God's purposes. Many early Christian writers held that either God caused some persons to fall ill or He did nothing to prevent such diseases from occurring. Secular medicine was thus widely viewed as working against God's divine plan for man and it took many centuries for the medical art to gain acceptance among the devout. Citing Arnobius (*Adversus gentes* 1.48) and Tatian (*Oratio Graecos* 18), Amundsen concludes that "while abortion, suicide, and euthanasia became sins, the prolonging of life did not become either a virtue or a duty." (See Amundsen, "The Phsycian's Obligation to Prolong Life," p. 27.)

21. Jones, trans., *The Doctor's Oath*, p. 55. For evidence on the possible influence of the Hippocratic Oath on early Jewish medical writers, see Fred Tosner and Sussman Muntner, "The Oath of Asaph," *Annals of Internal Medicine* 63 (1965): 317–20.

Conclusion

*The future belongs to those who shall have done
most for suffering humanity.*

—LOUIS PASTEUR

WE HAVE DISCOVERED not one but many diverse Greek and Roman philosophical and medical perspectives on abortion and euthanasia. Let us glance ret-
rospectively at some of the key findings and reflect briefly on their possible implications for a fuller understanding of the origins and character of Western
medical ethics. My remarks will encompass four broad areas: (1) the multiplicity
of ancient medical ethical perspectives; (2) the relationship of ancient physicians
to ancient philosophers; (3) the relationship of these physicians to their patients;
and (4) the relationship of physicians to the state.

DIVERSE MEDICAL ETHICAL PERSPECTIVES

From the evidence that we have examined, manifold and diverse Greco-Roman
ethical perspectives on the rightness or wrongness of abortion, euthanasia, and related topics have emerged. What does it mean?

One thing that it clearly means is that there is no such thing as *the* Greek or
Roman view on abortion, or *the* Greek or Roman view on euthanasia, or on when
humanhood begins and ends, or on what happens to a person when he dies, and so
on. Some contemporary scholars, like Langer and Mair, and several more of their
predecessors, like Lecky and Westermarck, have on the whole tended to lump together Greco-Roman perspectives on such vital bioethical and metaphysical questions. Differences in degree of approval or condemnation were admitted, but over-

all the impression was that the Greeks and Romans of pre-Christian antiquity generally concurred on these matters. Why? Ultimately, because of their very nearly shared values. But this tendency to construe Greco-Roman bioethical and related religious perspectives in monolithic and unitary terms is, I now suggest, mistaken.

In fact, philosophers, physicians, and laymen held a myriad of diverse views on these central questions of life and death. Some philosophers, like Pythagoras, categorically opposed abortion. Others, like Aristotle, did not. Some physicians, like the Hippocratic author of *On the Development of the Child*, performed abortions for almost any reason; Soranus, on the other hand, did not. Some laymen looked forward to divine personal immortality at death; others awaited dissolution and oblivion. And on and on. One can see at a glance that philosophers, physicians, and laymen were free to adopt diverse ethical perspectives. Furthermore, when they did so it appears likely that their views were often formulated quite independently of one another. For example, a patient did not necessarily adopt the eschatological perspective of his physician, no matter how much the latter was revered as a capable healer. Nor, I dare say, did the philosopher easily succeed in winning his physician friends over to his moral views on infanticide, no matter how much he otherwise may have been respected for his clear-headedness. This is not to deny that there were crosscurrents of influence on these and other ethical questions. Surely there were. But the freedom to form such diverse perspectives, with little or no interference from legal or religious authorities or institutions, went a long way toward creating a ripe climate for the ethical pluralism to which this study bears witness.

Incidentally, the multiplicity of ethical perspectives so far revealed was matched, it will be recalled, by a parallel diversity of scientific approaches to the practice of medicine. Hence, in the same fourth-century-B.C. Greek town one could typically find physicians who would and those who would not perform abortions; one could also find physicians who were and others who were not members of a particular medical sect, and so on. Thus it is fair to conclude that Greek culture, in particular, was indeed a rich and diverse one: as much or more so in medical and in ethical matters, it turns out, as it obviously was in its ever-changing and diverse forms of artistic expression as seen in Greek architecture, vase painting, and sculpture. Moreover, doesn't this societal toleration of a multiplicity of inventive approaches to art, to early science, and to ethics and philosophy in general at once epitomize much of the dynamism and strength of the Greek mind?

A related question may be raised as to whether the fifth- and fourth-century Greeks possessed a weaker sense of moral duty than has often been ascribed to them. This question is prompted by the fact that, in medically related matters at least, a plurality of conflicting ethical perspectives flourished alongside one another. And so it is not easy to discover a single, unified paradigm expressing the ancient physician's moral duty, although the Hippocratic Oath itself has been mistakenly viewed in those terms. For there were then several different approaches to the "proper" conduct of the physician-patient relationship, though some had more currency than others.

Yet, if there is an exception to this last claim, perhaps it occurs among the early Pythagorean, or Pythagorean-influenced, doctors. As I have argued, their steadfast commitment to the respect-for-life ethic led not only to rigorous dietary observances among the devout but also to rigorous, unitary, and unconditional medical ethical duties as well. The latter, as we saw, included the duty not to co-operate in abortion, infanticide, euthanasia, or suicide. These absolute moral constraints were formally predicated on the monolithic religious principle that God values each and every sentient creature without exception.

In addition, to a lesser extent Plato also comes close to furnishing a single moral paradigm of duty. For Plato searched for and apparently thought he had discovered the one right utopian social and moral principle from which a host of primary and secondary moral duties—many touching on matters of public health and medical care—were derivable. The principle to which I am referring, roughly speaking, expressed his view that whatever laws and customs were judged best for the smoothly functioning ideal state taken as a whole were also morally right acts in terms of the particular individual's welfare. The state came first for Plato not because the individual citizen or patient did not count. Rather, it was that, all things considered, the state counted *more*: its ongoing health and very survival were seen as a necessary condition for the minimal survival of any one or more of its citizens.

Moreover, the early modern historical view that detected a decisive Pythagorean influence on Greek culture is clearly mistaken. This view was tinged by eighteenth-century neo-Platonist thinking, according to which Hellenic and later Greek culture was seen as a highly synthetic whole uniquely informed by Pythagorean and neo-Pythagorean elements.[1] Yet that early modern view, now largely abandoned, is probably not entirely wrong, as some may argue.

For, to take but one example, while Edelstein is wrong in thinking that the Oath is an exclusively Pythagorean product, he is essentially right in tracing the distinctiveness of its uncompromising respect-for-human-life stand to Pythagorean influences. Further, I suggest that in many other spheres outside of medicine and ethics, the Greeks indeed owed much to the Pythagoreans, but clearly not everything. Therefore, it was truly an unfortunate exaggeration for earlier modern historians to ascribe to the Pythagoreans most of the credit for the manifold achievements of Greek culture in somewhat sweeping terms. Yet, as is sometimes the case even with historical exaggerations, there remains within them a possible glimmer of truth: the Pythagoreans, it seems, were in every sense a seminal and unique influence on Greek medicine and philosophy.

PHYSICIANS AND PHILOSOPHERS

In sizing up the relationship of ancient physicians to ancient philosophers, I have argued that, in essence, their feelings toward one another were both cooperative and antagonistic.

They were cooperative in the sense that both sought ultimately to plumb nature for some lasting insights into her universal laws. Many philosophers sought especially *to explain* phenomena through these laws in order to liberate the mind from ignorance. Most physicians sought *to use* the practical consequences of these laws in order to liberate the body from suffering.

Perhaps more important for clinicians and students of ethics, the intellectual relationship between physicians and philosophers was also antagonistic: both sought to suggest right ways to live. Hence, the authority of moral philosophers was implicitly challenged by doctors who—on primarily medical, not ethical, grounds—directed their clients to adjust their daily regimens in accord with their favored theories of good hygiene. Conversely, the authority of doctors was effectively scrutinized by philosophers, many of whom wondered aloud (as did Plato) whether doctors were really qualified to prescribe to the ordinary citizen intimate patterns of daily living that ideally presupposed a deep understanding of the ultimate values and ends of life.

This cooperative and antagonistic spirit has never vanished from the ranks of professional physicians and philosophers down to our own era. In the long run, this dynamic has played a constructive role in keeping each group and the public at large generally more alert to the potential problems and limitations that are engendered in these two complementary branches of humanistic and scientific endeavor.

In this connection, is it likely that part of the resourcefulness that marked the ancient physician-philosopher relationship resulted finally in each group reflecting somewhat more creatively than it previously had done on topics of life and death that formerly had belonged more exclusively to one group than to the other? That is, did some of the speculations of philosopher-scientists on such topics as when human life begins and ends, the meaning of death, the value of human life, and so on, possibly enrich the thinking of at least some of the more prominent and literate physicians on the role of their medical craft in preventing or prolonging life? Furthermore, did the widespread acquiescence of Greek and Roman physicians to their patients' requests for assistance in rendering abortions and hastening death possibly stimulate philosophers to address with greater urgency some of the moral implications of this conduct?

Personally, I do not doubt that there were crosscurrents of influence in both directions. More specifically, I raised in Part II the question of whether the views of various philosophers on the morality of abortion and euthanasia might have constituted at least one contributing cause to the eventual social acceptance of these practices in antiquity. I answer now in the affirmative. Admittedly, the evidence I have marshaled in the present study must, in all fairness, be called inconclusive on this question. I have furnished a detailed account of mainly four prominent philosophers on these topics, and the writings of many more remain forever irreclaimable in the ashes of history.

But of the four philosophers herein examined, it is worth noting that three argued in favor of abortion and infanticide under certain conditions (Plato, Aristotle, and Seneca). In addition, two endorsed the moral acceptability of voluntary euthanasia for the terminally or chronically ill (Plato and Seneca). These results surely add strength to the speculation that Greco-Roman philosophers played some role in fostering the dominant moral attitudes of a good many doctors and patients who felt that abortion and euthanasia were morally defensible. But I hesitate to say that this has been proved.

First, there is a formidable causal objection to contend with, one that the British philosopher David Hume so clearly defined.[2] That is, even if there existed sufficient evidence to show that most leading Greek or Roman philosophers judged abortion and euthanasia to be morally acceptable, one could not logically assert on this prior evidence alone that philosophers therefore succeeded in influencing the masses that these two practices were morally permissible. Much too much is taken for granted in such a hasty judgment, for (1) that B constantly follows A does not entail that A necessarily causes B and (2) there might be a variety of contributing causes for B, many of which we fail to perceive or distinguish.

Second, the possibility of a reverse assimilation of values cannot be fairly dismissed as a viable objection either. It is undeniable that on occasion the popular morals of the masses have, in subtle ways, infected the moral perspectives of academically trained philosophers or other leading experts.[3] I dare say this sort of thing goes on in our own epoch as it did in antiquity; it might be described as a trickle-up theory of social norms and values. Though I cannot stop here to debate the possible merits of such an interesting sociological theory, these preceding objections jointly constitute a real challenge to anyone attempting to gauge the historic influence of moral philosophers in shaping the medical or ethical values of a given culture, past, present, or future. Though I do not regard these objections as fatal, they nonetheless give serious pause to any thoughtful custodian of the history of ideas.

PHYSICIANS AND PATIENTS

There are two additional implications that come immediately to mind in view of my analysis of the moral responsibility of the physician toward his patients in responding to their requests for abortion or euthanasia. These are that the typical Greek or Roman doctor felt that he had neither (1) the absolute duty to prolong human life nor (2) the absolute duty to protect such life at any cost. I would like to speculate a bit on why this may have been so.

As for the absolute duty to *prolong* human life, I have already argued that the Hippocratic maxim " . . . First, do no harm," was really neutral on the question of whether a physician should assist in voluntary euthanasia. Furthermore, the average Greco-Roman physician was trained to assist the forces of nature in finding a natural resolution of patient discomfort and disease. This attitude followed in part from what I referred to in chapter 2 as the Hippocratic principle of natural healing. This principle recognized that the body possessed its own bio-

Figure 10. Detail, early fifth-century B.C. painted medallion from an Athenian drinking cup, attributed to Onesimos. Personal cleanliness in protecting and preserving health was practiced by educated Greeks and Romans, as this girl preparing to do laundry attests. Physicians taught that the body possessed its own curative powers. Reprinted by permission of Musées Royaux d'Art et d'Histoire, Brussels.

logical rhythms and curative powers (Fig. 10). The physician's job was to discover how these forces worked and then do nothing that would impede nature in her normal, curative course.

What is often missed, however, is that part of the Hippocratic physician's sense of the incalculable powers of nature as an indwelling force affecting the constitution of each and every patient rested on his accompanying awareness that death, too, represented a natural resolution to the human suffering generated by certain forms of disease. Of course, death was never greeted by the physician as a welcome visitor whenever his creative diagnostic and therapeutic skills proved equal to the challenge of a particular illness. But at other, less-fruitful times, to oppose nature in her normal cycle of generation and decay seemed the equivalent of hubris—especially when no known medical remedy existed.

To these considerations, also, I venture the following account. As the popular horror of death and the prospect of dwelling in a dank and unfriendly Hades eventually subsided—due in part to Aristotelian, Epicurean, and Stoic efforts to debunk the terrors of the afterworld—the very thought of assisting a patient in suicide or declining heroic measures to prolong the life of a suffering victim may have seemed somewhat less objectionable. For aside from the fact that death could then be more plausibly conceived by physician and patient alike as a refuge from untreatable pain and despair, there was also less cause to worry on religious grounds that the gods would thereby be offended or to worry that, as the earlier Pythagoreans had claimed, the suicide's soul would suffer a double penance in the next life. In a word, the prospect of death was just not that scary anymore.

As for the absolute duty to *protect* human life at all times, not only from diseases but from various members of the community who seek to prevent or end life (as in requests for abortion), the typical Greek or Roman physician felt unbound by such absolute constraints. In the case of requests for abortion, one cannot help but wonder whether part of the willingness of many physicians to grant abortions had something to do with their individual views on the status of the fetus within the moral community. Should the fetus be regarded as a person protected by the minimal moral and legal protections enjoyed by other children or by adults?

As we saw, the popular answer to this question by most citizens was no. In addition, except for the Pythagoreans, none of the philosophers that we examined held that human life began at the moment of conception in the relevant sense required here. Even though I did not find anywhere in the Hippocratic Collection an explicit position taken on this controversial issue by any one of the authors, it is very possible that the popular estimate of the fetus's low status may have carried over into medical appraisals of this matter, too. Also, there is the distinct possibility that various philosophical schools may have affected the thinking of physicians on this question as well, though which schools were most influential is hard to say.

Yet, although this stereotype has now been cast into doubt, one must beware of exaggerating the picture of the ancient physician-patient relationship in the opposite extreme. I, for one, think that a fair number of Greco-Roman physicians may well have recognized at least a presumptive or *prima facie* duty to protect human life in something like W. D. Ross's sense, though not in any absolute sense. That is, all things being equal, they would attempt to protect human life, though possibly to allow overriding reasons on a case-by-case basis for not doing so.[4] True, the average Greek physician probably did not swear to uphold the famous Oath of Hippocrates. He may never have even heard of it. But as a trained healer, wasn't it likely that his initial moral bias tended to favor the protection rather than destruction of human life?

In the special case of abortion, the moral issue additionally turned on whether the fetus possessed an incontestable right to be born. That such a right was routinely denied not only in philosophical circles but in religious and legal circles as well fostered a climate of institutional approval or inattention to abortion throughout most of antiquity. In fact, the respect-for-human-life ethic found few supporters. As I suggested at the close of the preceding chapter, it expressed a moral value that was all but ignored by most pagan physicians, even though they themselves may have been among its first authors. It remained for the early Christians to insist on that ethic's divine moral status and declare it the absolute standard of right conduct for doctor and patient alike.

PHYSICIANS AND THE STATE

We have seen that the Greeks were not the first ancient people to attempt to define the proper conduct of their physicians. The Babylonian Code of Hammurabi antedates the rise of Greek medical ethics by well over a thousand years. Moreover, the Assyrians, Persians, Hebrews, and Egyptians were shown to have made some efforts to formalize or clarify the duties of their physician-priests in regard to abortion or euthanasia.

Yet there was a marked difference in the Greek social and political conditions that accompanied the efforts of at least some fifth-century Hellenic physicians to begin inventing and adopting moral guidelines for the proper practice of medicine. That difference was that the Greek city-states, by and large, left their physicians alone. Greek physicians were virtually free to accept or reject patients and treat them in accordance with their own best judgment. The Greek states did not impose craft restrictions and additional legal regulations on their practitioners, unlike the states of Assyro-Babylonia, Persia, and Egypt, where the rulers busied themselves with such domestic affairs.

Hence, it is fair to ask what conditions may have been responsible for the doctor-initiated flowing of Greek medical ethics and etiquette? What would have caused at least some physicians to voluntarily invent or adopt various medical oaths or rules-of-craft conduct in the first place?

One possible answer is to attempt to explain this achievement as the fortuitous outcome of the so-called explosion of Greek genius, which is popularly associated with the philosophic, scientific, political, and artistic advances of the fifth-century Athenian golden age (see Appendix F). But it strikes me that the Greek love of abstract ideas and the cultural momentum of the golden age, however real these influences may have been on the general advance of Greek scientific medicine, supply all-too-ready answers to our query here—answers that finally explain very little.

More plausibly, I think the physician-initiated and voluntarily imposed Hippocratic norms can be explained as the partial result of a felt need on the part of some practitioners to bring more uniformity and integrity to the conduct of physicians as a whole—both toward each other and toward their patients.

Thus, we observed of the Hippocratic Oath that its covenant specifies some of the more important duties between established master-physicians and their junior partners whom they undertook to properly train. Similarly, the four Hippocratic works on etiquette also contained maxims that aimed at regularizing how physicians should act toward one another during professional consultations and in the marketplace. Such physician concerns can, of course, be properly understood from the altruistic standpoint of wishing to protect the patient's best interests—by sparing him, for example, from unpleasant bedside disputations between two doctors quarreling over the patient's proper treatment; or, typically, by sparing him from the abuses of would-be doctors or charlatans who had not been properly schooled in the trade secrets of the healing art.

Yet that is only part of the story. These identical medical concerns must also be frankly recognized for their egoistic content. They had the potential to protect the professional and business reputations of the ancient physicians themselves, who, after all, sought to sell their services to a trusting and respectful public.

Therefore, it is fair to conclude that the primary elements contributing to the emergence of Greco-Roman medical ethics and etiquette were twofold. First, there was the preexisting condition of freedom. Second, there was the willingness of some Greek physicians to respond to this freedom by accepting responsibility for their own professional conduct and that of their entire craft. Freedom brought with it the opportunity for medical experimentation and the chance for progressive advances in patient care. The very same freedom, however, also fostered opportunities for charlatanism, medical chicanery, and higher-than-acceptable risks of abuse or permanent injury to patients and their families who were seeking medical services. This latter prospect, in particular, struck a good many Greek and Roman physicians as morally unacceptable. It also left their craft open to hostile forms of public suspicion and criticism, some justified and some slanderous. This criticism and suspicion was bad for the business of ancient medicine; it represents a professional vulnerability from which medicine has not escaped to this day.

Discussion Questions

1. Is it accurate to construe the Hippocratic Oath as a strong indicator of the common moral duties observed by fifth- and fourth-century-B.C. Greek physicians? Why or why not?

2. Were philosophers of antiquity in general agreement on when human life, in the moral sense, begins? Are they in agreement today?

3. Did most laymen in antiquity think that the fetus had a right to life? Did most physicians? What about philosophers?

4. Do Greco-Roman physicians recognize a *prima facie* duty to protect human life?

5. Was the Hippocratic Oath widely known in the pre-Christian era?

NOTES

1. See, for example, Paul O. Kristeller, *Renaissance Thought: The Classic, Scholastic and Humanistic Strains*, rev. ed. (New York: Harper and Row, 1961).
2. David Hume, An Enquiry Concerning Human Understanding, sec. 4, pp. 1–2; sec. 5.
3. Kudlien, "Medical Ethics and Popular Ethics," pp. 109ff.
4. Ross, *The Right and the Good*, chap. 2, is instructive here.

Epilogue

Medical Ethics is too ancient and too essential a
reality in the lives of physicians, patients, and
society to be left entirely to the fortuitous currents
of philosophical fashion or the unsupported
assertions of clinicians.[1]

—EDMUND D. PELLEGRINO, M.D.

THE BIOMEDICAL REVOLUTION

As much as we may admire the therapeutic and ethical achievements of the Hippocratic physicians and their successors in Greece and Rome, most agree that the physician-patient relationship has undergone many significant changes since antiquity. Much of this change is due to the comparatively recent invention and application of automated medical technologies and experimental drug therapies in the treatment of disease. For example, in ever more instances, physicians can keep brain-dead patients "alive," or patients in persistent vegetative states functioning almost indefinitely through the use of respirator and related life-support technologies that sustain breathing and circulation. Many of these patients would have died of their afflictions straightaway in earlier, pretechnological times. In Aristotle's Athens, the average age of mortality was approximately forty.[2] What's more, this ethically perplexing state of affairs in critical care medicine has been realized by a vast array of new machines, including fully coordinated monitors, powerful radiologic and chemical therapies, microsurgical robotic techniques, customized artificial limbs and joints, as well as donor and mechanical organ substitutes.

In stark contrast, the ancient physician did not face the awesome problem of being able to prolong a patient's life indefinitely. He lived during a comparatively pretechnological period, when the latest advances in medical technology included new forms of bandaging, drug and dietary measures, pain-relieving surgical maneuvers, or the application of palpating techniques. He had no occasion, therefore, to agonize over whether his terminally ill kidney patient would be ready to receive a compatible donor organ in time to avert impending renal failure. Nor, obviously, did he have any care about many of the brand new ethical problems presented today by such controversial procedures as the formation of human life in a petri dish (in vitro fertilization). Nor was he faced with the counseling dilemmas brought on by genetic screening, including deciding whether to share or withhold sensitive genetic information to prospective parents regarding the health of their yet unborn offspring, based on what is often merely statistical, inconclusive evidence.

Nor, again, was the ancient physician bedeviled to the same degree as his modern counterpart by the option to prescribe an increasingly complex series of largely untested experimental drugs to consenting, terminally ill patients pleading for relief or cure at any cost. These are but a few of the many pressing ethical dilemmas that now confront contemporary teams of medical specialists trying to protect and save lives in medical centers across the country. Most, if not all, of these dilemmas involve fresh medical options and treatment strategies spawned by the biological, engineering, and medical revolutions that have converged in the twentieth and twenty-first centuries. As a result, nothing quite so exciting or unsettling has occurred before either in the history of medicine or in the evolution of medical ethics.

Given the unique technological character of contemporary medicine, some critics have objected that the Hippocratic medical tradition—its patient-care concepts and ethical principles in particular—is manifestly irrelevant. For the Hippocratic tradition came into being in comparatively primitive times vastly different from our own. These critics, therefore, conclude that the moral rules associated with the Hippocratic legacy are entirely inappropriate for contemporary ethical problem-solving. Specifically, some object to the strictures against abortion and voluntary euthanasia embodied in the Hippocratic Oath, since they are phrased in absolute terms, admitting no exceptions whatever. These two prohibitions, along with restrictions against infanticide and suicide which the Oath tacitly implies, need to be amended or abandoned, critics allege, in view of such biomedical developments as amniocentesis, fetal monitoring, brain scans, and heart-lung machines. Clearly, these and other technologies have greatly expanded the options of both clinician and patient.

Consequently, many thoughtful people both inside and outside of medicine now question whether all cases of abortion or voluntary euthanasia are morally wrong, as the Oath declares. What's more, landmark United States Supreme Court decisions like *Roe v. Wade* (1973), which, among other things, legalized abortion on request for virtually any reason during the first trimester of a woman's pregnancy,[3] unmistakably signal society's growing skepticism toward the correctness of some of the most renowned Hippocratic ideals.

In what follows, I will examine some selected developments of the biomedical revolution with an eye toward weighing the pertinence of the Hippocratic legacy to the demands and trends of the contemporary medical scene. In this connection, some of the controversies associated with RU-486, surrogate motherhood, physician-assisted suicide, advance directives, paternalism, animal experimentation, and gene therapy are especially deserving of comment.

Morning After/Abortion Pill: RU-486

It will be recalled from our exploration of contraception in chapter 6 that the ancients knew of no reliable methods of preventing childbirth other than abstinence or abortion.[4] Yet, the Greek gynecologist Soranus endorsed contraception, observing that it was abortifacients that destroyed "what has been conceived"; contraceptives he sensibly defined as not letting conception take place.[5] With the recent discovery of the antiprogestin drug RU-486 (mifepristone), sometimes called "the morning after abortion pill," a chemical compound has become available which induces abortion by blocking the implantation of the fertilized egg in the uterine wall. Therefore some regard RU-486 as an oral contraceptive.

One may inquire: Would this nonsurgical option be discouraged by the Hippocratic Oath? Unquestionably, for the Oath's opposition to abortion is founded on respect for developing human life, presumably from the moment of conception. If the conceptus (or preembryo) is unable to be implanted in the uterus due to the chemical effects of the RU-486 pill when it is taken shortly after intercourse, then the destruction of potential human life nonetheless occurs. Thus, whether RU-486 is linguistically construed as a last-chance contraceptive or a first-choice abortifacient is beside the point. The fact is that a future human life is annihilated and this the Oath opposes.

Exactly how to define RU-486 is much debated. Unlike standard contraceptives that block the comingling of sperm and egg, RU-486 is more akin to the intrauterine device (IUD). This latter device is popularly but mistakenly viewed as a form of contraception. Yet it turns out that both the IUD and RU-486 arguably function as different sorts of abortifacient. That is, rather than preventing ovulation (as do oral contraceptives), rather than preventing conception (as do spermicides, diaphragms, and condoms), RU-486 prevents the implantation of the fertilized egg in the uterine wall.[6] Yet a standard textbook definition states that only at the point of implantation does pregnancy occur (normally within the fifth to twelfth day following fertilization).[7]

While RU-486 has been available in France since 1988, it was approved for use in the United States by the Food and Drug Administration on September 28, 2000—after much medical testing and debate. It is speculated that as this chemical alternative to surgical abortion becomes widespread, it will likely expand the number of annual abortions occurring in America. Approximately 1.4 million pregnancies are terminated by abortion in the United States, 50 million worldwide, each year.[8] The likely increase in abortions will possibly occur because of the greater privacy and ease of use that the RU-486 pill would provide in comparison to the standard first-trimester abortion methods of dilation or suction curettage. This would certainly make RU-486 a much more attractive option than walking into an abortion clinic and having medically trained strangers end an unwanted pregnancy.

Furthermore, it is sobering to consider that before RU-486 entered the U.S. market (under the name Mileprex), a significant portion of all abortions in the United States were, in effect, used as a backup method of birth control. Even more telling, of the 1.4 million American women getting abortions each year, 44 percent have had at least one previous abortion.[9] Therefore, this already existing pattern of reproductive irresponsibility[10] strongly suggests that as physicians dispense RU-486 (limited to the first seven weeks of pregnancy), these little yellow pills will facilitate more abortions in America.

To be sure, the degree of blameworthiness associated with using RU-486 depends on the moral status accorded to the fetus, or in this case, the "conceptus" (a technical term for the fertilized egg of only a few weeks duration). It also depends indirectly on how pregnancy is defined. For example, if pregnancy is said to occur at implantation of the conceptus, and not merely at conception, then the RU-486 pill is arguably not morally objectionable. Why? Because it blocks implantation. But if, on the other hand, both pregnancy *and* the moral status of the fetus are said to occur precisely at the moment of conception, then RU-486 is condemnable. Again, for both RU-486 and IUDs, the finding of moral praise or blame in their use depends largely on that point in time at which the conceptus or fetus is accorded moral worth.

This conclusion, however, may be oddly narrow. Metaphysically, it is fair to ask: why not push our moral concern for potential human life further back still? If so, then even the unfertilized egg sloughed off during menstruation, or the sperm wasted in ejaculation, could be said to be wasted constitutive human life.

However, this argument is not compelling: it ignores the significance of the biologically transformational moment of conception. Conception marks the fragile starting point of cellular union and ongoing division that, under normal conditions, leads to newborn human life within about forty weeks. Whatever one may think personally about the morality of abortion, one fact is clear: Whether by surgical intervention or by chemical pill-taking, a potential human life is ended. The searing question of the moral status of that fetal life is ultimately a metaphysical matter that cannot be settled by scientific or legal data.

As we saw, the physician who prescribes RU-486 (let alone the patient who would take it), clearly violates the spirit of the Hippocratic Oath's injunction: "I will not give to a woman an abortive remedy. In purity and holiness I will guard my life and my art." Nevertheless, the offending physician and his possibly desperate patient will arguably be in good company. In 1994 the American Medical Association, through its Council on Ethical and Judicial Affairs, formally approved the practice of abortion. But it restricted this practice to occasions when it is performed for the purpose of protecting the health and welfare of the mother and carried out in accordance with the law and "good medical practices."[11] In doing so, the AMA affirmed and approved a procedure on which its "Statement of Principles, 1980" (see Appendix A) had remained peculiarly silent for well over a decade. Is it any wonder, then, that in contrast the Hippocratic Oath is viewed by feminists and libertarians as a pathetically paternalistic threat to reproductive rights, personal freedom, and self-determination? Then again, the Oath never was a manifesto for unrestrained personal liberty.

Surrogate Motherhood

More astonishing than the development of RU-486 is the revolutionary rise of the latest assisted reproductive technologies. As legal scholar Carmel Shalev observes in her fascinating book, *Birth Power: The Case for Surrogacy,* "whereas contraception makes it possible to choose *whether* to reproduce, the new reproductive technology makes it possible to choose *how* to reproduce."[12] Indeed, noncoital conception through in vitro fertilization (IVF), including the options of egg or sperm third-party donorship and embryo transfer (ET), have had at least three major impacts on human reproduction.

First, if contraception makes sex possible without reproduction, noncoital conception makes reproduction possible without sex.[13] Second, never in human history has reproductive freedom been greater: we are now providing a single person or a couple the leeway to choose not only with whom, but when, and by what means conception will take place.[14] Third, it is now possible through IVF and ET to redefine childrearing (in the extreme case) so that arguably five "parents" are involved: (a) the sponsoring *social mother and father,* who plan to legally adopt a newborn; (b) the *genetic mother,* who donates (or sells) her egg; (c) the *genetic father,* who donates his sperm; and (d) the *gestational surrogate mother* to whom the embryo is transferred from a petri dish via a syringe into her uterine lining, where it develops until birth. To the gestational surrogate mother, a birthing fee is paid (typically between $5,000 and $15,000) unless she declines as an altruistic gesture of friendship toward the adopting, usually infertile couple. In addition to these five parents, there is the omnipresent physician—most likely a fertility specialist—who may also help coordinate the surrogate arrangement among attorneys and medical social workers.

Critics have labeled various aspects of this assisted reproductive technology as dehumanizing to the newborn, exploitive of the gestational mother, and depersonalizing to the sacred traditions of the family. But are their objections valid?

These are difficult issues. To be sure, the role of the gestational surrogate mother goes far beyond the ancient expectations of the wet nurse. Typically, wet nurses nurtured orphaned or otherwise motherless or sick infants for a limited period of time, usually for a fee or in a barter arrangement. Indeed, as a result of the new noncoital reproductive technologies (IVF and ET), not only our concepts of motherhood and fatherhood but—more broadly—our notions of personhood, filial duty, romantic love, marriage, and the nuclear family have all begun to unloosen from their traditional moorings. As a result, countless moral and legal objections have arisen. Let us briefly explore three of these chief complaints.

One major objection to hiring gestational surrogate mothers via legal contracts is that this practice threatens to economically exploit poorer women. That is, the hiring "social parents" (who may or may not also be the "genetic parents") are usually economically affluent.[15] This is in contrast with the hired surrogate mother who is usually economically poorer. In the famed Baby M case (1987, 1988),[16] for example, William and Elizabeth Stern were in the stronger economic position; Mary Beth Whitehead and her husband, Richard, were in contrast economically struggling. This case became big news largely because the surrogate, Mrs. Whitehead, changed her mind after delivering Baby M. She further attempted to keep her genetically related newborn daughter (it was Mary Beth's egg and William Stern's sperm), thereby breaking her duly signed surrogacy contract. In response to ensuing developments (Whitehead "kidnaped" and hid Baby M in Florida), the New Jersey Supreme Court eventually became involved. In a ruling that has cast doubt on the legality and morality of all subsequent surrogate contracts, the high court declared that such contracts were unenforceable. That same court commented that such contracts could be highly exploitive of surrogate mothers like Mrs. Whitehead. Said the court, in part: "This is the sale of a child, or at the very least, the sale of a mother's right to her child. . . ."[17]

Predictably, feminists do not agree on this charge of exploitation. Shalev, for one, has criticized the New Jersey ruling, and I am inclined to agree with her. She insists that mentally competent and potential surrogate mothers are fully capable of evaluating an economic opportunity like hiring out as a gestational surrogate. If they sign up to rent their wombs, surrogates should be legally bound by their contracts subject to fair contractual remuneration, preliminary counseling, and legal review by opposing attorneys, among other stipulations.[18] To those dissenting feminists who protest that this arrangement exploits poorer women, Shalev answers that this amounts to a specious slippery slope and is inconsistent with other feminist ideals of equality. That is, this objection could block women from doing all sorts of lucrative yet potentially dangerous work. Hence, this particular objection fails. It invites precisely the sort of paternalistic double standards in employment that feminists must avoid.

A second objection is that surrogacy contracts tacitly promote a commercialization of the human procreative process, thereby promoting a commodification of human life that is repugnant. Again, on this view, a surrogate contract amounts to baby-selling.[19] If so, could one fairly conclude that the doctors and lawyers involved with arranging surrogate contracts are akin to pimps, and the gestational surrogate mothers are akin to high-tech prostitutes?

While this imagery is sensational and not a little amusing, the analogy of surrogates to prostitutes and doctors to pimps is hardly convincing. First, recreational sexual favors are not sold by the surrogate mother. Second, this objection ignores the humane element of the story, namely, that these surrogate arrangements bring about relief from psychological suffering to the childless couples. Furthermore, baby-selling is illegal in the United States and in virtually all Western countries. Yet, due to the negative publicity associated with the Baby M case, commercial surrogate contracts in the United States are now rarely pursued.[20] At any rate, the option of adopting a wayward or abandoned infant or older child comes much closer to that of the ancient value system of Hippocratic medicine, one that took the lives of children to be generally worth nurturing.

Lastly, there is the objection that the children born of surrogate contracts are likely to be harmed psychologically, spiritually, or socially. Will such children come to feel cheated out of a normal relationship with one or more of their genetic parents? Will they be stigmatized by society? Imagine, for example, situations in which their extraordinary origins are disclosed to future spouses, insurance companies, or employers. Ought such children be told their birth story at all? Some experts argue that children have a right, as part of their normal identity formation, to know who their genetic parents are.[21] In the aftermath of the Baby M case, I find that this third objection has merit. Indeed, the potential harm is not only likely to fall on the child, but may also extend to the adults who are forever joined biologically (if not legally) in the surrogate arrangement.

After much reflection, I concur with Cynthia Cohen's assessment. She writes: "As the rate of reproductive technologies accelerates, the ability to provide ethical safeguards for the creation and use of the new reproductive technologies diminishes. This may be the persuasive reason to provide some form of direction and regulation of the new reproductive technologies that incorporates *defensible* ethical limits to their use."[22] Unfortunately, the Hippocratic medical literature offers no real guidance on how to regulate or defend surrogate motherhood. How could it, given the pretechnological setting in which it was spawned? For similar reasons, the scriptural traditions of Judaism and Christianity lend little specific guidance. Increasingly, we are on our own.

Physician-Assisted Suicide

If the beginning of human life perplexes doctors and nurses, how human life should end is no less daunting a problem. In a landmark 1997 decision, the United States Supreme Court ruled unanimously that terminally ill patients possess no accepted legal right to assistance in the act of committing suicide. In 1994, a physician-assisted suicide Death with Dignity Act had been adopted in a referendum (Proposition 16) by the citizens of Oregon. Due to relentless legal challenges, all of which were eventually overcome in the Oregon courts, this law only became activated in 1998. Of note, the U.S. Supreme Court also declared in its 1997 ruling that individual states were free to ban physician-assisted suicide if they wished.[23]

Currently, the federal legislature is also in the process of registering its views on this issue. For example, on October 12, 1999, the United States House of Representatives passed a measure that would, in effect, overturn Oregon's physician-assisted suicide law. This it would do by making it illegal for physicians to prescribe the required lethal drug. But even if this Oregon law survives such legislative challenges (which, to me, seems likely), the issue of whether doctors or nurses or pharmacists should help dying patients quit life transcends mere legal maneuvers—just like the preceding issues of abortion or surrogate motherhood.

These are, after all, moral issues: courts and legislatures, with the best of intentions, have sometimes lost their moral footing. For that reason, ordinary citizens and health care workers must remain vigilant.

As it stands, Oregon's physician-assisted suicide law is the only such measure in the nation. It provides that a competent, terminally ill adult may obtain from her doctor lethal drugs by which to quit life, provided that two doctors certify she is of sound mind and has fewer than six months to live. It stipulates that after the dying patient signs a single-page consent form, the doctors may prescribe—but *never* administer—the poisonous drugs.[24]

In view of the sensitive circumstances associated with medical care at the end of life, the American Medical Association, through its Council on Ethical and Judicial Affairs, has taken a firm stand against physician-assisted suicide. In 1992, the AMA issued an opinion harshly condemning this practice. It called such acts a breach of the physician's duty to care for and comfort the patient, even if cure is admittedly beyond reach.[25]

> It is understandable, though tragic, that some patients in extreme duress—such as those suffering from a terminal, painful, debilitating illness—may come to decide that death is preferable to life. However, allowing physicians to participate in physician-assisted suicide would cause more harm than good. Physician-assisted suicide is fundamentally incompatible with the physician's role as healer, would be difficult or impossible to control, and would pose serious societal risks. Instead of participating in physician assisted suicide, physicians must aggressively respond to the needs of patients at the end of life. Patients should not be abandoned once it is determined that cure is impossible. Patients near the end of life must continue to receive emotional support, comfort, care, adequate pain control, respect for patient autonomy, and good communication.[26]

To be sure, physician-assisted suicide is too complex a moral and psychological issue to be settled here.[27] Even so, it seems only fair to balance the AMA's condemnation, and the Supreme Court's rejection, with at least two historically powerful arguments in its favor.

First, there is the argument from autonomy associated with the British utilitarian John Stuart Mill (1806–1873). This argument asserts that as autonomous individuals, we have a basic right to direct our own lives so long as we do not harm others.[28] Facing death and dying is also a part of our lives. Therefore, terminally ill individuals ought to be able to determine when, under what circumstances, and for how long they wish to endure their frequently burdensome illnesses. Their autonomy in ending their lives is permissible and requires society's noninterference in this personal decision.

Second, there is the argument from mercy associated with the Scottish philosopher David Hume (1711–1776). This argument is part of a larger skeptical challenge to what Hume deemed the superstitious constraints of religion. It asserts that out of mercy, individuals who are ceaselessly suffering may rightly end their lives. The terminally ill person may be so wracked with irremediable pain that he feels useless and miserable. Therefore, out of consideration for his own fading "chance for happiness," it is morally acceptable to quit life.[29]

Both of these proeuthanasia arguments have faced serious objections, religious and secular. Yet they remain among the most influential arguments in favor of the alleged right to die. In my view, an even more ominous question is whether such a right to die, if recognized, would gradually evolve into a duty to die, especially in a society in which "outsourcing," pragmatism, and ageism increasingly prevail.

Advance Directives

Given the importance of trying to carry out the patient's wishes during a life-threatening illness or emergency—especially if the patient becomes mentally incapacitated—nearly all fifty states have passed legislation authorizing the use of so-called advance medical directives. Thanks to the Patient Self-Determination Act (implemented December 1, 1991), all competent adult patients must be informed of their rights to make medical decisions and to initiate advance directives when they are admitted to a health care facility in the United States. Influenced by "living will" legislation adopted by California (the Natural Death Act, 1976), advance directives respond, in part, to the fact that with nearly 80 percent of all Americans dying in hospitals or other medical facilities, the process of dying has become for many patients and their families more feared than death itself.[30]

Recall that these legal instruments furnish patients with the opportunity to inform future caregivers that specified medical measures should, or should not, be taken to prolong their lives. In effect, living wills, in conjunction with advance directives and durable powers of attorney, are legal tools capable of halting heroic measures in hopeless situations—in conformity with the patient's express wishes. More controversially, some advance directives may authorize the cessation of artificially delivered hydration and nutrition, even though these omissions are morally, if not legally, objectionable on grounds that they violate minimally humane standards of care.[31] At any rate, almost all provide the opportunity to say "do not resuscitate" if the (usually) aged patient suffers a major stroke, heart attack, or other serious setback—assuming their medical condition is thereby rendered futile.

For the patient who reaches such a critical stage, such advance directives amount to voluntary *passive* euthanasia. Living wills usually contain language similar to: "If I am permanently unconscious or there is no reasonable expectation for my recovery from a seriously incapacitating or lethal illness or condition, I do not wish to be kept alive by artificial means."[32] As we saw in chapter 7, the Hippocratic doctors and their heirs were similarly disinclined to prolong the lives of their hopelessly suffering patients. Therefore, it is mistaken to infer that such advance directives violate the spirit or letter of Hippocratic medicine per se. Indeed, these living wills and related instruments—precisely because they allow death without killing the patient through direct action—conform to the Hippocratic insight that human life is too precious to subject its bearer to prolonged agony. Ideally, treatment should never be turned into torture, from the Hippocratic perspective.

Furthermore, the ethics of medicine today, as in antiquity, remains vulnerable to the influences of popular culture and religious sentiment. Twenty-first-century physicians, like the patients they serve, hold a myriad of personal views on end-of-life issues. Hence, they are decidedly not, like the rare Oath-taker who swore to Apollo, of one and only one mind. Thus, while influenced by contemporary medical laws and customs, a considerable range of latitude is left to the modern physician's conscience and conduct. In this regard, doctors today have much in common with the majority of their Greek and Roman forebears: most ancient healers felt unfettered by the single-minded imperatives of the Hippocratic Oath (if they ever heard of it at all), and so ignored its provisions as they saw fit.

Yet some contemporary critics object to what they describe as the overbearing paternalism toward patients that the Hippocratic writings project. The ancient idea that, all things considered, the doctor knows what is best for his patient's welfare is an assumption increasingly at odds with the consumer-oriented public marketplace of health care services. Indeed, the well-established patient rights movement in America, and doubtless the rise of feminism, have sought to render that paternalistic attitude obsolete. Focusing primarily on liberty rights, the movement asserts that normally it is the patient-consumer's right to know the full truth about his or her diagnosis, treatment, and prognosis in plain language. (See Appendix B.) It also emphasizes the right of the patient to be told frankly of viable alternatives to the therapy his or her physician is prescribing.[33] Such candor serves the purpose, among other alleged benefits, of involving the patient more directly and honestly in the selection of the most effective, affordable, and therapeutically appropriate treatment.

Preventive Medicine

This uproar over patient rights in the past thirty years has occurred against the backdrop of a seemingly ossified Hippocratic value system, one in which the physician unabashedly claims to possess superior judgment and evinces an avuncular attitude and demeanor that is intended to be beyond reproach. Obviously, the twin effects of the consumer rights movement stemming in part from the anti-establishment impulses of the late 1960s, and, more recently, from the introduction of managed care medicine and the need to quell the spiraling costs of medicine, have called into question these paternalistic tendencies.

For example, in the Hippocratic Oath it is proclaimed: "I will apply dietetic measures for the benefit of the sick according to my ability and judgment" (see P3, p. 84). But in *Decorum*, the physician is advised to "reveal nothing of the patient's future or present condition, for many patients on account of this have taken a turn for the worse."[34] This last bit of advice no doubt originally applied to patients with more serious afflictions. However, the paternalistic stance of Hippocratic medicine—now often spurned—is unmistakable. In ancient Rome, Galen went so far as to suggest that the patient should be encouraged to admire his physician like a god, since this reverential attitude would likely speed the healing process!

Hippocratic medicine has also been faulted for its narrow tendency to define medical care mainly in terms of emergency treatment.[35] On this view, it allegedly overlooks the allied function of medicine as a body of knowledge and battery of services equally useful for the maintenance of health and the prevention of disease. Recall that in the decade of the 1970s, "preventive medicine" received renewed emphasis through such efforts as public information advertising, voluntary health screening, and community education aimed at encouraging sound health habits.

As to the charge that the Hippocratic tradition ignores preventive medicine, it is simply mistaken to construe ancient physicians as narrow-minded healers who disregarded the importance of keeping their patients well through proper diet, exercise, rest, and hygiene. In fact, the patient was encouraged whenever possible to accept responsibility for the balance and maintenance of his bodily constitution. Detailed guidelines of sound regimen were, in fact, regularly issued and recorded in the medical literature. Typical of this preventive health orientation is the advice of the fourth-century-B.C. physician Diocles of Carustus. He writes: "The cultivation of health begins with the moment a man wakes up."[36] Note, too, that it was usually within the conceptual milieu of a holistic approach to health care, one that stressed the importance of both mental and physical factors in regaining and preserving well-being, that the ancient physician and his patient worked. That contemporary medicine and nursing has returned with new appreciation to the ancient concept of holistic health, and that it has also rediscovered the value of preventive medicine, serves to remind us of the basic wisdom of the Hippocratic tradition. Indeed, even a restrained form of paternalism is reinsinuating itself into a congeries of issues today, from end-of-life care to the eligibility criteria for organ transplant recipients.

Yet, in contrast to the ancient Greek or Roman physician who typically worked alone or with a student helper, the modern attending physician typically functions in the hospital setting as a member of a coordinated team of primary and secondary caregivers. Though the attending physician is customarily in charge of the case, he may arrive at a diagnosis and implement a treatment plan in collaboration with medical and nursing specialists from a wide array of technical backgrounds. So the specialist in internal medicine, faced with a difficult case, might draw upon the expertise of a hematologist, radiologist, ophthalmologist, dermatologist, or neurologist before settling on a final diagnosis. Of course, registered nurses, physical therapists, lab technicians, paramedics, and medical social workers may also contribute vital services. Thus, the ancient model of solo doctoring is increasingly rare.

While all this is so, it is equally true that seeking diagnostic advice from other medically trained practitioners was never opposed by the Hippocratic authors. Just the opposite: it was explicitly encouraged. Unlike charlatans, good physicians are described by these writers as being able to recognize their own limitations and harboring respect for the sometimes superior knowledge of their colleagues without feelings of jealousy. For example, the Hippocratic author of *Precepts* emphatically states: "A physician does not violate etiquette even if, being in difficulties on occasion over a patient and uncertain owing to inexperience, he should urge the calling in of others in order to learn by consultation the truth about the case."[37] It was further acknowledged that medical consultations could produce irritating consequences on occasion, just as they may today. Therefore, with an eye to proper decorum and the desire not to alarm the patient uppermost in his mind, that same author prudently admonishes the consulting doctors to ". . . never quarrel or jeer at one another."

Despite the openness of the Hippocratic physician to diagnostic assistance from peers, it is true that he was, in general, distrustful of medical assistance and advice being rendered from mere family members, well-intentioned laymen, and others *outside* the medical fraternity. For one thing, laymen were said to be bad at following orders; for another, they were usually the first to blame the doctor if the patient took a turn for the worse.[38] Also, specialized nurses (midwives excepted), physical therapists, lab technicians, social workers, and related support personnel stand without any real parallel in the ancient setting. But this hardly seems a fatal indictment of Hippocratic medicine when taken in context. Rather, it points to the frankly simpler administration and understanding of the healing arts at that time. Given the strictly laissez-faire, unregulated, and self-sufficient fashion in which medicine then was practiced, it would have been entirely unnatural to involve anything like an orchestrated medical team in the treatment of acute injury or illness. Essentially, what would have been gained—therapeutically, financially, or otherwise—in a vocational framework largely bereft of specialization and institutionalization?

Nor can it be ignored that countless other developments characteristic of the current biomedical revolution, from animal experimentation to gene therapy, appear to be without any real analogue in the ancient world. Let us turn briefly to each of these two developments.

Animal Experimentation

Is it fair to say that animal experimentation played no role in the investigations of ancient medicine? After all, the practice of vivisection—defined as the cutting of live animals in order to observe and analyze their inner organs and bodily functions—was known to the Greeks as early as the sixth century B.C. In fact, Alcmaeon of Croton (fl. 500 B.C.) used vivisection in his study of animal physiology. By so doing, he correctly inferred the function of the optic nerve by cutting into the viscera and recording the animal's resulting blindness.[39] But it may be objected that these earliest animal studies by Alcmaeon and others were observations only: no theoretical hypotheses were being tested against the empirical evidence gathered by the anatomist's probing tools. Nor was there a rigorous review, or expansion within a larger theoretical framework, of the observational data so typical of comprehensive animal research studies today.

What's more, several leading philosophers, including Aristotle, Pythagoras, and Seneca, held conflicting opinions concerning ethical standards for the humane treatment of animals.[40] As for the Hippocratic authors, they took no clear stand for or against animal experimentation as a method for advancing medical knowledge. In general, Greek and Roman physicians viewed animals as exploitable for human purposes. Emblematic of their orientation (and contributing to it), Aristotle taught that animals existed within a hierarchy of nature; humans resided at the top of this hierarchical scale since humans alone possessed reason. "Now if nature makes nothing incomplete, and nothing in vain," Aristotle reasoned in his *Politics*, "the inference must be that she has made all animals for the sake of man."[41]

In contrast, Pythagoras rejected this strict hierarchy of fixed kinds of species. He opposed both animal experimentation and meat eating and personally practiced vegetarianism. Pythagoras asserted that all living things are kindred. One recalls that he also asserted that the human soul, at the moment of death, transmigrates into other kinds of animals. Indeed, Iamblichus (A.D. 250–325) ascribed to Pythagoras the view that one ought not to sacrifice animals to the gods, nor by any other means injure animals, but ". . . observe most solicitous justice toward them."[42]

In addition, the statesman and Stoic philosopher Seneca (4 B.C.–A.D. 65) also practiced vegetarianism briefly in his youth, feeling that this practice was more respectful of the lives of animals. Yet he failed to adhere to this discipline. Near the end of his life, however, he expressed in a letter to his nephew, Lucilius, a profound sympathy for the Pythagorean teaching that all animals are interrelated and so should be treated humanely.[43]

It remained for the Hippocratic-inspired physician Galen (A.D. 129–199), the most renowned and influential healer of the Roman Empire, to be the first to carry vivisection into the realm of methodological experimentation. For example, Galen performed serial sections of the spinal cord. This he did in order to demonstrate the connections between nerves and the bodily regions they affected. He thereby demonstrated that surgical intervention to control specific bodily functions could result in a deeper understanding of the processes of physiological phenomena.[44]

In part owing to the antimaterialistic and otherworldly focus of early Christian teaching, animal experimentation came to a halt during the medieval period. It was not until Andrea Vesalius's 1543 publication of *De humani corporis fabrica*—the first anatomical study based on detailed, direct dissections of the human body—that Galen's long accepted but flawed animal-based human anatomical system fell into disfavor. In sum, animal experimentation proved to be an invaluable technique for physiological study from the days of Alcmaeon, Aristotle, and Galen to its revival in the Renaissance by men like Vesalius, continuing to the early modern discoveries of William Harvey's (1578–1657) human circulatory system and Louis Pasteur's 1885 discovery of a vaccine for rabies.[45] Thus, it may be fairly concluded that the ancients initiated in very limited form the practice of animal experimentation, which in its full fruition became a hallmark method of Western medical inquiry.

Furthermore, it marks a curious and ironic turn that Pythagorean-inspired condemnations against destroying animal life for mere human ends—a condemnation now fully embraced by some internationally based animal rights activists—have recently captured the attention of the World Medical Association (WMA). This professional association has fought back publicly against what it views as law-breaking animal rights extremists. This has been done, in part, by publishing a powerful set of ethical principles that proudly affirms that "advances in biomedical research have dramatically improved the quality and prolonged the duration of life throughout the world. However, the ability of the scientific community to continue its efforts to improve personal and public health is being threatened by a movement to eliminate the use of animals in biomedical research." (See Appendix E.)

In sum, the WMA advocates striking a balance between respecting the welfare of animals used for research while, at the same time, condemning the uncivil or illegal harassment of legitimate health scientists by zealous animal rights activists. With an estimated seventeen to twenty-two million research animals sacrificed in the caged wheels of biomedical progress annually in the United States alone, and with the results of these studies benefitting both human and veterinary animal science,[46] it is likely that the original conflicting views of Pythagoras and Aristotle will continue to excite controversy in brand new ways well into the new millennium.

Gene Therapy

Just as the use of animal experimentation helped establish the groundwork of rational medicine through careful observation and analogical reasoning, so, too, the advent of molecular biology in the 1960s, and the introduction of recombinant deoxyribonucleic acid (DNA) techniques in the early 1970s, have introduced a revolutionary approach to conquering human disease: gene therapy.[47] Simply defined, gene therapy involves the insertion of beneficial genes into the cells of patients.[48] In contrast, genetic diagnosis involves trying to determine which gene or genes are part of the causal process that bring about a specific disease. According to Professor Inder Verma of The Salk Institute, "by inserting the new therapeutic gene into the nucleus of a cell, one will either eliminate the defect, ameliorate the defect, slow down the progression of the disease, or in some [beneficial] way interfere with the disease."[49] Currently, gene therapy is being used in an effort to treat approximately fifteen diseases. Researchers have identified up to five thousand genes that may be linked to at least four hundred diseases, including breast cancer, cystic fibrosis, Huntington's disease, and sickle cell anemia. Also, genetic screening tests are available or under development for many of these diseases, even though, tragically, no cures now exist for the vast majority.[50] In fact, geneticists estimate that there are three thousand to five thousand genes that either cause or predispose humans to various diseases (along with indeterminate environmental factors). Hence, the prospect for genetic cures to many significant maladies currently wreaking havoc on the human animal opens a Pandora's box of hopes and fears.

Before examining some of these puzzling ethical and biotechnological concerns, it is tempting to inquire: Are there ancient origins to gene therapy, as there were in the emergence of animal experimentation? The answer is no, not in any straightforward sense.

As we saw in chapter 2, one can locate within the nascent atomic theories of the materialists Leucippus (ca. 440 B.C.) and Democritus (460–370 B.C.) the ontological notion that disease is caused by the size, shape, and arrangement of indestructible atoms found within the spaces and pores (i.e., void) of the human body. In addition, one can also locate in the philosophy of the ancient atomists a deterministic lawlike gestalt similar to that assumed by modern science and, by extension, the Human Genome Project (HGP). This international research project aims to identify and sequence the roughly 100,000 human genes comprising the genetic blueprint of man. So while this goal is logically compatible with the deterministic bent of the ancient atomists, the dissimilarities between the detailed architecture of gene therapy and the primitive outlines of ancient atomic theory are overwhelming. Indeed, it is most doubtful that ancient physicians or philosophers ever contemplated the gene therapy juggernaut.

Nevertheless, if Plato's utopian vision in his *Republic* of breeding the best possible citizens by secretive, eugenically fashioned marriages is any guide, it is germ-line gene therapy, not somatic, that would have best served his scheme.[51] To clarify, somatic gene therapy aims to cure disease in the individual only. In contrast, germ-line gene therapy aims at repairing or strengthening the individual's reproductive cells so that his future offspring would also be protected. Plato recognized that nature and nurture shaped the growth and development of each individual and that this could influence future generations of citizens. Therefore, his utopian city-state ideally aimed to regulate the familial, educational, commercial, and military institutions of society.

Karl Popper, in his book *The Open Society and Its Enemies,* roundly condemned Plato's eugenic program as despotic and manipulative.[52] In Popper's view, Plato fiendishly sacrificed individual liberties for the alleged greater glory of the state. For example, his rigged marriage lottery cheated the Guardian class out of forming procreative bonds based on individual attraction and choice. Surely Popper is right: his warning against social and biological tyranny echoes into the halls of science in the twenty-first century.

Wishing to distance himself from the scientism and butchery embodied by a select core of German physicians during World War II (50 percent of whom joined the Nazi Party), and perhaps mindful of the excesses of Plato's philosopher-kings, Nobel laureate James D. Watson sounded this alarm shortly after he became the director of the Human Genome Project:

The power of the information to be gained from mapping and sequencing projects raises concerns about how it will be used. There is no avoiding the fact that arguments drawn in part from eugenics have been politically misused in the past, most egregiously by the Nazis but also elsewhere in Europe and North America. Indeed, the specter of coercive government eugenics programs persists even today in the statutes still on the books in several nations. . . . The only way to ensure that history does not repeat itself is for the scientific and medical communities to remain constantly vigilant for abuses of genetics.[53]

Philosopher Arthur Dyck has questioned whether Watson's warning is adequate. He writes: "What Watson is calling for is akin to insisting that the best bet for avoiding atrocities is to have the foxes alone watch out for what happens to the chickens!"[54]

Upon reflection, Dyck's criticism strikes me as overly harsh for at least two reasons. First, the United States Congress, aware of the need to be fully informed of the social and personal issues associated with the HGP, has from the start mandated that millions of dollars of funding be earmarked for humanistic research into the most pressing ethical, legal, and social problems likely to be generated by this remarkable project. This significant funding commitment, constituting the largest amount of money ever allocated for bioethical research (5 percent of the annual HGP budget), signals an admirably responsible public admission of the likely hornets' nest of problems that the HGP will unleash.[55]

Second, the United States government has also required that Institutional Review Boards (IRBs) be impaneled to monitor any organizations receiving federal funds for genetic research. Nonscientists, including lawyers and philosophers, as well as citizens from other professions, serve on these boards. These nonscientist members will help ensure even-handed scrutiny, candor, and fairness in the administration of this cutting-edge technology.

Even so, at this point gene therapy is no panacea. There remain serious, recalcitrant problems associated with the effective delivery of the therapeutic gene into the nucleus of the target cell. Assuming this and related problems are resolved, a good many diseases will eventually be eligible for some sort of genetic intervention. If so, the resulting ethical problems will hold profound implications for the future evolution of man, medicine, and morality. Among the most challenging problems are these:

(1) Who should receive gene therapy?
(2) Would there be pressure to submit to gene therapy, or discrimination if one declined?
(3) In applying gene therapy to human embryos, would informed consent be ignored?
(4) How would gene therapy affect our concept of the moral status of the fetus?

(5) Would altering a person's genes, whether for therapeutic or enhancement purposes, change the essential identity of the self?

(6) Would germ-line gene therapy lead to the biological creation of a "master race"?

(7) What will the legal and psychosocial impacts of gene therapy be for current and future generations?

To date, few firm answers exist to these knotty bioethical questions. Nor is there any way to stuff the genomic genie back into the proverbial lamp. Yet, as LeRoy Walters has observed, not all of these troubling questions are unique to gene-therapy interventions.[56] For example, in the case of organ transplants, the question of who ought to receive such therapy is similarly raised. So, too, issues of informed consent arise in bioethical explorations of the suitability of surgery for fetuses, infants, or other minor children.

In essence, unlike human organs, which are uniquely owned by each patient, the human gene pool may be said to belong transcendentally to all the global community of nations. Hence, the need for an *informed public* is imperative. This is especially true for any democratic society wishing to reach a fair informed consensus on these gripping issues—issues that inescapably link the origins and character of individual human experience to our evolving idea of humanity.

THE HIPPOCRATIC OATH REVISITED

In view of the preceding sampling of modern health care trends toward high-tech medicine generally, including the patient rights movement, preventive health measures, the new reproductive technologies, biomedical animal experimentation, gene therapy options, hospital team care, and the heated debate over physician-assisted suicide, it is hard to resist the conclusion that contemporary medicine differs in markedly striking ways from that antique brand of healing known to Homer, Hippocrates, Aristotle, and Galen. But do all these changes amount to a difference in the degree or in the kind of medicine that is or should be practiced today?

If the kind of medicine being practiced today is radically different, should we not then resolutely, and once and for all, set aside the Hippocratic Oath (let alone the larger Hippocratic writings with which it is loosely associated) as " . . . a museum piece, an amiable but useless custom?"

These are the provocative words of the physician and medical educator, Carleton B. Chapman. In a *New York Times* feature story focusing on the Hippocratic Oath's role in American medical school education, Chapman is quoted as saying: "For centuries the Oath has been viewed sentimentally and uncritically by the medical profession as its ethical standard and has, rather paradoxically, served as a barrier to the development of an adequate and comprehensible ethical statement for the profession."[57] Also, in the United States few, if any, graduating classes of medical students are required to recite the Oath anymore, and almost no students are required to study it. So, what, if anything, can be said in favor of the Hippocratic Oath or the Hippocratic writings on etiquette in view of such alleged deficiencies?

That the Oath and the name of Hippocrates may still remain in the popular mind the highest symbol of the physician's dedication to healing, or that it may continue to encourage a fundamental bond of trust between the patient, the physician, and the medical profession, matters not. For if this popular impression is predicated on a romantic vision of Hippocratic medicine, which—we now know—was at best rarely adopted in antiquity and, in addition, has now largely been replaced by more serviceable medical codes in our own epoch, then there is little consolation to be derived from such misplaced popular enthusiasm. Ultimately, such enthusiasm is based not on an ignorance of the past but on a misunderstanding of the real moral and medical needs of the present and future. In fact, I would insist that it is our duty to set aside the Hippocratic Oath entirely, if it can be plausibly demonstrated that its moral and humanitarian ideals have substantially outlived their usefulness.

But has this happened? Far from it. In fact, I shall argue that the Oath, and the reform movement in medicine from which it partly derived, is still surprisingly relevant to contemporary medical ethical concerns. This is not to say that the Oath is flawless. It is not to say that one could never be completely justified in overruling its rigidly conceived duties. I readily grant that many significant changes have been introduced into the physician-patient relationship during the biomedical revolution of the twentieth century. But I further contend that the net effect represents an overall change in the degree rather than in the kind of basic moral awareness that is still needed on the part of health professionals in order to ensure that the most humane medical services possible will continue to be provided in the decades to come.

In my opinion, the Oath remains surprisingly relevant in at least two respects. First, it continues to center the attention of society on a basic core of perennial medical ethical issues constituting virtually ineliminable categories of legitimate moral concern that we ignore only at our own peril.

Second, it affirms the importance of the graduate physician's covenant (or public promise) to be professionally committed to and so morally responsible for: (a) the physical and psychological welfare of patients who trustingly, and often naively, seek medical relief from their assorted maladies; and (b) the technical competence and moral integrity of himself as well as his or her medically trained peers.

In the remaining pages, I would like to explore briefly these two contemporary contributions that the Oath continues to make.

PERENNIAL ISSUES

The Hippocratic Oath may certainly be credited with usefully focusing the attention of Western medicine on at least five central medical ethical issues. These core issues are: (1) patient confidentiality; (2) abortion; (3) euthanasia; (4) truth-telling; and (5) justice in the distribution of health services. In my opinion, this list serves to highlight, though it far from exhausts, crucial areas of personal and institutional conduct that no comprehensive medical code for physicians or other health professionals can legitimately ignore. To do so would amount to a crass desertion of among the most fundamental medical ethical concerns of our own, or any other, humane era.

Incidentally, if the Oath's stricture against surgery strikes the modern reader as unforgivably foolish (see P5, p. 84), as indeed it may, given the many outstanding surgical achievements of the twentieth century, this defect is to my mind decisively outweighed by the more progressive features of the Oath that remain substantially pertinent. It should be accepted for what it is: an anachronism. Even so, the reservations of the Oath against surgery are at least understandable when one recalls the general crudeness of surgical techniques in antiquity, many applications of which killed more patients than were cured. (Recall, too, that the Oath never forbade cautery or bone-setting explicitly.) For that matter, one cannot help noticing that the issue of unnecessary surgery is still being debated on several fronts by surgeons and their qualified critics in our own time and place (e.g., the heart bypass or the hysterectomy).

In any case, the ethical topics (1)–(5) above addressed by the Oath and supplemented in the related writings on etiquette deserve a fair hearing; let us consider some aspects of them now in the fuller context of late twentieth– and twenty-first-century developments.

Confidentiality

The Oath implies an intelligent concern for the confidentiality of the patient's prior medical history, prescribed treatment, and personal life. It states, in part: "Whatever I may see or hear in the course of treatment . . . I will keep to myself, holding such things shameful to be spoken about" (see P7, p. 84). However, some critics fault the Oath on this. They take the utilitarian position that *sometimes* a greater good would accrue to a greater number of people in society if physicians were willing to inform law enforcement officials about any suspicious details of a given patient's mental or physical health. For example, couldn't some crimes be prevented if psychiatrists were legally required to alert local authorities about any patients in their care reportedly having homicidal dreams? And what about patients who arrive at emergency rooms bearing unexplained cuts or wounds?

Proponents of such overriding exceptions to the confidentiality rule face the burden of devising a sound referral criterion that would ensure that no patients could be singled out arbitrarily. Obviously, any such criterion could lead to unintended abuses. There is always the possibility of misjudging the true nature of the patient's present condition (or his past or future conduct). Thus, it is fair to conclude that, at very least, the presumptive duty of the physician to preserve the pri-

vacy of his patient's affairs is admirably defended by the Oath. If exceptions are
to be granted, and conceivably this may be necessary to do on rare occasions,
every precaution must be adopted to promote evenhandedness and a sound rationale for doing so.

In addition, there is general agreement that due to the central computeriza-
tion of medical data and managed care "information sharing," the ability to protect the patient's medical files from insurance companies, the government, and
current or future employers is truly a formidable task. Although federal legislation is being introduced in the United States to remedy some of these potential in-
trusions, only a respectful Hippocratic commitment will fortify the physician-patient relationship against these intrusive social pressures. Significantly, the AMA's
Principles of Medical Ethics (see Appendix A, article 4), the AHA's A Patient's
Bill of Rights (see Appendix B, articles 5–6), the Declaration of Geneva (see Appendix C), and the Code for Nurses (see Appendix D) all pledge to preserve patient privacy and confidentiality against such bureaucratic assaults. However, with
the medical insurance industry demanding to know what heretofore had been considered the private details of the patient's health record on threat of not paying
doctors for their services, it will, in my view, take strongly sanctioned patient privacy laws modeled on the Hippocratic commitment of confidentiality to halt this
Orwellian trend.

Abortion and Euthanasia

As we have seen, the Hippocratic Oath also relevantly centers our attention on the
value and respect we may or may not ascribe to human life. This it does by pro-
nouncing its twin strictures against abortion and euthanasia in uncompromising
language. As individuals, we may well challenge the absolutist position that the
Oath takes in opposing these acts. For example, some may plausibly argue that
when the mother's physical or psychological condition is seriously threatened by
the fetus, abortion is then morally justified. Or, in reference to euthanasia, some
may argue that when a terminally ill patient is suffering torturous pain of such
magnitude that (a) no drug will any longer furnish relief and (b) the patient pleads
to have his life ended, active voluntary euthanasia via a lethal injection is morally
justified. Whether these or numerous other dissenting positions on abortion and
euthanasia turn out to make more moral sense than the Oath's position will depend ultimately on the specifics of each case and the soundness of the reasons advanced pro or con. The simple point here is that, minimally, by condemning these
acts the Hippocratic Oath succeeds in dramatically calling our attention to two
crucial matters of moral choice. These two issues are no less important for us to
clarify and deal with today than they were in the Athens of Socrates.

So here, too, I conclude that the Oath provisionally serves as a reliable introductory guide to moral considerations that are inextricably linked to the most
momentous medical dilemmas we face; namely, judgments affecting who shall

live and who shall die. The Oath proclaims a bias favoring life and the living for which no apology need be made.

Truth-Telling

Regarding the physician's duty to be truthful, the Oath-taker pledges: "I will come for the benefit of the sick, remaining free of all intentional injustice, of all mischief . . ." (see P6, p. 84). This paternalistic principle implies that the doctor ought to do whatever he thinks will benefit the sick person in his care. Also he should not lie, for this would be a form of mischief. He should carry out his course of treatment in a forthright, physician-knows-best manner " . . . according to my ability and judgment," as the Oath says (P3).

Yet, elsewhere in the Hippocratic writings on etiquette, as we saw earlier at *Decorum* 16, the physician is urged not to reveal to his patients any gloomy assessment of their illnesses without careful forethought about the possible demoralizing effects it could have on them. The result is that on the one hand there is the moral duty not to lie; this the entire Oath, being a public promise, presupposes. On the other hand, this very duty sometimes comes into conflict with the moral rule not to knowingly harm the patient (which P3 of the Oath also underscores).

Regrettably, the Oath neither acknowledges nor resolves this problem of a possible conflict of duty. Being the kind of compactly worded religious or guild document that it is, one could not fairly expect it to address every conceivable difficulty that might arise. But I suspect that the rule against intentionally harming the patient was routinely allowed to override the competing rule against deception in those instances where the brutal truth was judged by the more caring doctors to be much too shattering for a particular patient to bear.

For better or worse, this discretionary withholding of information is no longer the trend. Telling the patient the unadorned truth is the norm in American medical circles. In the original 1973 version of the AHA's A Patients's Bill of Rights, there appeared to be a willingness to yield to the paternalistic principle of not harming the patient when this principle conflicted with the patient's right to know about his complete medical condition. But in the revised 1992 version (see Appendix B, article 2), this loophole is dropped. Indeed, this version is emphatic in insisting that the competent patient "is encouraged to obtain" and discuss with his physician all current information on his diagnosis, treatment, and prognosis. It is evident, therefore, that the paternalistic inclinations of the earlier Hippocratic writers to sometimes allow shading the truth to protect the patient from psychological harm has been overridden by the supposed advantages of openness and candor. Whether this impulse toward full disclosure is now driven more by legal and economic rather than ethical and spiritual concerns I will leave for others to judge. Doubtless, all of these factors are involved in setting hospital guidelines for giving or withholding from patients a full account of their medical maladies and prognoses.

In an unexpected wrinkle to the Hippocratic duty to be truthful, the *Archives of Internal Medicine* recently published a report detailing a worrisome and growing exception to this general endorsement of honesty. The *Archives* reported that hypothetically, at least, "many physicians approve of deceiving insurance companies or health maintenance organizations (HMOs) to secure payment for treatment," especially when their patients cannot obtain the medical care they need any other way.[58]

But this report is flawed, in my opinion. It is overly narrow, involving only 169 internists in eight American cities. Even so, it is admittedly suggestive of a Robin Hood–like siege mentality on the part of up to 58 percent of the 169 doctors surveyed. That is, 58 percent were willing to lie in the case of patients suffering from the more serious conditions, such as breast cancer, heart disease, or costly chronic illnesses. In contrast, fewer than 3 percent indicated that they would lie for a patient seeking mere cosmetic surgery by redescribing the patient's condition as if it were noncosmetic in order to recover surgical fees for, say, a nose job. But what if this reported willingness on the part of clinicians to deceive health maintenance organizations (HMOs)—self-rationalized as "good guy" patient advocacy—were to become widespread in the culture of American medicine? If so, these maverick doctors would be going far beyond the mere violation of a long-standing Hippocratic ideal. At worst, they would be adopting a twisted logic of fraud and deceit while at the same time economically enriching their own practices.

Distributive Justice

Next there is the question of the quality of justice in the delivery and distribution of healthcare services. In other words, who shall get what portion of the healthcare pie, given that there are limited medical resources to go around and many more people in need?

As we saw in the immediately preceding section, the Hippocratic Oath pledges the doctor to remain free of all intentional injustice. Also, that same paragraph (P6) requires *equal treatment* of patients regardless of their sex, background, or social class " . . . be they free or slaves." In the same paragraph, the physician pledges to abstain from any and all sexual relations with his patients "both female and male persons," again, regardless of their social class (see P6, p. 84). Given the tide of sexual harassment complaints and lawsuits in the United States arising in part from Title VII of the Civil Rights Act of 1964 and reinforced by the Equal Employment Opportunity Commission since 1980, and given the intimate nature of the doctor-patient relationship and its appropriately formal boundaries, the Oath's prohibition against sexual relations is astonishingly prescient.[59] Unfortunately, some studies published during the past decade suggest that, particularly among psychiatrists and psychologists, this Hippocratic standard has sometimes been ignored. Although not widespread, such "dual role" conduct is obviously immoral; it ruinously transforms the physician-patient relation from the professional to the personal. All pretense of healing and trust are thereby dissolved.

Such a profound commitment to equal treatment of the sick and fair play toward the weak and vulnerable expressed a supreme egalitarian ideal that was, for the most part, uncharacteristic of Greek and Roman thinking. It remains a noble ideal by no means entirely realized in our own epoch. It expresses a humane value reaffirmed more broadly by the World Medical Association's Declaration of Geneva (see Appendix C). This declaration of principles states, in part: "I will not permit considerations of religion, nationality, race, party politics, or social standing to intervene between my [medical] duty and any patient." Again, the robust foresight of the Hippocratic Oath and the progressive reinterpretation of some of its central values to better serve the contemporary medical setting, here on both a national and international scale, are unmistakable.

However, some important qualifications must be added. First, that the ancient Oath-taker admirably pledged to treat all of his patients equally (once he took them on) is not the same as saying that he charitably pledged to treat all those who sought his medical services. He could decline to treat whomever he wished. In fact, the now-idealized notion that the high-minded physician has an additional duty to care for the sick, penniless, and downtrodden as part of an implicit debt owed to his community or to his God based on feelings of personal gratitude and mercy was never a native Greek or Roman idea. Not until the emergence of Judeo-Christian values in the late Roman Empire did this particular vision of charitable medical care for the needy and poor begin to take root.[60] Even then, it was a practice especially encouraged by the advent of the early Christian hospitals, which were relatively few in number.[61] Still, this does not deny that the pre-Christian doctors rendered their medical services free of charge from time to time. But such occurrences were infrequent and were usually calculated to enhance future business prospects or personal reputations.[62]

Second, as Robert Veatch has observed, the modern ideal of providing general access to medical services for all those in need may, in reality, conflict with fulfilling the familiar Hippocratic duty of doing what will most benefit the patient's health.[63] This constitutes a serious moral and economic dilemma. It is one that has not yet been fully acknowledged in the latest contemporary medical codes, nor was it even remotely anticipated by the Oath of Hippocrates. The seriousness of the dilemma turns on the following consideration: As the limited supply, growing demand, and rising costs associated with many types of high-tech, life-sustaining therapies such as kidney dialysis, neonatal intensive care, and open-heart surgery become increasingly parasitic on our nation's economy, this conflict of duty may well lead to a new form of economic triage, according to which those who could not personally pay for certain costlier maladies would simply be economically doomed to die of them. In the United States, most citizens are painfully aware of the rising costs of medical care, and they continue to harbor doubts about reversing this trend.

Indeed, it is fair to ask whether in the future all who need access to various medical facilities and resources in order to remain alive and well, and who arguably deserve some measure of medical care whether they are rich or poor in fact will be granted *equally* the treatment they require. There is reason to think that a balanced solution can be reached only when the notion of prolonging or preserving human life at any cost is critically examined by every one of our major social institutions. Philosopher Daniel Callahan has suggested that a human life may be said to have reached its fair limit in the aging process when the individual has had the opportunity to experience a significant portion of those life goals meaningful to him or her over a maturing span of time.[64] Possibly this or some similar notion will be adopted, for better or worse, in the new millennium as the limits of human life and health care are more fully realized.

Physician Erich Loewy has also raised serious questions concerning the collective wisdom of our current health care priorities. Comparatively speaking, he has mischievously dubbed many of the debates within contemporary bioethics as "rich man's ethics."[65] His stunning point is that until the poor and disenfranchised in the United States (and elsewhere) receive the basic medical attention they so desperately need, to worry about the esoteric implications of recombinant DNA therapy, or to debate ad nauseam the psycholinguistic subtleties of free informed consent is to misplace our collective energies. What clinicians, nurses, social workers, and the general public ought to do is become socially active in the push for universal health care coverage. If Loewy is right, as I am inclined to agree, only then will medical ethics and bioethics merge into an international movement for social justice.

PROFESSIONAL COMMITMENT

Whatever the future of international bioethics, on a more modest scale the Hippocratic Oath remains relevant to contemporary medicine by affirming the importance of the physician's covenant. This covenant formally inaugurates the trustee relationship between physician and patient on which all responsible medicine is ultimately founded. Yet it will be helpful to reconsider just what such an agreement means in modern terms.

Historically, it will be recalled that the second paragraph of the Oath served to: (a) bind the medical student to his teacher; (b) pledge the student to acquire and preserve the highest moral and technical standards of his art; and (c) require the student to remain vigilant so that the knowledge of his craft is extended only to those who are judged morally and intellectually fit (see P2, pp. 83–84). Beyond this, a crucial social implication of the covenant was that it symbolized a public promise—what we would properly call a professional promise or commitment—to guard the welfare of patients along with the integrity of medicine itself against all major forms of abuse. This especially refers to forms of abuse that can originate from within the medical ranks. Such misconduct usually took the form of intellectual dishonesty or economic and moral wrongdoing. Today, the practice of medicine is also evidently vulnerable to these same human weaknesses. But most of these incidents have been vastly reduced since antiquity owing to the consistently higher caliber of medical students plus the rigorous standards imposed by both the state and the profession on the entire medical enterprise.

Yet any such intellectual dishonesty, I imagine, included such deeds as these: regularly declining to seek consultations from medical peers though in serious doubt of a patient's proper diagnosis; losing touch with new therapeutic discoveries that might prove helpful while at the same time pretending to stay abreast of one's art; treating patients suffering from unfamiliar diseases, injuries, or complaints about which one knows little; and refusing to share with other practitioners effective cures of one's own that could help *their* patients regain health.

To be sure, economic and moral abuses are closely intertwined. Economic wrongdoing is almost always the direct or indirect result of some moral defect. Moreover, an assortment of intellectually dishonest behaviors of the sort described above are usually associated with even more fundamental moral deficiencies—notably lying (to oneself or others). Still, in order to further expand our analysis, it will be convenient to speak about a few of the more recurrent economic abuses that have plagued medicine over the centuries. These include: charging for services that are not, in fact, rendered; overcharging for services that are; concocting fictional diagnoses and remedies in order to secure extra business from unsuspecting patients who are really not ill; intentionally not curing patients as expeditiously as they might be cured in order to bilk them; and selling remedies or treatments that one knows in advance either will not work as described or will not work well enough to do any good. This lurid list of misanthropic acts is, of course, all quite illegal and universally regarded as unethical in our own day. In antiquity, however, this was not always so; medicine was largely unregulated and doctors were never licensed. Yet, even now, such abuses doubtless occur from time to time, despite far stricter legal and professional codes.

It is a strange fact that medicine, by its very nature, is such an intimate enterprise that no finite account of its conceivable moral abuses could claim to be exhaustive or fully descriptive of its potential for wrongdoing. Nor need we consider in detail all the possible personal injuries or deaths that would be visited on innocent persons if individual doctors, or the societies to which they belonged, ever lost their moral footing. The medical agenda of Nazi Germany immediately comes to mind, but other historical examples could be cited as well.[66] On a purely individual scale, we saw that the Hippocratic Oath explicitly condemned as morally wrong having sexual relations with patients; treating patients unequally, based on their unequal social background or their sex; aiding in abortion or active euthanasia; gossiping about or otherwise spreading news of patients' personal affairs; and, in effect, intentionally committing any act that might inflict harm, mischief, or injustice of any sort.

The point is that this concise catalogue of moral prohibitions was originally intended to heighten the young doctor's awareness of, and commitment to, the noblest ideals at which medicine and its most trusted servants could aim. Currently, some may choose to quarrel about the particular details of the acts that the Hippocratic Oath condemns. And one can only applaud recent efforts toward a thoughtful reinterpretation and further refinement of the Oath's humanistic ideals. But few deny the admirable intent and relevance of the covenant itself, which finally transcends in importance any list of particular deeds. It stands as a public commitment to personal professional competence and moral rectitude. At the same time, it constitutes a solemn promise to one's professional peers to keep medicine free from scoundrels, charlatans, and crooks.

In the broadest sense, therefore, the covenant expresses the personal desire and resolve to make oneself and one's profession the very best that both can be. To be a professional, in this sense, is to profess competence and personal integrity not merely at the moment of entry into the ranks of trained healers, but every day of one's working life.

Discussion Questions

1. Would the Hippocratic Oath condemn the use of the morning-after/abortion pill RU-486? Why or why not? Would it oppose the use of contraceptives generally?
2. Describe how up to five "parents" could find themselves biologically or legally involved in a surrogate contract to produce a child. In your opinion, is surrogate motherhood damaging to such offspring? Are such contracts morally acceptable?
3. Why can't the moral issue of physician-assisted suicide be settled finally by the U.S. Supreme Court? Is "death with dignity" definable morally?
4. Does the Hippocratic tradition of medical ethics accept or condemn advance directives? How could advance directives be abused?
5. Is it fair to characterize Hippocratic medicine as bereft of any concern for preventive health guidelines? Why is preventive health such an important ethical issue today?
6. What contribution, if any, did the ancient Greek and Roman physicians make to animal experimentation as a basis for medical science?
7. Does gene therapy have any discernible roots in ancient medicine? Will gene therapy inevitably lead to the development of a master race?
8. Is the Hippocratic Oath, in part or in whole, still relevant to contemporary medical practice? Why or why not?
9. Write a contemporary version of the Hippocratic Oath that you could accept. What would be the function of your oath? What obstacles would it likely face?

NOTES

1. Edmund D. Pellegrino, "The Metamorphosis of Medical Ethics: A 30-Year Retrospective," *Journal of the American Medical Association*, 269, no. 9 (1993): 1158.
2. John M. Riddle, *Contraception and Abortion from the Ancient World to the Renaissance* (Cambridge, MA: Harvard University Press, 1992), p. 14.
3. Some conveniently forget that the U.S. Supreme Court's ruling fell short of granting an absolute right to abortion. The Court ruled, in part: "The right to privacy encompasses a woman's decision whether or not to terminate her pregnancy [but] a woman's right to terminate her pregnancy is not absolute." *Roe v. Wade*, 410 US 113 (1973), p. 154.

4. Riddle, *Contraception and Abortion*, pp. 44–46. Riddle speculates that the pomegranate, taken orally in the right quantity (which he does not provide) may have worked as a birth control method of "limited effectiveness." This is doubtful, in my opinion, given the thin evidence and dubious biochemistry. My point concerning reliability still stands.
5. See chapter 6, subhead "Contraception."
6. Anita L. Allen, "Abortion: Legal and Regulatory Issues," in *EB 1995*, vol. 1, p.18.
7. Ruth Macklin, "Abortion: Contemporary Ethical Perspectives," in *EB* 1995, vol. 1, p. 14.
8. Allen, "Abortion: Legal and Regulatory Issues," pp. 18–19. See also Nancy N. Dubler and Anita White, "Fertility Control: Legal and Regulatory Issues," in *EB* 1995, vol. 2, pp. 840–843.
9. Steven Waldman, Elise Ackerman, and Rita Rubin, "Abortions in America," *US News and World Report*, 19 January 1998), p. 22. The basic facts on abortion in America are these: Forty-three percent of American women will have at least one abortion in their lifetime (p. 20); and roughly 1.4 million have abortions each year, 89 percent before the 12th week of gestation, 82 percent are unmarried or separated, and 44 percent have had a least one *previous* abortion (p. 22). The authors observe: ". . . 25 years after *Roe v. Wade*, abortions are safe, legal, and not rare" (p. 20).
10. Few statistics exist that show why American women obtain abortions. In the last comprehensive survey (1987), "76 percent said they were concerned about how having a baby could change their lives; 15 percent had problems with their relationship or wanted to avoid single parenthood"; 13 percent cited the health of the fetus; 7 percent cited the health of the mother; and 1 percent cited rape or incest. Even for most abortions occurring in the 20th week or later, "the health of the fetus or mother was a relatively minor consideration in the decision. . . ." (Ibid., pp. 15, 31.)
11. AMA Council on Ethical and Judicial Affairs, 1994, Opinion 2-01. According to Allan Rosenfield and Sara Iden, for the last hundred years, American doctors "have tended to place the value of the life of the mother above that of the fetus . . . there has been general agreement [since *Roe v. Wade*] that abortion is permissible in those cases where the health of the mother is seriously compromised by a pregnancy." (See Allan Rosenfield and Sara Iden, "Abortion: Medical Perspectives," in *EB 1995*, vol. 1, p. 4.)
12. Carmel Shalev, *Birth Power: The Case for Surrogacy* (New Haven, CT: Yale University Press, 1989), p. 15.
13. Ibid., pp. 15–16.
14. Ibid.
15. Cynthia B. Cohen, "Reproductive Technologies: Ethical Issues," in *EB* 1995, vol. 4, p. 2237.
16. New Jersey Superior Court, *Matter of Baby M* 217 N.J. Super. 313.525A.2nd 1128; see also New Jersey Supreme Court, *Matter of Baby M* 584 A 2nd 1227 (N.J. 1988). Cited in Gregory E. Pence, *Classic Cases in Medical Ethics*, 2nd ed. (New York: McGraw Hill, 1995), p. 476.
17. Pence, *Classic Cases*, p. 130.
18. Shalev, *Birth Power,* chap. 8, pp. 152–66 ("Woman as Economic Being").
19. Pence, *Classic Cases*, p. 139.
20. Ibid., p. 145.
21. Cohen, "Reproductive Technologies: Ethical Issues," p. 2236.
22. Ibid., p. 2239.

23. In this June 1997 unanimous decision, the U.S. Supreme Court reviewed *Compassion in Dying v. Washington* 79 F.3d 790, 9th Cir 1996 and *Quill v. Vacco* 80 F.3d 71b, 2nd Cir. (1996). See also G. I. Annas, "The Promised End—Constitutional Aspects of Assisted Suicide," *New England Journal of Medicine* 335 (1996): 684–87.

24. S. H. Verhovek, "Oregon Chafes at Measure to Stop Assisted Suicides," *New York Times*, 29 October 1999, sec. A1, p. 18.

25. Alexander Morgan Capron, "Death and Dying: Euthanasia and Sustaining Life; Professional and Public Policies," in *EB* 1995, vol. 1, p. 579.

26. For the full statement, see *Journal of the American Medical Association* 267 (1993): 2229–33. See also Pat Phillips, "End-of-Life Care Movement Growing," *Journal of the American Medical Association* 278 (1997): 967–70.

27. On the psychiatric puzzles associated with a request to die, see Philip R. Muskin, "The Request to Die: Role for a Psychodynamic Perspective on Physician-Assisted Suicide," *Journal of the American Medical Association* 279 (1998): 323–28. On the growing medicalization and institutionalization of death in America, see Tania Salem, "Physician-Assisted Suicide: Promoting Autonomy or Medicalizing Suicide?" *The Hastings Center Report* 29, no. 3 (1999): 30–36.

28. J. S. Mill, "On Liberty," in *Matters of Life and Death*, ed. Tom Regan, 2nd ed. (New York: McGraw Hill, 1986), chap. 1, p. 66.

29. David Hume, "On Suicide" (1783) in *Hume on Religion*, ed. Richard Wolheim (New York: World Publishing, 1963), pp. 253–59.

30. *U.S. President's Commission for the Study of Ethical Problems in Medicine and Biomedical and Behavioral Research, 1983. Deciding to Forego Life-Sustaining Treatment: A Report on the Ethical, Medical and Legal Issues in Treatment Decisions* (Washington, D.C.: U.S. Government Printing Office), pp. 17–18.

31. See Missouri Department of Health, *Cruzan v. Director* 110 S.Ct. 2841–92 (1990).

32. *U.S. President's Commission*, 1983, p. 55.

33. One looks in vain for the parallel notion of the rights of persons, whether in the role of patients or otherwise, in the ancient moral or legal literature. The whole concept of rights, especially when construed to entail accompanying duties owed by others to the bearer of those rights, is a rather recent moral and legal development originating in seventeenth-century European thought. Nonetheless, it would be mistaken to suppose that the ancient physician was blatantly insensitive to the need of securing his patient's consent before starting treatment. The looming medical principle was that Nature was the master healer. Most physicians realized that for psychological, if not moral, reasons, the desired cure was most likely to result if the patient were made to feel a cooperative partner who assisted Nature and the physician by following the prescribed therapy.

34. Hippocrates *Decorum* 16.

35. Kenneth Vaux, *Biomedical Ethics: Morality for a New Medicine* (New York: Harper and Row, 1974), p. 9.

36. Cited by Sigerist, *History of Medicine*, vol. 2, p. 238.

37. Hippocrates *Precepts* 8.

38. Hippocrates *Decorum* 18.

39. James C. Whorton, "Animal Research: Historical Aspects," in *EB 1995*, vol. 1, p. 143.

40. Kerry S. Walters and Lisa Portness. *Ethical Vegetarianism: From Pythagoras to Peter Singer* (New York: SUNY Press, 1999), pp. 11–25, 253–60.

41. Aristotle *Politics* 1.5, 8, cited by Walters and Portness, *Ethical Vegetarianism,* p. 254. See also John Scarborough, *Facets of Hellenic Life* (Boston, MA: Houghton Mifflin, 1976), p. 326.

42. Iamblichus, *On the Pythagorian Life*, trans. K. S. Guthrie. Cited by Walters and Portness, *Ethical Vegetarianism*, p. 14.

43. Seneca *Lucilium-Epistulae Morales,* trans. Richard M. Gummere (New York: G. P. Putnam's, 1925), vol. 3, pp. 241–45, Epistle 58.

44. Whorton, "Animal Research: Historical Aspects," pp. 143–44.

45. Ibid., p. 144.

46. Paul Carrick, "Environmental Ethics and Medical Ethics: Some Implications for End-of-Life Care," part 2, *Cambridge Quarterly of Healthcare Ethics* 8, no. 2 (1999): 253.

47. W. French Anderson and Theodore Friedman, "Gene Therapy: Strategies," in *EB* 1995, vol. 2, p. 9.

48. Leon Jaroff, "Fixing the Genes," *Time*, 11 January 1999, p. 68.

49. Ibid., p. 144.

50. Anderson and Friedman, "Gene Therapy Strategies," p. 908. A resulting epistemic dilemma is that we have genetic diagnoses in most cases, without cures. For this reason, many patients decline genetic screening. It is doubtful that this unsatisfactory situation will resolve soon.

51. Plato *Republic* 6, 7, 9, 14.

52. Karl Popper, *The Open Society and Its Enemies*, vol. 1, 5th ed. (Princeton, NJ: Princeton University Press, 1966), chaps. 5 and 6.

53. James D. Watson, Cook Deagan, and Robert Mullan, "The Human Genome Project and International Health," *Journal of the American Medical Association* 263, no. 24 (1990): 3324.

54. Arthur J. Dyck, "Eugenics in Historical and Ethical Perspective," in *Genetic Ethics: Do the Ends Justify the Genes?* eds. John F. Kilner, Rebecca D. Pentz, and Frank E. Young (Grand Rapids, MI: William B. Eerdmans Publishing Company, 1997), p. 30.

55. National Institutes of Health, "The Human Genome Project: New Tools for Tomorrow's Health Research," rev. ed. (Bethesda, MD: U.S. Department of Health and Human Services, 1992), p. 18.

56. For a comprehensive discussion of the bioethical issues, see LeRoy Walters, *Journal of Clinical Ethics* 2 (1991): 267–74; and Eric Juengst and LeRoy Walters, "Gene Therapy: Ethical and Social Issues," in *EB 1995*, vol. 2, pp. 914–20.

57. Lawrence K. Altman, "The Doctor's World," *New York Times*, 1 May 1979, sec. C1.

58. Brenda C. Coleman, "Many Doctors Would Lie to Help Patients," *Harrisburg Patriot News,* 25 October 1999), sec. A5.

59. See, for example, Equal Employment Opportunity Commission (EEOC), "Sexual Harassment Regulations," 29 CRF § 1604.11 (1980).

60. Actually, a case could be made that some free medical attention to the needy and hopelessly ill was dispensed by priest-physicians in pre-Christian times at the Temples of Asclepius at locations like Epidaurus on mainland Greece. There were four hundred Asclepian temples by Aristotle's time. But such free care was, at any rate, the exception rather than the rule. It is also arguable whether what the patient usually received was medical treatment at all or rather superstitious ritual therapies epitomized by the famed dream-healing process or incubation sleep (judged by Hippocratic standards, at least). It remains true, however, that charity was not a firmly embedded pagan value.

61. It was not until A.D. 39 that Fabiola, a wealthy Roman widow, founded the first Christian hospital, and as late as A.D. 431 Saint Augustine regarded them as a novelty. Alan T. Marty, who has argued convincingly that public hospitals were *not* uniquely Christian institutions in antiquity, asserts that they spread more rapidly in the Eastern Byzantine world "because of the energy and scholarship of the disciples of Nestorius [the fifth-century Patriarch of Constantinople]. . . . By the middle of the sixth century, however, hospitals were more securely established and their property duly safeguarded." (See Alan T. Marty, "The Pagan Roots of Western Hospitals," *Journal of Surgery, Gynecology, and Obstetrics* 133 [1971]: 1019–22 passim.)

62. Even so, *Precepts* 6 furnishes us with an inviting glimpse of the Hippocratic physician at his best. The author writes: "I urge you not to be too unkind, but to consider carefully your patient's superabundance or means. Sometimes give your services for nothing, calling to mind a previous benefaction or present satisfaction. And if there be an opportunity of serving one who is a stranger in financial straits, give full assistance to all such. For where there is love of man, there is love of the art." See Jones, trans., *Hippocrates*, vol. 1, p. 319. See also chapter 5.

63. Robert M. Veatch, "Codes of Medical Ethics: Ethical Analysis," in *EB*, vol. 1, p. 177.

64. Daniel Callahan, *Setting Limits: Medical Goals in an Aging Society* (New York: Simon and Schuster, 1987). See also Paul Carrick, "Environmental Ethics and Medical Ethics: Some Implications for End-of-Life Care," part 1, *Cambridge Quarterly of Healthcare Ethics* 8, no.1 (1999): 112–15.

65. Erich H. Loewy, *Textbook of Healthcare Ethics* (New York: Plenum, 1996), p. 16.

66. The effectiveness of professional codes of ethics against the coercive powers of the modern state is explored by Jack S. Boozer in his article, "Children of Hippocrates: Doctors in Nazi Germany," *The Annals of the American Academy of Political and Social Sciences* 450 (July 1980): 83–97.

Principles of Medical Ethics

American Medical Association
Revised, 1980

The medical profession has long subscribed to a body of ethical statements developed primarily for the benefit of the patient. As a member of this profession, a physician must recognize responsibility not only to patients, but also to society, to other health professionals, and to self. The following principles adopted by the American Medical Association are not laws, but standards of conduct that define the essentials of honorable behavior for the physicians.

I. A physician shall be dedicated to providing competent medical service with compassion and respect for human dignity.

II. A physician shall deal honestly with patients and colleagues, and strive to expose those physicians deficient in character or competence, or who engage in fraud or deception.

III. A physician shall respect the law and also recognize a responsibility to seek changes in those requirements which are contrary to the best interests of the patient.

IV. A physician shall respect the rights of patients, of colleagues, and of other health professionals, and shall safeguard patient confidences within the constraints of the law.

V. A physician shall continue to study, apply, and advance scientific knowledge, make relevant information available to patients, colleagues, and the public, obtain consultation, and use the talents of other health professionals when indicated.

    VI. A physician shall, in the provision of appropriate patient care, except in emergencies, be free to choose whom to serve, with whom to associate, and the environment in which to provide medical services.

    VII. A physician shall recognize a responsibility to participate in activities contributing to an improved community.

A Patient's Bill of Rights

American Hospital Association 1973, Revised 1992

INTRODUCTION

Effective health care requires collaboration between patients and physicians and other health care professionals. Open and honest communication, respect for personal and professional values, and sensitivity to differences are integral to optimal patient care. As the setting for the provision of health services, hospitals must provide a foundation for understanding and respecting the rights and responsibilities of patients, their families, physicians, and other caregivers. Hospitals must ensure a health care ethic that respects the role of patients in decision making about treatment choices and other aspects of their care. Hospitals must be sensitive to cultural, racial, linguistic, religious, age, gender, and other differences as well as the needs of persons with disabilities.

The American Hospital Association presents A Patient's Bill of Rights with the expectation that it will contribute to more effective patient care and be supported by the hospital on behalf of the institution, its medical staff, employees, and patients. The American Hospital Association encourages health care institutions to tailor this bill of rights to their patient community by translating and/or simplifying the language of this bill of rights as may be necessary to ensure that patients and their families understand their rights and responsibilities.

BILL OF RIGHTS

These rights can be exercised on the patient's behalf by a designated surrogate or proxy decision maker if the patient lacks decision-making capacity, is legally incompetent, or is a minor.

1. The patient has the right to considerate and respectful care.

2. The patient has the right to and is encouraged to obtain from physicians and other direct care givers relevant, current, and understandable information concerning diagnosis, treatment, and prognosis.

Except in emergencies when the patient lacks decision-making capacity and the need for treatment is urgent, the patient is entitled to the opportunity to discuss and request information related to the specific procedures and/or treatments, the risks involved, the possible length of recuperation, and the medically reasonable alternatives and their accompanying risks and benefits.

Patients have the right to know the identity of physicians, nurses, and others involved in their care, as well as when those involved are students, residents, or other trainees. The patient also has the right to know the immediate and long-term financial implications of treatment choices, insofar as they are known.

3. The patient has the right to make decisions about the plan of care prior to and during the course of treatment and to refuse a recommended treatment or plan of care to the extent permitted by law and hospital policy and to be informed of the medical consequences of this action. In case of such refusal, the patient is entitled to other appropriate care and services that the hospital provides or transfer to another hospital. The hospital should notify patients of any policy that might affect patient choice within the institution.

4. The patient has the right to have an advance directive (such as a living will, health care proxy, or durable power of attorney for health care) concerning treatments or designating a surrogate decision maker with the expectation that the hospital will honor the intent of that directive to the extent permitted by law and hospital policy.

Health care institutions must advise patients of their rights under state law and hospital policy to make informed medical choices, ask if the patient has an advance directive, and include that information in patient records. The patient has the right to timely information about hospital policy that may limit its ability to implement fully a legally valid advance directive.

5. The patient has the right to every consideration of privacy. Case discussion, consultation, examination, and treatment should be conducted so as to protect each patient's privacy.

6. The patient has the right to expect that all communications and records pertaining to his/her care will be treated as confidential by the hospital, except in cases such as suspected abuse and public health hazards when reporting is permitted or required by law. The patient has the right to expect that the hospital will

emphasize the confidentiality of this information when it releases it to any other parties entitled to review information in these records.

7. The patient has the right to review the records pertaining to his/her medical care and to have the information explained or interpreted as necessary, except when restricted by law.

8. The patient has the right to expect that, within its capacity and policies, a hospital will make reasonable response to the request of a patient for appropriate and medically indicated care and services. The hospital must provide evaluation, service, and/or referral as indicated by the urgency of the case. When medically appropriate and legally permissible, or when a patient has so requested, a patient may be transferred to another facility. The institution to which the patient is to be transferred must first have accepted the patient for transfer. The patient must also have the benefit of complete information and explanation concerning the need for, risks, benefits, and alternatives to such a transfer.

Declaration of Geneva

World Medical Association
Amended, 1994

At the time of being admitted as a member of the medical profession:

I solemnly pledge myself to consecrate my life to the service of humanity;

I will give to my teachers the respect and gratitude which is their due;

I will practice my profession with conscience and dignity;

The health of my patient will be my first consideration;

I will respect the secrets which are confided in me, *even after the patient has died*;

I will maintain by all the means in my power, the honor and the noble traditions of the medical profession;

My colleagues will be my sisters and brothers;

I will not permit considerations of age, disease or disability, creed, ethnic origin, gender, nationality, political affiliation, race, sexual orientation, or social standing to intervene between my duty and my patient;

I will maintain the utmost respect for human life from its beginning even under threat and I will not use my medical knowledge contrary to the laws of humanity. I make these promises solemnly, freely, and upon my honor.

Code for Nurses

International Council of Nurses 1953, Revised 2000

PREAMBLE

Nurses have four fundamental responsibilities: to promote health, to prevent illness, to restore health, and to alleviate suffering. The need for nursing is universal.

Inherent in nursing is respect for human rights, including the right to life, to dignity and to be treated with respect. Nursing care is unrestricted by considerations of age, color, creed, culture, disability or illness, gender, nationality, politics, race, or social status.

Nurses render health services to the individual, the family and the community and coordinate their services with those of related groups.

1. NURSES AND PEOPLE

The nurse's primary professional responsibility is to people requiring nursing care.

In providing care, the nurse promotes an environment in which the human rights, values, customs, and spiritual beliefs of the individual, family, and community are respected.

The nurse ensures that the individual receives sufficient information on which to base consent for care and related treatment.

The nurse holds in confidence personal information and uses judgment in sharing this information.

The nurse shares with society the responsibility for initiating and supporting action to meet the health and social needs of the public, in particular those of vulnerable populations.

The nurse also shares responsibility to sustain and protect the natural environment from depletion, pollution, degradation, and destruction.

2. NURSES AND PRACTICE

The nurse carries personal responsibility and accountability for nursing practice and for maintaining competence by continual learning.

The nurse maintains a standard of personal health such that the ability to provide care is not compromised.

The nurse uses judgment regarding individual competence when accepting and delegating responsibility.

The nurse at all times maintains standards of personal conduct which reflect well on the profession and enhance public confidence.

The nurse, in providing care, ensures that use of technology and scientific advances are compatible with the safety, dignity, and rights of people.

3. NURSES AND THE PROFESSION

The nurse assumes the major role in determining and implementing acceptable standards of clinical nursing practice, management, research, and education.

The nurse is active in developing a core of research-based professional knowledge.

The nurse, acting through the professional organization, participates in creating and maintaining equitable social and economic working conditions in nursing.

4. NURSES AND COWORKERS

The nurse sustains a cooperative relationship with coworkers in nursing and other fields.

The nurse takes appropriate action to safeguard individuals when their care is endangered by a coworker or any other person.

Animal Use in Biomedical Research

World Medical Association 1989

Adopted by the Forty-first World Medical Assembly in Hong Kong, September 1989, the World Medical Association Statement on Animal Use in Biomedical Research includes principles that affirm not only the need to respect the welfare of animals used for research but also the continued use of animals in biomedical research as essential. It specifically condemns the harassment of scientists by animal rights activists.

PREAMBLE

Biomedical research is essential to the health and well-being of every person in our society. Advances in biomedical research have dramatically improved the quality and prolonged the duration of life throughout the world. However, the ability of the scientific community to continue its efforts to improve personal and public health is being threatened by a movement to eliminate the use of animals in biomedical research. This movement is spearheaded by groups of radical animal rights activists whose views are far outside mainstream public attitudes and whose tactics range from sophisticated lobbying, fund raising, propaganda and misinformation campaigns to violent attacks on biomedical research facilities and individual scientists.

The magnitude of violent animal rights activities is staggering. In the United States alone, since 1980, animal rights groups have staged more than 29 raids on

U.S. research facilities, stealing over 2,000 animals, causing more than 7 million dollars in physical damages and ruining years of scientific research in the process. Animal activist groups have engaged in similar activities in Great Britain, Western Europe, Canada, and Australia. Various groups in these countries have claimed responsibility for the bombing of cars, institutions, stores, and the private homes of researchers.

Animal rights violence has had a chilling effect on the scientific community internationally. Scientists, research organizations, and universities have been intimidated into altering or even terminating important research efforts that depend on the use of animals. Laboratories have been forced to divert thousands of research dollars for the purchase of sophisticated security equipment. Young people who might otherwise pursue a career in biomedical research are turning their sights to alternative professions.

Despite the efforts of many groups striving to protect biomedical research from animal activism, the response to the animal rights movement has been fragmented, under-funded, and primarily defensive. Many groups within the biomedical community are hesitant to take a public stand about animal activism because of fear of reprisal. As a result, the research establishment has been backed into a defensive posture. Its motivations are questioned, and the need for using animals in research is repeatedly challenged.

While research involving animals is necessary to enhance the medical care of all persons, we recognize also that humane treatment of research animals must be ensured. Appropriate training for all research personnel should be prescribed and adequate veterinary care should be available. Experiments must comply with any rules or regulations promulgated to govern human handling, housing, care, treatment, and transportation of animals.

International medical and scientific organizations must develop a stronger and more cohesive campaign to counter the growing threat to public health posed by animal activists. Leadership and coordination must be provided.

The World Medical Association therefore affirms the following principles:

1. Animal use in biomedical research is essential for continued medical progress.
2. The WMA Declaration of Helsinki requires that biomedical research involving human subjects should be based on animal experimentation, but also requires that the welfare of animals used for research be respected.
3. Humane treatment of animals used in biomedical research is essential.
4. All research facilities should be required to comply with all guiding principles for humane treatment of animals.
5. Medical Societies should resist any attempt to deny the appropriate use of animals in biomedical research because such denial would compromise patient care.
6. Although rights to free speech should not be compromised, the anarchistic element among animal rights activists should be condemned.

7. The use of threats, intimidation, violence, and personal harassment of scientists and their families should be condemned internationally.
8. A maximum coordinated effort from international law enforcement agencies should be sought to protect researchers and research facilities from activities of a terrorist nature.

Historical Chronology: Ancient Medicine and Culture

This chronology, while instructive, makes no claim to be exhaustive. Standard dates are used.

MEDICAL DEVELOPMENTS		PHILOSOPHY AND TECHNOLOGY	
B.C.		**B.C.**	
2500	Egyptian surgery depicted at Saqquarah	3000	Writing Invented
1727	Code of Hammurabi includes guidelines for medical practices, including eye surgery and permissible fees	2860–2565	Great Pyramids built
		624–545	Thales of Miletus
		611–546	Anaxamander
1700	Edwin Smith Papyrus describes medical and surgical practices in Egypt	586–526	Anaximenes
		581–479	Pythagoras
1700	Contraceptives in use in Egypt	544-484	Heraclitus
		490–430	Empedocles
ca. 1500	Leprosy reported in Egypt and India	485–415	Protagoras
		470–399	Socrates
1500	Embers Papyrus	460–370	Democritus
1300	Berlin Papyrus	428–347	Plato
ca. 725	Homer refers to highly developed battlefield surgery	384–322	Aristotle
		350	Theater of Epidaurus

ca. 650	Asclepius's healing cult begins	341–270	Epicurus
ca. 650	Epilepsy described in Babylonian text	312	First Roman Aqueduct *Aqua Appia* (11 miles)
600	Postmortem C-section (Lex regia)	307	Ptolemy Soter opens library and museum at Alexandria, Egypt
ca. 522	Democedes founds medical school at Athens	300	Euclid's *Elements*
500	Alcmaeon, Greek physician	287–212	Archimedes
ca. 490	Hemlock drug developed	99	Central heating in Rome
469–399	Hippocrates of Cos	99–55	Lucretius, poet and Epicurean
430–427	Plague in Athens	4 B.C.–A.D. 65	Seneca, statesman and Stoic
ca. 265	Romans' first contact with Greek medicine via prisoners of war		
ca. 212	Diocles of Carystus, Greek physician		
99-55	Scribonius Largus, Greek physician		
90	Asclepiades, Greek physician, practices nature healing in Rome		

A.D.

A.D.

23	Birth of Pliny the Elder, Roman writer on natural history	21	Roman baths opened
40	Celsus's *On Medicine*	50	Romans learn about soap from the Gauls
98–138	Soranus of Ephesus, Greek physician	121–180	Marcus Aurelius, Stoic and Roman emperor
129–199	Galen, Greek physician	ca. 285	Papyrus of Alexander describes 5 machines: cogwheel, pulley, lever, screw, wedge
164–180	Plague in Roman Empire		
350	First hospitals in Eastern Roman Empire	354	Birth of St. Augustine of Hippo
390	Fabiola founds a hospital in Rome		
512	Illustrated edition of Discorides' *De Materia Medica*		

LITERARY ARTS

B.C.

ca. 725	Homer
ca. 650	Hesiod
581	Sappho
525–456	Aeschylus
518–438	Pindar
485–424	Herodotus
496–406	Sophocles
484–406	Euripides
190–159	Terence
106–43	Cicero
70–19	Virgil
65–8	Horace
43	Birth of Ovid

A.D.

47–120	Plutarch
58–138	Juvenal

POLITICS AND RELIGION

B.C.

3760	First year of Jewish calendar
2780	Imhotep, Egyptian Pharaoh
1500	Moses leads Hebrews out of Egypt
776	Olympic games first recorded
753	Founding of Rome
ca. 600	Egyptian *Book of the Dead*
461–430	Age of Pericles
448–433	Rebuilding of Acropolis
431–404	Peloponnesian War
323	Alexander the Great dies
100–44	Gaius Julius Caesar
31	Caesar Augustus, first Roman emperor
20 B.C.–A.D. 50	Philo Judaeus
ca. 4	Birth of Jesus

A.D.

31	Egypt becomes a Roman province
58	St. Paul's *Letters to the Corinthians*
70	Romans destroy Jewish Temple in Jerusalem
313	Christianity legalized in Roman Empire
410	Alaric sacks Rome
476	Fall of Roman Empire

SELECT BIBLIOGRAPHY

These are among the principal works that were consulted. They are divided into separate sections of books and articles. A still useful list of primary source material may be found in Miriam Drabkin, "A Select Bibliography of Greek and Roman Medicine," *Bulletin of the History of Medicine* 2, no. 4 (1942): 399–408.

BOOKS

Ackernecht, Edwin H. *A Short History of Medicine.* New York: Ronald Press, 1955.

Allbutt, Clifford T. *Greek Medicine in Rome.* London: MacMillan Ltd., 1921.

Amundsen, Darrel W. *Medicine, Society and Faith in the Ancient and Medieval Worlds.* Baltimore: Johns Hopkins University Press, 1996.

Ariès, Philippe. *The Hour of Our Death.* Translated by Helen Weaver. New York: Knopf, 1981.

Aristotle. *Historia Animalium.* Translated by D. W. Thompson. Vol. IV of *The Works of Aristotle*, edited by J. A. Smith and W. D. Ross. 11 vols. Oxford: Clarendon Press, 1910.

———. *The Basic Works of Aristotle.* Edited by Richard McKeon. New York: Random House, 1941.

———. *Politics.* Translated by H. Rackham. Loeb Classical Library. Cambridge, MA: Harvard University Press, 1969.

Asimov, Isaac. *Asimov's Chronology of the World: The History of the World from the Big Bang to Modern Times.* New York: Harper Collins, 1991.

Barker, Ernest. *The Politics of Aristotle.* Oxford: Oxford University Press, 1946.

Beauchamp, Tom L. and Seymour Perlin, eds. *Ethical Issues in Death and Dying.* New Jersey: Prentice-Hall, 1978.

Bourke, Vernon J. *History of Ethics.* 2 vols. New York: Image Books, 1970.

Bowra, C. M. *The Greek Experience.* New York: Mentor Books, 1959.

Breasted, James H. *The Edwin Smith Surgical Papyrus.* 2 vols. Chicago: University of Chicago Press, 1930.

Burnet, John. *Early Greek Philosophy.* New York: Macmillan, 1980.

Callahan, Daniel. *Setting Limits: Medical Goals in an Aging Society.* New York: Simon and Schuster, 1987.

Chadwick, John and W. N. Mann. *The Medical Works of Hippocrates.* Oxford: Blackwell Scientific Publications, 1950.

Choron, Jacques. *Death and Western Thought*. New York: Macmillan, 1963.
———. *Suicide*. New York: Charles Scribner's Sons, 1972.
Cohn-Haft, Louis. *The Public Physicians of Ancient Greece*. Smith College Studies in History, Vol. 42. Northampton, MA, 1956.
Copleston, Frederick. *A History of Philosophy*. Vol. 1, pt. 2, *Greece and Rome*. New York: Image Books, 1962.
Cornford, Francis M. *Plato's Cosmology: The Timaeus of Plato*. New York: Bobbs-Merrill, 1937.
———. *From Religion to Philosophy*. New York: Harper, 1957.
de Coulanges, Numa D. Fustel. *The Ancient City: A Study of the Religion, Laws and Institutions of Greece and Rome*. Garden City, NY: Doubleday, 1956.
DeVogel, C. J. *Pythagoras and Early Pythagoreanism*. The Netherlands: Royal Van Gorcum Ltd., 1966.
Diels, Hermann. *Die Fragmente der Vorsokratiker*. Berlin: Weidmann, 1903.
———. *Die Handschriften der antiken Ärzte*. Vol. I, *Hippokrates und Galenos*. Berlin: n.p., 1905.
The Dinkard: The Original Pahlavi Text. Translated by Ratanshan Erachshah Kohiyar under the editorship of Peshotan dastur Behramjee Sanjana. Bombay: Duftur Ashkara Press, 1874–91.
Dodds, E. R. *The Greeks and the Irrational*. Berkeley: University of California Press, 1968.
Dover, K. J. *Greek Popular Morality: In the Time of Plato and Aristotle*. Los Angeles: University of California Press, 1974.
Durant, Will. *The Story of Civilization*. Vol. 2, *The Life of Greece*. New York: Simon and Schuster, 1939.
———. *The Story of Civilization*. Vol. 3, *Caesar and Christ*. New York: Simon and Schuster, 1944.
Edelstein, Ludwig. *Peri Aerōn und die Sammlung der hippokratischen Schriften*. Berlin: Weidmann, 1931.
———. *Ancient Medicine: Selected Papers of Ludwig Edelstein*. Edited by Owsei Temkin and Lilian C. Temkin. Baltimore: Johns Hopkins University Press, 1967.
Edelstein, Ludwig and Emma J. Edelstein. *Asclepius: A Collection and Interpretation of the Testimonies*. 2 vols. Baltimore: Johns Hopkins University Press, 1945.
Entralgo-Laín, P. *Doctor and Patient*. Translated by F. Partridge. New York: McGraw Hill, 1969.
Frankena, William K. *Ethics*. Foundations of Philosophy Series. Englewood Cliffs, NJ: Prentice-Hall, 1963.
Freeman, Kathleen. *Ancilla to the Pre-Socratic Philosophers: A Complete Translation of the Fragments in Diels, Fragmente der Vorsokratiker*. Oxford: Basil Blackwell, 1948.
Galen. *On the Natural Faculties*. Translated by Arthur J. Brock. Loeb Classical Library. Cambridge, MA: Harvard University Press, 1916.
Gardner, Helen. *Art Through the Ages*. Edited by Horst de la Croix and Richard G. Tansey. 6th ed. New York: Harcourt Brace Jovanovich, 1975.
Garrison, Fielding H. *An Introduction to the History of Medicine*. 4th ed. Philadelphia: W. B. Saunders Company, 1929.
Gordon, Benjamin Lee. *Medicine Throughout Antiquity*. Philadelphia: F. A. Davis, 1949.
The Greek Historians: The Complete and Unabridged Works of Herodotus, Thucydides, Xenophon, and Arrian. Edited by Francis R. B. Godolphin. 2 vols. New York: Random House, 1942.

Grun, Bernard. *The Timetables of History: A Horizontal Linkage of People and Events*. 3rd rev. ed. New York: Simon and Schuster, 1991.

Hamilton, Edith. *Mythology*. New York: New American Library, 1969.

Hart, H. L. A. *Punishment and Responsibility*. Oxford: Oxford University Press, 1968.

Hartman, Edwin. *Aristotelian Investigations: Substance, Body, and Soul*. Princeton: Princeton University Press, 1977.

Heidel, W. A. *Hippocratic Medicine: Its Spirit and Method*. New York: Columbia University Press, 1941.

Hesiod. *The Works and Days, Theogony, The Shield of Herakles*. Translated by Richard Lattimore. Ann Arbor: University of Michigan Press, 1965.

Hicks, R. D. *Stoic and Epicurean*. New York: Russell and Russell, 1962.

Himes, Norman E. *Medical History of Contraception*. Baltimore: Williams and Wilkins Co., 1936.

Hippocrates. *Oeuvres completes d'Hippocrate*. Translated by Emile Littré, 10 vols. Paris: Javal et Bourdeaux, 1939–61.

———. *On Intercourse and Pregnancy*. Translated by Tage Ellinger. New York: Henry Schuman, Inc., 1952.

———. *Hippocrates*. Translated and edited by W. H. S. Jones. 4 vols. Cambridge, MA: Harvard University Press, 1962.

Homer. *The Iliad of Homer*. Translated by Richard Lattimore. Chicago: University of Chicago Press, 1961.

———. *The Odyssey of Homer*. Translated by Richard Lattimore. New York: Harper and Row, 1967.

Jacobovits, Immanuel. *Jewish Medical Ethics: A Comparative and Historical Study of the Jewish Religion's Attitude and Its Practice*. New York: Bloch Publishing Co., 1975.

Jones, W. H. S. *The Doctor's Oath*. Cambridge: Cambridge University Press, 1924.

Jonsen, Albert R. *The Birth of Bioethics*. New York: Oxford University Press, 1998.

Jonsen, Albert R., Mark Siegler, and William J. Winslade. *Clinical Ethics: A Practical Approach to Ethical Decisions in Clinical Medicine*. 4th ed. New York: McGraw Hill, 1998.

Kahn, Charles. *Anaximander and the Origins of Greek Cosmology*. New York: Columbia University Press, 1960.

Kilner, John F., Rebecca D. Pentz, and Frank E. Young, eds. *Genetic Ethics: Do the Ends Justify the Genes?* Grand Rapids, MI: William B. Eerdmans Publishing Company, 1997.

Kristeller, Paul O. *Renaissance Thought: The Classic, Scholastic and Humanistic Strains*. Rev. ed. New York: Harper and Row, 1961.

Kudlien, Fridolf. *Die Sklaven in der griechischen Medizin der klassischen und hellenistischen Zeit*. Forschungen zur antiken Sklaverei, II. Wiesbaden: Steiner, 1968.

Kurtz, Donna and John Broadman. *Greek Burial Customs*. Ithaca, NY: Cornell University Press, 1971.

Laertius, Diogenes. *Lives of Eminent Philosophers*. 2 vols. Loeb Classical Library. Cambridge, MA: Harvard University Press, 1959.

Largus, Scribonius. *Compositiones*. Edited by Georg Helmreich. Leipsig: Teubner, 1887.

Lecky, William E. *History of European Morals: From Augustus to Charlemagne*. 2 vols. London: Longmans, Green and Co., 1905.

Leiser, Burton M. *Liberty, Justice, and Morals: Contemporary Value Conflicts*. New York: Macmillan, 1973.

Lewin, Louis. *Die Gifte in der Weltgeschichte*. Berlin: J. Springer, 1920.

Liddell, H. G. and R. Scott. *Greek–English Lexicon*. Abridged. Oxford: Clarendon Press, 1972.

Lipton, Robert Jay. *The Nazi Doctors: Medical Killing and the Psychology of Genocide*. New York: Basic Books, 1986.

Loewy, Erich H. *Textbook of Healthcare Ethics*. New York: Plenum Press, 1996.

Lucretius. *On the Nature of Things*. Translated by H. A. I. Munro. London: Bell, 1913.

Lyons, Albert S. and Joseph R. Petrucelli. *Medicine: An Illustrated History*. New York: Harry N. Abrams, Inc., 1978.

MacDowell, D. M. *Athenian Homicide Law in the Age of the Orators*. Manchester: University of Manchester Press, 1963.

MacIntyre, Alasdair. *A Short History of Ethics*. New York: Macmillan, 1976.

Majno, Guido. *The Healing Hand: Man and Wound in the Ancient World*. Cambridge: Cambridge University Press, 1975.

Margolis, Joseph. *Negativities: The Limits of Life*. Columbus, OH: Charles E. Merrill Publishing Co., 1975.

Michell, Humfrey. *The Economics of Ancient Greece*. 2nd ed. Cambridge, U.K.: W. Heffer, 1963.

Moon, R. O. *The Relation of Medicine to Philosophy*. New York: Longmans, Green, and Co., 1909.

Needham, Joseph. *A History of Embryology*. 2nd rev. ed. New York: Abelard-Schuman, 1959.

Neuburger, M. *The History of Medicine*. London: Oxford University Press, 1910.

Nilsson, Martin. *A History of the Greek Religion*. Translated by F. J. Fielden. 2nd ed. New York: Norton, 1964.

Oates, Whitney J. *The Stoic and Epicurean Philosophers*. New York: Random House, 1940.

Oates, Whitney J. and Eugene O'Neill, Jr., eds. *The Complete Greek Drama*. 2 vols. New York: Random House, 1938.

Pauly, August. *Pauly's Real-Encyclopädie der classischen Altertumswissenschaft*. 82 vols. Stuttgart: J. B. Metzler, 1893–1974.

Pence, Gregory E. *Classic Cases in Medical Ethics*. 2nd ed. New York: McGraw Hill, 1995.

Peters, F. E. *Greek Philosophical Terms: A Historical Lexicon*. New York: New York University Press, 1967.

Plato. *The Collected Dialogues of Plato*. Edited by Huntington Cairns and Edith Hamilton. New York: Random House, 1966.

———. *The Republic*. Translated by Francis M. Cornford. London: Oxford Press, 1973.

———. *The Laws*. Translated by Trevor J. Saunders. New York: Penguin Books, 1976.

Popper, Karl. *The Open Society and Its Enemies*. 5th ed., vol. 1. Princeton: Princeton University Press, 1966.

Porter, Roy, ed.. *Cambridge Illustrated History of Medicine*. Cambridge: Cambridge University Press, 1996.

Regan, Tom, ed. *Matters of Life and Death*. New York: Random House, 1980. Second ed., New York: McGraw Hill, 1986.

Riddle, John M. *Contraception and Abortion from the Ancient World to the Renaissance*. Cambridge, MA: Harvard University Press, 1992.

————. *Eve's Herbs: A History of Contraception and Abortion in the West.* Cambridge, MA: Harvard University Press, 1997.

Robinson, John Mansley. *An Introduction to Early Greek Philosophy.* New York: Houghton Mifflin, 1968.

Rohde, Edwin. *Psyche.* Translated by W. B. Hillis. 8th ed. London: Paul Treuch Trubner, Ltd., 1925.

Rosen, George. *Madness in Society: Chapters in the Historical Sociology of Mental Illness.* Chicago: University of Chicago Press, 1968.

Ross, David. *Aristotle.* New York: Harper and Row, 1974.

Ross, W. D. *The Right and the Good.* Oxford: Clarendon Press, 1930.

Sandbach, F. H. *The Stoics.* New York: W. W. Norton, 1975.

Saunders, J. B. *The Transitions from Ancient Egyptian to Greek Medicine.* Lawrence, KS: University of Kansas Press, 1963.

Scarborough, John. *Facets of Hellenic Life.* Boston: Houghton Mifflin, 1976.

Schleiner, Winifred. *Medical Ethics in the Renaissance.* Washington, D.C.: Georgetown University Press, 1995.

Seneca. *Moral Essays.* Translated by John W. Basore. 3 vols. Loeb Classical Library. London: William Heinemann, Ltd., 1932.

————. *Ad Lucilium Epistulae Morales.* Translated by Richard M. Gummere. 3 vols. Loeb Classical Library. Cambridge, MA: Harvard University Press, 1962.

Shalev, Carmel. *Birth Power: The Case for Surrogacy.* New Haven, CT: Yale University Press, 1989.

Siegel, Rudolph E. *Galen's System of Physiology and Medicine.* New York: Krager Press, 1968.

Sigerist, Henry E. *A History of Medicine,* 2 vols. New York: Oxford University Press, 1951 and 1961.

Singer, Charles. *Greek Biology and Greek Medicine.* London: Oxford University Press, 1922.

Singer, Charles and E. Ashworth Underwood. *A Short History of Medicine.* 2nd ed. Oxford: Oxford University Press, 1952.

Snell, Bruno. *The Discovery of the Mind: The Greek Origins of European Thought.* Translated by T. G. Rosenmeyer. New York: Harper and Row, 1960.

Sophocles. *The Oedipus Plays of Sophocles.* Translated by Paul Roche. New York: Mentor, 1958.

Soranus. *Soranus' Gynecology.* Translated by Owsei Temkin. Baltimore: Johns Hopkins University Press, 1956.

Suzuki, D. and Knudtson, P. *Genethics: The Clash Between the New Genetics and Human Values.* Cambridge, MA: Harvard University Press, 1989

Taylor, A. E. *A Commentary on Plato's Timaeus.* London: Oxford University Press, 1928.

Temkin, Owsei. *Galenism: The Rise and Decline of a Medical Philosophy.* Ithaca: Cornell University Press, 1973.

————. *Hippocrates in a World of Pagans and Christians.* Baltimore: Johns Hopkins University Press, 1991.

Theophrastus. *Inquiry into Plants.* Translated by Arthur Hort. 2 vols. Loeb Classical Library. Cambridge, MA: Harvard University Press, 1961.

Vaux, Kenneth. *Biomedical Ethics: Morality for the New Medicine.* New York: Harper and Row, 1974.

Vermeule, Emily. *Aspects of Death in Early Greek Art and Poetry*. The Sather Classical Lectures, vol. 46. Los Angeles: University of California Press, 1974.

Walters, Kerry S. and Lisa Portness. *Ethical Vegetarianism: From Pythagoras to Peter Singer.* New York: SUNY Press, 1999.

Westermarck, Eduard A. *The Origins and Development of the Moral Ideas*. 2 vols. London: Macmillan and Co., 1906–8.

Wolheim, Richard, ed. *Hume on Religion*. New York: World Publishing, 1963.

Zaner, Richard M. *Ethics and the Clinical Encounter.* New Jersey: Prentice Hall, 1988.

Zeller, Eduard. *The Stoics, Epicureans, and Sceptics*. New York: Russell and Russell, Inc., 1962.

The Zend-Avesta. Translated by James Darmester, 3 vols. Oxford: Clarendon Press, 1880–83. Reprint, Westport, CT: Greenwood Press, 1972.

Zimmern, Alfred E. *The Greek Commonwealth*. 2nd rev. ed. Oxford: Clarendon Press, 1915.

ARTICLES

Allen, Anita L. "Abortion: Legal and Regulatory Issues." In *Encyclopedia of Bioethics*, edited by Warren T. Reich. 4 vols. New York: Simon and Schuster Macmillan, vol. 1 (1995): 18.

Altman, Lawrence K. "The Doctor's World." *New York Times*, 1 May 1979, C1.

Amundsen, Darrel W. and Gary Ferngren. "History of Medical Ethics: Ancient Near East." In *Encyclopedia of Bioethics*, edited by Warren T. Reich. 4 vols. New York: The Free Press, vol. 2 (1978): 880–83.

————. "History of Medical Ethics: Ancient Greece and Rome." In *Encyclopedia of Bioethics*, edited by Warren T. Reich. 4 vols. New York: The Free Press, vol. 3 (1978): 930–37.

————. "The Liability of the Physician in Classical Greek Legal Theory and Practice." *Journal of the History of Medicine and Allied Sciences* 32 (1977): 172–203.

————. "The Liability of the Physician in Roman Law." In *International Symposium on Society, Medicine and Law*, edited by H. Karplus. Amsterdam: Elsevier, 1973.

————. "Medicine and the Birth of Defective Newborns: Approaches of the Ancient World." In *Euthanasia and the Newborn: Conflicts Regarding Saving Lives*, edited by Richard C. McMillan, Tristram H. Engelhardt, and Stuart F. Spicker. Boston: D. Reidel, 1987: 3–22.

————. "The Ninth Circuit Court's Treatment of the History of Suicide by Ancient Jews and Christians in Compassion in *Dying v. State of Washington*: Historical Naivete or Special Pleading?" *Issues in Law and Medicine* 13 (1998): 365–423.

————. "The Physician's Obligation to Prolong Life: A Medical Duty without Classical Roots." *Hastings Center Report* 8 (1978): 23–30.

————. "Romanticizing the Ancient Medical Profession: The Characterization of the Physician in the Graeco–Roman Novel." *Bulletin of the History of Medicine* 48 (1974): 320–37.

————. "The Significance of Inaccurate History in Legal Considerations of Physician-Assisted Suicide." In *Physician-Assisted Suicide,* edited by Robert F. Weir. Bloomington, IN: Indiana University Press, 1997: 3–32.

Anderson, W. French and Theodore Friedman. "Gene Therapy: Strategies." In *Encyclopedia of Bioethics*, edited by Warren T. Reich. 4 vols. New York: Simon and Schuster Macmillan, vol. 2 (1995): 907.

Annas, George J. and Michael A. Grodin, eds. "Historical Origins of the Nuremberg Code." In *The Nazi Doctors and the Nuremberg Code: Human Rights in Human Experimentation*. New York: Oxford University Press, 1992: 121–44.

Annas, G. J. "Human Rights and Health—the Universal Declaration of Human Rights at 50." *New England Journal of Medicine* 339 (December 1998): 1778–81.

——————. "The Promised End—Constitutional Aspects of Assisted Suicide. *New England Journal of Medicine* 335 (1996): 684–87.

Berry, R. M. "The Genetic Revolution and the Physician's Duty of Confidentiality: The Role of the Old Hippocratic Virtues in the Regulation of the New Genetic Intimacy." *Journal of Legal Medicine* 18 (1997): 401–41.

Biggarts, J. H. "Cnidus v. Cos." *Ulster Medical Journal* 41 (1971): 1–9.

Biggs, Robert. "Medicine in Ancient Mesopotamia." *History of Science* 8 (1969): 94–105.

Blume, E. "Hippocratic Oath Versus Managed Care: Physicians Caught in Ethical Squeeze." *Journal of the National Cancer Institute* 89 (1997): 543–45.

Bok, Sissela. "Death and Dying: Euthanasia and Sustaining Life." In *Encyclopedia of Bioethics*, edited by Warren T. Reich. 4 vols. New York: The Free Press, vol. 1 (1978): 268–77.

Boozer, Jack S. "Children of Hippocrates: Doctors in Nazi Germany." *The Annals of the American Academy of Political and Social Sciences: Reflections on the Holocaust* 450 (1980): 83–97.

Bulger, R. E. "Use of Animals in Experimental Research: A Scientist's Perspective." *Anatomical Record* 219 (1987): 215–20.

"Caesarean Section." *Encyclopaedia Brittanica* 4 (1971).

Callahan, Daniel. "Bioethics." In *Encyclopedia of Bioethics*, edited by Warren T. Reich. 4 vols. New York: Simon and Schuster Macmillan, vol. 1 (1995): 247–56.

Cambell, M. C. "The Oath: An Investigation of the Injunction Prohibiting Physician-Patient Sexual Relations." *Perspectives in Biology and Medicine* 32 (1989): 300–8.

Capron, Alexander Morgan. "Death and Dying: Euthanasia and Sustaining Life: Professional and Public Policies." In *Encyclopedia of Bioethics*, edited by Warren T. Reich. 4 vols. New York: Simon and Schuster Macmillan, vol. 1 (1995): 579.

Carrick, Paul. "Environmental Ethics and Medical Ethics: Some Implications for End-of-Life Care." Part 2, *Cambridge Quarterly of Healthcare Ethics* 8, no. 2 (1999): 253.

Clouser, K. Danner. "Biomedical Ethics: Some Reflections and Exhortations." *The Monist* 60 (1977): 47–61.

Cohen, Cynthia B. "Reproductive Technologies: Ethical Issues." In *Encyclopedia of Bioethics*, edited by Warren T. Reich. 4 vols. New York: Simon and Schuster Macmillan, vol. 4 (1995): 2237.

Coleman, Brenda C. "Many Doctors Would Lie to Help Patients." *Harrisburg Patriot News*, 25 October 1999, A5.

Crawley, A. E. "Foeticide." In *Encyclopedia of Religion and Ethics*, edited by James Hastings. 13 vols. New York: Charles Scribner's Sons, vol. 6 (1966): 54–57.

Daube, David. "The Linguistics of Suicide." *Philosophy and Public Affairs* 1 (1972): 387–437.

Degnin, Francis D. "Levinas and the Hippocratic Oath: A Discussion of Physician-Assisted Suicide." *Journal of Medicine and Philosophy* 22 (1997): 99–123.

DeLacy, P. H. "Epicurus." In *Encyclopedia of Philosophy*, edited by Paul Edwards. 8 vols. New York: Collier Press, vol. 3 (1967): 3–5.

Dickstein, E., J. Erlen, and J. A. Erlen. "Ethical Principles Contained in Currently Professional Medical Oaths." *Academic Medicine* 66 (1991): 622–24.

Diller, H. "Zur Hippokratesauffassung des Galen." *Hermes* 68 (1933): 167–81.

Dubler, Nancy N. and Anita White. "Fertility Control: Legal and Regulatory Issues." In *Encyclopedia of Bioethics*, edited by Warren T. Reich. 4 vols. New York: Simon and Schuster Macmillan, vol. 4 (1995): 840–43.

Edelstein, Ludwig. "Hippocrates." *The Oxford Classical Dictionary*, edited by N. G. L. Hammond and H. H. Scullard. 2nd ed. Oxford: Clarendon Press (1970): 518–19.

Emanuel, E. J. "The History of Euthanasia Debates in the United States and Britain." *Annals of Internal Medicine* 121 (1994): 793–802.

Engelhardt, H. T. "Germ-line Genetic Engineering and Moral Diversity: Moral Controversies in a Post-Christian World." *Social Philosophy and Policy* 13 (1996): 47–62.

Feen, Richard H. "The Historical Dimensions of Infanticide and Abortion: The Experience of Classical Greece." *Lincare Quarterly* 51 (1984): 248–54.

Ferngren, Gary. "A Roman Declamation on Vivisection." *Transactions and Studies of the College of Physicians*, N.S. 4 (1982): 272–90.

———. "The Status of Defective Newborns from Late Antiquity to the Reformation." In *Euthanasia and the Newborn: Conflicts Regarding Saving Lives*, edited by Richard C. McMillan, Tristram H. Engelhardt, and Stuart F. Spicker. Boston: D. Reidel, 1987: 47–64.

Flacelière, Robert. "Medicine." In *The Praeger Encyclopedia of Ancient Greek Civilization*. New York: Frederick A. Praeger, 1967: 288–90.

Flew, Anthony. "Immortality." In *Encyclopedia of Philosophy*, edited by Paul Edwards. 8 vols. New York: Collier Press, vol. 4 (1967): 139–50.

Frankena, William K. "The Ethics of Respect for Life." In *Respect for Life: In Medicine, Philosophy, and the Law,* edited by Stephen Barker. Baltimore: Johns Hopkins University Press, 1975.

Fye, Bruce W. "Active Euthanasia: An Historical Survey of Its Conceptual Origins and Introduction into Medical Thought." *Bulletin of the History of Medicine* 62 (1978): 492–502.

Gourevitch, Danielle. "Suicide among the Sick in Classical Antiquity." *Bulletin of the History of Medicine* 43 (1969): 501–18.

Gracia, Diego. "The Structure of Medical Knowledge in Aristotle's Philosophy." *Sudhoffs Archiv* 62, no. 1 (1978): 1–36.

Hähnel, R. "Der künstliche Abortus in Altertum." *Archiv für Geschichte der Medizin* 29 (1936): 224–55.

Hall, K. "Intensive Care Ethics in Evolution." *Bioethics* 11 (1997): 241–45.

Hall, T. S. "Idiosyncrasy: Greek Medical Ideas of Uniqueness." *Sudhoffs Archiv* 58, no. 3 (1974): 283–302.

Hallie, Phillip. "Stoicism." In *Encyclopedia of Philosophy*, edited by Paul Edwards. 8 vols. New York: Collier Press, vol. 8 (1967): 19–22.

Healy, G. B. "Can We Be Faithful to the Hippocratic Oath in the Era of Managed Care?" *Archives of Otolaryngology* 124 (1998): 497–98.

Hellegers, André E. "Abortion: Medical Aspects." In *Encyclopedia of Bioethics,* edited by Warren T. Reich. 4 vols. New York: The Free Press, vol. 1 (1978): 1–5.

Henderson, C. F. "A Short History of the Use of Animals in Vaccine Development and Quality Control." *Developments in Biological Standardization* 86 (1996): 3–10.

Hirzel, Rudolf. "Der Selbstmord." *Archiv für Religionswissenschaft* 11 (1908): 75–104.

Jaeger, Werner. "Aristotle's Use of Medicine as a Model of Method in His Ethics." *Journal of the History of Science* 77 (1957): 54–61.

Jaroff, Leon. "Fixing the Genes." *Time*, 11 January 1999, 68.

Juengst, Eric and LeRoy Walters. "Gene Therapy: Ethical and Social Issues." In *Encyclopedia of Bioethics*, edited by Warren T. Reich. 4 vols. New York: Simon and Schuster Macmillan, vol. 2 (1995): 914–20.

Kalish, Richard. A. "Death, Attitudes Toward." In *Encyclopedia of Bioethics*, edited by Warren T. Reich. 4 vols. New York: The Free Press, vol. 1 (1978): 286–90.

Kaufman, M. R. "Early Greek Concepts of Mind and 'Insanity.'" *Psychiatric Quarterly* 40 (1966): 1–33.

Khushf, G. "Why Bioethics Needs the Philosophy of Medicine: Some Implications of Reflection on Concepts of Health and Disease." *Theoretical Medicine* 18 (1997): 145–63.

Kibre, Pearl. "Hippocratic Writings in the Middle Ages." *Bulletin of the History of Medicine* 18, no. 4 (1945): 371–412.

Konold, Donald. "Codes of Medical Ethics: History." In *Encyclopedia of Bioethics*, edited by Warren T. Reich. 4 vols. New York: The Free Press, vol. 1 (1978): 162–70.

Kudlien, Fridolf. "Medical Ethics and Popular Ethics in Greece and Rome." *Clio Medica* 5 (1970): 91–121.

———. "The Old Greek Concept of 'Relative Health.'" *Journal of the History of Behavioral Sciences* 9 (1973): 53–59.

———. "Medicine as a 'Liberal Art' and the Question of the Physician's Income." *Journal of the History of Medicine* 31 (1976): 448–59.

Lain-Entralgo, Pedro. "The Ethics of Diagnosis in Ancient Greek Medicine." In *The Ethics of Diagnosis*, edited by Jose Luis Peset and Diego Gracia. Boston: Kluwer, 1992: 13–18.

Langer, William L. "Infanticide: A Historical Survey." *History of Childhood Quarterly: The Journal of Psychohistory* 1 (1974): 363–65.

Lidz, J. W. "Medicine as Metaphor in Plato." *Journal of Medicine and Philosophy* 20 (1995): 527–41.

Longrigg, James. "Philosophy and Medicine: Some Early Interactions." *Harvard Studies in Classical Philology* 67 (1963): 147–75.

MacKinney, Loren C. "Medical Ethics and Etiquette in the Early Middle Ages: The Persistence of Hippocratic Ideals." *Bulletin of the History of Medicine* 26 (1952): 1–31.

Macklin, Ruth. "Abortion: Contemporary Ethical Perspectives," In *Encyclopedia of Bioethics*, edited by Warren T. Reich. 4 vols. New York: Simon and Schuster Macmillan, vol. 1 (1995): 14.

Mair, A. W. "Life and Death: Greek." In *Encyclopedia of Religion and Ethics*, edited by James Hastings. 13 vols. New York: Charles Scribner's Sons, vol. 8 (1966): 25–31.

Marketos, S. G., A. A. Diamandopoulos, and C. B. Moschos. "Is the Hippocratic Oath an Anachronism?" *World Health Forum* 16 (1995): 77–78.

McDonald, Kim A. "Studies of Women's Health Produce a Wealth of Knowledge on the Biology of Gender Differences." *Chronicle of Higher Education*, 25 June 1999, A19–22.

Merikas, George. "Hippocrates: Still a Contemporary." *Humane Medicine* 8 (1992): 212–18.

Miller, Fred. "Epicurus on the Art of Dying." *The Southern Journal of Philosophy* 14, no. 2 (1976): 169–77.

Moffic, H. Steven, John Coverdale, and Timothy Bayer. "The Hippocratic Oath and Clinical Ethics." *Journal of Clinical Ethics* 1 (1990): 287–89.

Moissides, M. "Le Malthusianisme dans l'Antiquité Greque." *Janus* 36 (1932): 169–79.

Moravcsik, Julies. "Ancient and Modern Conceptions of Health and Medicine." *Philosophy and Medicine* 1 (1976): 337–48.

Moseley, Kathryn L. "The History of Infanticide in Western Society." *Issues in Law and Medicine* 1 (1986): 345–61.

Muskin, Philip R. "The Request to Die: Role for a Psychodynamic Perspective on Physician-Assisted Suicide." *Journal of the American Medical Association* 279 (1998): 323–28.

Nadelson, Carol C. and Malkah T. Notman. "Women: Research Issues." In *Encyclopedia of Bioethics*, edited by Warren T. Reich. 4 vols. New York: Simon and Schuster Macmillan, vol. 5 (1995): 2572–76.

Nittis, Savas. "The Hippocratic Oath in Reference to Lithotomy: A New Interpretation with Historical Notes on Castration." *Bulletin of the History of Medicine* 7 (1939): 719–28.

———. "The Authorship and Probable Date of the Hippocratic Oath." *Bulletin of the History of Medicine* 8 (1940): 1012–21.

Noonan, John T. "An Almost Absolute Value in History." In *The Morality of Abortion*, edited by John T. Noonan. Cambridge, MA: Harvard University Press, 1970.

Novak, David. "Judaism." In *Encyclopedia of Bioethics*, edited by Warren T. Reich. 4 vols. New York: Simon and Schuster Macmillan, vol. 3 (1995): 1301–8.

Nutton, V. "Beyond the Hippocratic Oath." *Clio Medica* 24 (1993): 10–37.

———. "What Is an Oath?" *Journal of the Royal College of Physicians of London* 29 (1995): 518–24.

Oliver, James H. "An Ancient Poem on the Duties of a Physician." *Bulletin of the History of Medicine* 7 (1939): 315–23.

Orr, R. D., M. Pang, E. D. Pellegrino, and M. Siegler. "Use of the Hippocratic Oath: A Review of Twentieth Century Practice and a Content Analysis of Oaths Administered in Medical Schools in the U.S. and Canada in 1993." *Journal of Clinical Ethics* 8 (1997): 377–88.

Pellegrino, E. D. and A. A. Pellegrino. "Humanism and Ethics in Roman Medicine: Translation and Commentary on a Text of Scribonius Largus." *Literature and Medicine* 7 (1988): 22–38.

Pellegrino, Edmund D. "The Hippocratic Oath and Clinical Ethics." *Journal of Clinical Ethics* 1 (1990): 290–91.

———. "Medical Ethics: Entering the Post-Hippocratic Era." *Journal of the American Board of Family Practice* 1 (1988): 230–37.

———. "The Metamorphosis of Medical Ethics: A 30-Year Retrospective." *Journal of the American Medical Association* 269 (1993): 1158–62.

———. "Rethinking the Hippocratic Oath." In *Last Rights? Assisted Suicide and Euthanasia Debated*, edited by M. M. Uhlmann. Washington, D.C.: Ethics and Public Policy Center, 1998: 256–61.

————. "Toward a Virtue-Based Normative Ethics for the Health Professions." *Kennedy Institute of Ethics Journal* 5 (1996): 253–77.

Penella, R. J. and T. S. Hall. "Galen's 'On the Best Constitution of Our Body': Introduction, Translation, and Notes." *Bulletin of the History of Medicine* 47 (1973): 282–96.

Pernick, Martin S. "Back from the Grave: Recurring Controversies over Defining and Diagnosing Death in History." Edited by Richard M. Zaner. Boston: Kluwer, 1988: 17–74.

Phillips, Pat. "End-of-Life Care Movement Growing." *Journal of the American Medical Association* 278 (1997): 967–70.

Post, S. G. "History, Infanticide, and Imperiled Newborns." *Hastings Center Report* 18 (1988): 14–17.

Prioreschi, P. "The Hippocratic Oath: A Code for Physicians, about a Pythagorean Manifesto." *Medical Hypotheses* 44 (1995): 447–62.

Reiser, Stanley J. "Critical Care in an Historical Context." In *Ethics and Critical Care Medicine*, edited by John C. Moskop and Loretta Kopelman. Boston: D. Reidel, 1985: 215–24.

————. "Medical Ethics Reflected in Codes of Ethics: The Hippocratic Oath and the 1980 AMA Code Compared." *Texas Medicine* 87 (1991): 77–81.

————. "Responsibility for Personal Health: A Historical Perspective." *Journal of Medicine and Philosophy* 10 (1985): 7–17.

Rich, Ben A. "Postmodern Medicine: Deconstructing the Hippocratic Oath." *University of Colorado Law Review* 65 (1993): 77–136.

Rosalki, Jonathan. "The Hippocratic Contract." *Journal of Medical Ethics* 19 (1993): 154–56.

Rose, Herbert J. "Dead, Disposal of the." In *The Oxford Classical Dictionary*, edited by N. G. L. Hammond and H. H. Scullard. Oxford: Clarendon Press, 2nd ed. (1970): 314–15.

Rosen, George. "History in the Study of Suicide." *Psychological Medicine* 1 (1971): 267–85.

Rosner, Fred and Sussman Mutner. "The Oath of Asaph." *Annals of Internal Medicine* 63 (1965): 317–20.

Sakula, A. "In Search of Hippocrates: A Visit to Kos." *Journal of the Royal Society of Medicine* 77 (1984): 686–88.

Salem, Tania. "Physician-Assisted Suicide: Promoting Autonomy or Medicalizing Suicide." *The Hastings Center Report* 29, no. 3 (1999): 30–36.

Sandulescu, C. "Primum Non Nocere: Philological Commentaries on a Medical Aphorism." *Acta Antiqua Hungarica* 13 (1965): 359–68.

Schuller, D. E. "The 'Business' of Medicine: Hippocratic or Hypocritical?" *Annals of Allergy, Asthma, and Immunology* 77 (1996): 28–32.

Scott, P. A. "Aristotle, Nursing and Health Care Ethics." *Nursing Ethics* 2 (1995): 279–85.

Shuster, E. "The Nuremberg Code: Hippocratic Ethics and Human Rights." *Lancet* 351 (1998): 974–77.

Singer, Charles and Arthur Peck. "Zoology." In *The Oxford Classical Dictionary*, edited by N. G. L. Hammond and H. H. Scullard. Oxford: Clarendon Press, 2nd ed. (1970): 1148–50.

Smith, D. C. "The Hippocratic Oath and Modern Medicine." *Journal of the History of Medicine and Allied Sciences* 51 (1996): 484–500.

Solmsen, Friedrich. "The Vital Heat, the In-Born Pneuma and the Aether." *The Journal of Hellenic Studies*, no. 77 (1957): 119–23.

Strachan, J. C. G. "Who *Did* Forbid Suicide at *Phaedo* 62 B?" *Classical Quarterly* 20 (1970): 216–20.

Temkin, Owsei. "Greek Medicine as Science and Craft." *Isis* 33 (1953): 213–25.

———. "Health and Disease." In *Dictionary of the History of Ideas*, edited by Philip P. Wiener. 4 Vols. New York: Charles Scribner's Sons, vol. 2 (1973): 395–407.

———. "The Idea of Respect for Life in the History of Medicine." In *Respect for Life: In Medicine, Philosophy, and the Law*, edited by Stephen Barker. Baltimore: Johns Hopkins University Press, 1975.

———. "The Almighty God." In *Hippocrates in a World of Pagans and Christians*. Baltimore: Johns Hopkins University Press, 1991: 86–93.

Tichtchenko, P. "Resurrection of the Hippocratic Oath in Russia." *Cambridge Quarterly of Healthcare Ethics* 3 (1994): 49–51.

Veatch, Robert M. "Codes of Medical Ethics: Ethical Analysis." In *Encyclopedia of Bioethics,* edited by Warren T. Reich. 4 vols. New York: The Free Press, vol. 1 (1978): 171–79.

———. "Medical Codes and Oaths; History; Ethical Analysis." In *Encyclopedia of Bioethics,* edited by Warren T. Reich. 4 vols. New York: Simon and Schuster Macmillan, vol. 1 (1995): 1419–35.

———. "Should We Study the Hippocratic Oath?" *Journal of Clinical Ethics* 1 (1990): 291–92.

Verhovek, S. H. "Oregon Chafes at Measure to Stop Assisted Suicides." *New York Times*, 29 October 1999, A1, 18.

Vlastos, Gregory. "Isonomia." *American Journal of Philology* 74, no. 4 (1953): 337–66.

Waldman, Steven, Elise Ackerman, and Rita Rubin. "Abortions in America." *US News and World Report*. January 19 (1998): 22.

Warren, Mary Anne. "On the Moral and Legal Status of Abortion." *The Monist* 57 (1973): 43–61.

Watts, W. J. "Ovid, the Law and Roman Society on Abortion." *ACTA Classica* 16 (1973): 89–101.

Weissler, A. M. "The Hippocratic Ethic in a Contemporary Era of Clinical Uncertainty." *Mayo Clinic Proceedings* 66 (1991): 966–67.

Whorton. "Animal Research: Historical Aspects." In *Encyclopedia of Bioethics,* edited by Warren T. Reich. 4 vols. New York: Simon and Schuster Macmillan, vol. 1 (1995): 143–44.

Wilson, John A. "Medicine in Ancient Egypt." *Bulletin of the History of Medicine* 36 (1962): 114–23.

Winau, R. "The Hippocratic Oath and Ethics in Medicine." *Forensic Science International* 69 (1994): 285–89.

York, G. K. "Is Hippocrates Obsolete?" *Journal of the Royal Society of Medicine* 91 (1998): 164–65.

Zaner, Richard M. "Justice and the Individual in the Hippocratic Tradition." *Cambridge Quarterly of Healthcare Ethics* 5 (1996): 511–18.

INDEX